D0712106

AMA: VOICE OF AMERICAN MEDICINE

AMA

VOICE OF AMERICAN MEDICINE

JAMES G. BURROW

THE JOHNS HOPKINS PRESS

1963

Printed in the United States of America
Distributed in Great Britain by Oxford University Press, London
Library of Congress Catalog Number 63–15347

PREFACE

ALTHOUGH THE AMERICAN MEDICAL ASSOCIATION has moved from political obscurity in the nineteenth century into the sharp limelight of the 1960's, its evolution as a political force has received little attention in books devoted to the social sciences. Professor Oliver Garceau's scholarly work, *The Political Life of the American Medical Association* (1941), deals largely with the structural mechanisms of organized medicine and the processes of policy formation, while Morris Fishbein's centennial history gives greatest emphasis to the organization's scientific activities. This work supplements rather than duplicates other studies in describing the AMA's response to the social and political challenges of the twentieth century.

As the Association's political problems increase in the 1960's, so also does the strength of its growing membership. Including over 195,000 of the nation's 269,000 physicians, the AMA has established itself as the voice of American medicine. While its actions are often criticized within the profession from which important groups have occasionally risen to oppose its policies, the AMA continues to draw varying measures of support from most of its membership. Dissenting forces within the organization have found few channels for effective expression, and the Association's views are generally regarded in the United States and abroad as those of American physicians.

Compensating for the excessive burdens of research has been my awareness of the rising public interest in medical problems, growing public confusion about the Association's policies, and the increasing political importance of the organization itself. I am convinced that the Association's heroic struggles throughout much of the century are too important to ignore as well as the less impressive aspects of its record in some decades. The present volume embodies the results of independent investigation and makes no attempt to espouse the particular interest of any group.

I wish to acknowledge my indebtedness to various groups and individuals who have assisted in lightening the load of research. At the Association's headquarters several members of the staff co-operated in generously supplying useful materials. At the National Archives in the Agricultural and General Services Branch of the National Resources Records Division, Mr. Harold T. Pinkett, Miss Helen Finneran, and Mr. Stanley W. Brown aided research in the records of the Bureau of Agricultural and Industrial Chemistry. The staffs of the Vanderbilt Medical School, the University of Tennessee College of Medicine, and the University of Arkansas Medical School also assisted, and H. B. Everette, M.D., of Memphis, generously allowed use of his extensive records acquired through more than two decades of service in the House of Delegates.

I am especially indebted to several others who read portions of the manuscript and offered valuable criticisms. Jean A. Curran, M.D., of Boston, provided many useful suggestions and much encouragement, and Dr. Charles T. Gaisser of Florence, Alabama, greatly assisted with problems of interpretation. The criticisms offered by Dr. Richard H. Shryock of Philadelphia, and Louis Lasagna, M.D., of Baltimore, were also helpful. To Dr. Fred A. Shannon of the University of Illinois, I owe an immeasurable debt for guidance and advice while preparing a large part of this study as a doctoral dissertation and for helpful suggestions later in revising and enlarging it. Mr. John Gallman and Mrs. Margaret U. Chambers of the Johns Hopkins Press have supplied valuable assistance, and Mr. John H. Kyle, formerly editor, gave me much encouragement. Mrs. G. E. Allen of Memphis greatly assisted in reducing the clerical imperfections of the manuscript. I am also grateful to the American Philosophical Society for two grants which largely financed the closing phases of research. My greatest debt, however, is to Robin, my wife, whose faith and encouragement never failed. The organization herein described assumes no responsibility for this study, and I am fully responsible for any errors either of fact or interpretation.

James G. Burrow
Highland Park, Illinois

CONTENTS

Chapter 1

THE NINETEENTH CENTURY BACKGROUND

THE SMALL GROUP OF PHYSICIANS that assembled in the city of New York in 1846 to consider the formation of what was later to be the American Medical Association faced problems far removed from those that agitated the American public. This was an age of sectional jealousies and Manifest Destiny. The war was under way that resulted in the annexation of another considerable part of Mexico. Although annexation schemes were breeding increased bitterness over the slavery question, there was hope that other divisive issues could be settled in such a way as to reduce sectional friction. Large parts of the North had already been willing to acquiesce in the annexation of Texas when Oregon was included in the same bargain, and in 1846 the South found hope in the prospects of lower import duties under the Walker tariff.

The unconcern of the American people over the problems of the medical profession was shared by a considerable number of practitioners themselves. Professional apathy that had contributed to the defeat of earlier organizational efforts also restricted the size and representative character of the New York session that had as its principal object the establishment of a national organization to raise the standards of medical education. A little over half of the approximately 100 delegates who attended came from the state of New York, and about two-thirds of the medical colleges sent no representatives.[1] The next session that met the

[1] N. S. Davis, *History of the American Medical Association from Its Organization up to January, 1855*, S. W. Butler, ed. (Philadelphia: Lippincott, Grambo and Co., 1855), pp. 31–39; N. S. Davis, *History of Medical Education and Medical Institutions in the United States from the First Settlement of the British Colonies to the Year 1850* (Chicago: S. C. Griggs & Co., Publishers, 1851), pp. 124–25; a brief sketch of the origin of the AMA is found in Henry Burnell Shafer, *The American Medical Profession, 1783–1850* (No. 417 of Studies in

following year, however, attracted greater interest and brought together 239 representatives from 22 states and the District of Columbia who assembled in Philadelphia on May 5. This meeting, which officially organized the American Medical Association, set May 2, 1848, as the date for its first annual session in Baltimore.[2]

Divided House of Healing

Many forces obstructed the Association's efforts to improve the standards of medical education as the new organization moved into the second half of the nineteenth century. Sectarian medical bodies that multiplied on the American scene generally resisted its efforts. The healing world not only embraced conventional practitioners, but homeopaths, eclectics, and before the end of the century, many other cults.[3] Disciples of Samuel

---

History, Economics and Public Law [New York: Columbia University Press, 1936]), pp. 237–40 and a short account of the life of Nathan Smith Davis, "The Father of the American Medical Association" is given by Nathan Smith Davis III in Morris Fishbein [ed.], *A History of the American Medical Association,* 1847–1947 (Philadelphia: W. B. Saunders Company, 1947), pp. 3–16. See also pp. 603–6.

[2] Davis, *History of AMA,* pp. 117, 40–52.

[3] The AMA referred to all nonconformist healers as "sectarian." Its Judicial Council has defined this term to include any practitioner who "follows a dogma, tenet or principle based on the authority of its promulgator to the exclusion of demonstration and practice." *The Journal of the American Medical Association* (Chicago: The American Medical Association, 1924) 82 (June 14, 1924), 1952. The *Journal* in the text, refers to *The Journal of the American Medical Association.* The *Journal* is referred to hereafter in the footnotes as *JAMA* with volume and year. Since most of the articles in *JAMA* and in other AMA publications are committee reports and the like, the references in most cases are limited to the publication and page number. Homeopathy was established upon the idea that ". . . diseases or symptoms of diseases are curable by those particular drugs which produce similar pathologic effects upon the body (*similia similibus curantus*); second, that the dynamic effect of drugs is heightened by giving them in infinitesimally small doses, which are to be obtained by carrying dilution and trituration to an extreme limit; third, the notion that most chronic diseases are only manifestations of suppressed itch or 'Psora,'" Fielding H. Garrison, *An Introduction to the History of Medicine* (4th ed.; Philadelphia: W. B. Saunders Company, 1929), p. 438. Garrison's definition is cited in W. A. Newman Dorland, with the collaboration of E. C. L. Miller, *The American Illustrated Medical Dictionary* (20th ed.; Philadelphia: W. B. Saunders Company, 1944), p. 680, but very inaccurately. Eclecticism is defined as "A system of medicine which treats disease by the application of single remedies to known pathologic conditions, without reference to nosology, special attention being given to developing indigenous plant remedies." Leslie Brainerd Arey and others, eds., *Dorland's*

Hahnemann, the founder of homeopathy, established the American Institute of Homeopathy in 1844, nearly twenty years after the movement reached the United States, and a year after its founder's death in France. The growth of this form of practice is illustrated by the organization of the International Hahnemannian Association in 1880, the Southern Homeopathic Association in 1885, and the Missouri Valley Homeopathic Medical Association before the end of the century.[4] The eclectic movement, which emphasized a variety of botanical preparations for the cure of illnesses, stood out as a revolt against the alleged overuse of mercury, antimony, harsh purgatives, and a few other remedies. While originating with Samuel Thomson, who patented his medical mixtures first in 1813, a large part of the movement had passed far beyond his control before Alva Curtis, leader of one faction, established his own school at Columbus, Ohio, in 1836, and before an older group, founded by Wooster Beach, brought to the banks of the Ohio six years later what soon became known as the Eclectic Medical Institute of Cincinnati. The founding of the American Eclectic Medical Association in 1848 by elements of the Beach and Curtis factions, and its revival in 1870 after thirteen years of inactivity, demonstrated the tenacity of this movement.[5]

Illustrated Medical Dictionary (23rd ed.; Philadelphia: W. B. Saunders Company, 1957), p. 426. A fuller account of the divergent beliefs of older irregular medical groups is given in L. E. Jones and John M. Scudder, *The American Eclectic: Materia Medica and Therapeutics* (Cincinnati: Moore, Wilstach, Keys & Co., Printers, 1858), I, 9–33. For a defense of the position that homeopathy "is a supplement to 'regular' medicine and not a substitute for it," see Linn J. Boyd, *A Study of the Simile in Medicine* (Philadelphia: Boericks and Tafel, 1936), p. 26, and for a defense of the eclectic system see A. F. Stephens, "The Eclectic School of Medicine," *The Twentieth Century Magazine* (November, 1910), pp. 121–26. Abraham Flexner, the eminent authority on medical education, contended that homeopaths, eclectics, physiomedicals, and osteopaths might rightly be considered as sectarian rather than fraudulent practitioners since they all believe that "anatomy, pathology, bacteriology, [and] physiology must form the foundation of medical education," but regarded chiropractors and mechano-therapists as no more than "unconscionable quacks." Abraham Flexner with an introduction by Henry S. Pritchett, *Medical Education in the United States and Canada* (The Carnegie Foundation for the Advancement of Teaching, Bulletin No. 4 [New York, 1910]), p. 158. In charging that conventional practitioners laid undue stress on chemical compounds and surgery, these groups, with some justification, considered regular doctors as sectarian.

[4] Boyd, *Simile in Medicine,* p. 36; *Medical and Surgical Register of the United States and Canada,* 1898 (5 ed.; Detroit: R. L. Polk & Co., Publishers, 1898), pp. 46, 58, 62, 59.

[5] *Twenty-Eighth Annual Announcement and Catalogue* (1872–1873), in the *Eclectic Medical Journal,* XXXII, No. 1 (January, 1872), 3; Samuel Thom-

To the rival healing groups that developed before the founding of the AMA, the last half of the century added others. In 1874, Andrew T. Still, a frontiersman, claiming title to a lost diploma from a Southern medical school allegedly destroyed in the Civil War, instituted the practice of osteopathy at Macon, Missouri. Later he moved to Kirksville where he established the American School of Osteopathy in 1892. Daniel D. Palmer of Davenport, Iowa, started the chiropractic movement in 1895, as much to his own profit as to the dismay of those interested in reducing medical chaos.[6] The full launching of Christian Science came with the publication of Mary M. Glover's (later Eddy) *Science and Health* in 1875. A few medical men even supported the Anti-Vivisection Society which began in 1883, and continued as a source of annoyance to the AMA.[7]

While experiments in electro- and hydrotherapy did not assume the nature of distinct sectarian practice, they illustrate some of the forces that created further disunity in American medicine. Benjamin Rush began experimentation with hydrotherapy near the end of the eighteenth century, but not until John Bell of Philadelphia popularized its use nearly fifty years later did it gain much notice. The groups exploiting the electrical mysteries as a cure for ailments established the American

---

son, *A Narrative of the Life and Medical Discoveries of Samuel Thomson . . .* (8th ed.; Columbus, Ohio: Pike, Platt, & Co., Agents, 1832), pp. 191–92, 261–62; Frederick C. Waite, "American Sectarian Medical Colleges before the Civil War," *Bulletin of the History of Medicine,* XIX (February, 1946), 150–54; *Life and Medical Discoveries of Samuel Thomson and A History of the Thomsonian Materia Medica* (The Lloyd Library of Botany, Pharmacy and Materia Medica, Bulletin No. 11, 1909, Reproduction Series, No. 7 [Cincinnati, Ohio: J. U. & C. G. Lloyd]), p. 53.

[6] Arthur Grant Hildreth, *The Lengthening Shadow of Dr. Andrew Taylor Still* (Mason, Missouri: Arthur Grant Hildreth publisher, 1938), pp. 12, 30; Louis S. Reed, *The Healing Cults: A Study of Sectarian Medical Practice: Its Extent, Causes, and Control* (The Committee on the Costs of Medical Care, Publication No. 16 [Chicago: University of Chicago Press, 1932]), pp. 107–8. Morris Fishbein discusses several medical sects in *The Medical Follies: An Analysis of the Foibles of Some Healing Cults* (New York: Boni & Liveright, 1925). Osteopathy emphasizes the "normal structural relationship" of the body as the greatest factor in preserving its well-being while chiropractic theory attributes disease largely to the improper functioning of the nervous system. Arey and others, *Dorland's Illustrated Medical Dictionary,* pp. 1069, 300. Much of conventional medicine's opposition to osteopathy has passed as this system has considerably broadened its theory and training. Reed, *The Healing Cults,* pp. 107–8.

[7] Reed, *The Healing Cults,* pp. 76–78; Polk, *Medical and Surgical Register* (1898), 5 ed., p. 47. Christian Science is not defined in Arey and others, *Dorland's Illustrated Medical Dictionary.*

Electro-Therapeutic Association in 1891, and the National Society of Electro-Therapeuticists, which was of probably a little later origin.[8] The use of electricity in medical practice attracted a growing number of physicians whose reputations were not seriously endangered by their extravagant claims about its healing virtues.

The divided state of the healing world produced several intersectarian associations that further accentuated the divisive trends. Appealing to all groups employing physical methods for the treatment of disease, the American Association of Physio-Medical Physicians and Surgeons appeared in 1883, the American Association of Physicians and Surgeons in 1894, and the American Medical Union five years later. Sponsors of the latter organization consisted of twenty practitioners who, opposing the exclusive policies of the AMA, sought "to secure the repeal of all medical statutes based on the principles of despotic paternalism."[9] Intersectarian groups, bearing pretentious titles, reflected more the extravagant dreams of their founders than their numerical strength. Such organizations often deliberately withheld membership figures, but a high mortality rate indicates their insignificance. Only the name of the American Association of Physio-Medical Physicians and Surgeons appears in the second edition of the *American Medical Directory* of 1909.[10]

The American Medical Association opposed all sectarian groups and began early to rid its ranks of nonconforming elements. At the Philadelphia session of 1855, it condemned the mingling of homeopathy with standard medical practice and announced that schools mixing the teaching of homeopathy with scientific medicine should not be supported by the profession. The AMA brought strong pressures against medical so-

[8] J. H. Kellogg, *Rational Hydrotherapy* (Battle Creek, Mich.: Modern Medicine Pub. Co., 1923), pp. 32, 35; Polk, *Medical and Surgical Register* (1898), 5th ed., pp. 49, 60. A brief account of the rise of electrotherapeutics is given in Geo. M. Beard and A. D. Rockwell, *A Practical Treatise on the Medical and Surgical Uses of Electricity* (6th ed.; revised by A. D. Rockwell [New York: William Wood & Company, Publishers, 1888]), pp. 198–215. For a discussion of other types of treatments such as heliotherapy (use of sunlight), thermotherapy (use of heat), and crounotherapy (use of mineral waters), see Wilhelm Winterniz, assisted by Alois Strasser and B. Buxbaum, "Hydrotherapy, Thermotherapy, Heliotherapy, and Phototherapy," Augustus A. Eshner, trans., (In Vol. 9 of *A System of Physiologic Therapeutics* [Philadelphia: P. Blakiston's Son & Co., 1902]), and E. Heinrich Kisch, "Balneology and Crounotherapy," in the same volume.

[9] Polk, *Medical and Surgical Register* (1898), 5th ed., pp. 46, 48–49; *Polk's Medical Register and Directory of North America,* 1906 (9th ed.; Detroit: R. L. Polk & Co., 1906), p. 67.

[10] *American Medical Directory* (1909), 2nd ed., p. 8.

cieties that tolerated sectarian practitioners. At the session in Washington, D. C., in 1870, it called upon the Massachusetts Medical Society to expel from its membership all homeopaths and eclectics. As the Massachusetts society complied, the sincerity of the Association's threat was not tested until 1882, when the Judicial Council, created in 1873 to consider judicial and ethical questions, decided against further representation of delegates from the New York State Medical Society because of its connection with homeopathic groups.[11] The AMA was less successful in its attempt to deal with problems involving the relationship of practitioners of traditional and sectarian medicine, which remained largely unsolved throughout the century.[12]

While divisive forces in the healing world separated practitioners of physical and spiritual therapy and isolated them into numerous groups with conflicting theories and methods, other influences in conventional medicine itself promoted organizational divisions along lines of color, geography, and specialization. These organizations did not generally arise out of antipathy for the American Medical Association, yet they tended to create a centrifugal movement which partially offset the Association's work for unification. The impetus for the organization of Negro physicians came largely as a by-product of the AMA's own action. In 1870, ostensibly on grounds of lower educational requirements, it debarred the National Medical Society of the District of Columbia, a Negro organization, as well as two Negro hospitals from representation. Yet despite this move, a quarter of a century elapsed before ostracized Negro physicians established the National Medical Association.[13]

The vastness of the United States encouraged the rise of regional organizations. One of these, the Aesculapian Society of the Wabash Valley, organized in 1846, was older than the AMA and outlasted the century.[14] The Northern Tri-State Medical Association that included many physicians in Indiana, Michigan, and Ohio was organized in 1874. The next year marked the beginning of the Tri-State Medical Society of

[11] Fishbein, *History of AMA,* pp. 62, 79, 83, 105–8. The action against the toleration of sectarian principles of instruction was caused by the installation of a new chair of homeopathy at the University of Michigan by the state legislature.

[12] For the Association's difficulty in dealing with the matter see *The Transactions of the American Medical Association* (Philadelphia, 1876), XXVII, 48; *ibid.* (1878), XXIX, 39–40, 44.

[13] Fishbein, *History of AMA,* pp. 80, 84; *American Medical Directory* (1914), 4th ed., p. 66.

[14] *Polk's Medical Register and Directory* (1906), 9th ed., I, 69.

Vincennes, Indiana, which became the Mississippi Valley Medical Association in 1883. The Medical Society of the Missouri Valley followed in 1888; the Tri-State Medical Society of Iowa, Illinois, and Missouri in 1891; the Tri-State Medical Society of the Carolinas and Virginia in 1898; and the Ohio Valley Medical Association the next year.[15] These regional bodies appear to have generally maintained cordial relations with the American Medical Association. The Mississippi Valley Medical Association adopted its Code of Ethics in 1886, and three physicians who filled its highest office also served as president of the AMA between 1894 and 1901.[16] While the AMA always looked with favor on the establishment of county, district, and state organizations, it appeared somewhat fearful of the rise of interstate bodies that threatened to draw portions of the profession from its orbit of influence.

The Association also watched the growth of specialization in the profession with much concern, as the increasing complexity of medical science brought into existence many specialized medical organizations that had the divisive effect of de-emphasizing the common interests of physicians. As early as 1883, Nathan S. Davis saw in the multiplication of specialized bodies a serious threat to the Association's strength.[17] Among the rising number of these organizations were the American Ophthalmological Society, 1864; the American Otological Society, 1867; the American Neurological Association, 1875; the American Gynecological Society and American Dermatological Association, 1876; the American Laryngological Association, 1879; the American Surgical Association, 1880; the American Climatological Association, 1883; and several others before the end of the century.[18] When the Congress of American

[15] *Ibid.*, p. 89; *American Medical Directory* (1914), 4th ed., p. 66; Mississippi Valley Medical Association, *Transactions* (1899), I, 1–2; *JAMA*, 22 (March 31, 1894), p. 483.

[16] Mississippi Valley Medical Association, *Transactions* (1899), I, 2; see table in introductory material; Fishbein, *History of AMA*, p. 1190.

[17] Fishbein, *History of AMA*, p. 111. The Association gave some encouragement to the movement for specialization early in its history when in 1849 the assembly divided the annual sessions into six sections for the performance of its scientific work. *Ibid.*, pp. 1092–93.

[18] *American Medical Directory* (1914), 4th ed., pp. 64–65. In 1882 the address of President S. D. Gross to the American Surgical Association indicated some ill-feeling toward the AMA. He stated that "If it be said that we are striking a blow at the American Medical Association, we deny the soft impeachment. On the contrary, we shall strengthen that body by rousing it from its Rip Van Winkle slumbers, and infusing new life into it. We can hurt no society now in existence or, likely to come into existence." American Surgical Association, *Transactions*, Vol. 1, p. xxii.

Physicians and Surgeons was created in 1887, ostensibly representing all of these specialized bodies, Davis believed that it was a deliberate attempt to weaken the AMA and create another rival organization. The *New Orleans Medical and Surgical Journal* also called attention to the threat.[19]

Actually the divisions arising from color, geography, and specialization did not exhaust the possible lines of cleavage. While of no great significance, the National Woman Physicians' Association established in 1887 found justification for existence on the basis of sex. The American Order of the Guild of the Misericordia, partially composed of physicians, was a benevolent society created to aid areas struck by catastrophe. The organization of the International Medical Missionary Society in 1881 illustrated the combination of scientific knowledge with Christian evangelistic zeal.[20] Other organizations arose representing railway surgeons, physicians and surgeons attached to state prisons and institutions for the insane, and medical men in the federal military services.

Medical Education

While troubled by the real or potential rivalry of other medical organizations, the status of medical education provided the Association with another grievance. The rapid increase in the number of medical colleges devoted to the advancement of some therapeutic system and the laxity of their standards continued as a threat to scientific medicine well into the twentieth century. Such an "open shop" also made the ascendancy of the AMA over the realm of healing extremely difficult. Sectarian practice contributed both to the number and weakness of many schools. John Shaw Billings, formerly with the Surgeon General's Bureau and a national figure, described this situation before the British Medical Association in 1886:

> You have nineteen portals of entrance to the profession and have not found it easy to keep them all up to standard. In America we have over

[19] Fishbein, *History of AMA,* p. 135. The *Journal* charged in 1887 that the aggregate membership of the nine specialized bodies then co-operating in this organization did not exceed 350. *JAMA,* 9 (November 5, 1887), 598. The first meeting of the congress was in 1888, the year which the *American Medical Directory* gives as the date of its origin. See 4th ed. (1914), p. 66.

[20] Polk, *Medical and Surgical Register* (1890), 2nd. ed., pp. 63, 57–58; Polk, *Medical and Surgical Register* (1898), 5th ed., p. 58.

eighty gates, a number of turnstiles and a good deal of ground in unenclosed common.[21]

Nonconforming schools, however, were by no means solely responsible for the low educational standards. Training offered even by some of the more firmly established institutions including the University of Pennsylvania School of Medicine, the College of Physicians and Surgeons of Columbia University, University of the City of New York Medical Department, Jefferson Medical College, and Harvard University Medical Department fell below the peaks of scientific advance.[22] The Committee on Medical Education of the AMA referred to schools of conventional teaching when it reported in 1867 that:

> The curriculum of instruction should be materially, if not completely, reformed. It has undergone no thorough improvement except in a very few of the schools, during the last half century. It is, in fact, essentially the same now as it was at the death of Dr. [Benjamin] Rush, in 1813.[23]

When Charles Eliot became president of Harvard in 1869 (the year that the institution provided its first microscope for medical students), his early effort to institute written examinations for medical degrees met opposition from the director of the medical school who asserted with little exaggeration that a majority of the students could hardly write.[24] Of the theses required and accepted for graduation, Samuel D. Gross, a leading medical educator, then at Jefferson Medical College in Philadelphia, wrote in 1876:

> . . . it is not too much to say that not one in fifty affords the slightest evidence of competency, proficiency, or ability in the candidate for graduation. Often, indeed, they were not even composed by him.[25]

[21] Quoted in Fielding H. Garrison, *John Shaw Billings: A Memoir* (New York: G. P. Putnam's Sons, 1915), p. 256. See also William Frederick Norwood, *Medical Education in the United States before the Civil War* (Philadelphia: University of Pennsylvania Press, 1944), pp. 416–21.

[22] For references to the older and stronger medical institution before the Civil War see Norwood, *Medical Education,* p. 433, and Frederick Clayton Waite, *The Story of A Country Medical College* (Montpelier: Vermont Historical Society, 1945). For accounts of separate institutions see Norwood, *Medical Education,* pp. 63–218 especially, and Francis R. Packard, *History of Medicine in the United States* (2 vols.; New York: Paul B. Hoeber, Inc., 1931), II, 737–821.

[23] AMA, *Transactions* (1867), XVIII, 365.

[24] Helen Clapesattle, *The Doctors Mayo* (Minneapolis: The University of Minnesota Press, 1951), p. 21; Charles Eliot, *Harvard Memories* (Cambridge: Harvard University Press, 1923), pp. 28, 35.

[25] S. D. Gross, *American Medical Literature* (Philadelphia, 1876), pp. 55–57, quoted in Shafer, *American Medical Profession,* p. 176.

Many schools, established at a time when legal requirements were all but non-existent, likewise virtually waived entrance and exit requirements for medical students who were captured in the rivalry of enrollment.

Although the AMA was established to raise medical educational standards, the Committee on Medical Education confessed twenty years later that all the Association's efforts toward that end had "failed to produce any very important practical results . . . ," but noted some gradual improvement.[26] Only a few days before the session of 1867 heard these discouraging words, 24 delegates from 18 colleges in 11 states and the District of Columbia attended a conference in Cincinnati beginning May 3, called by the AMA in an effort to initiate a real movement of reform. They adopted numerous resolutions regarding such matters as higher entrance requirements, lengthening the term and increasing the required years of study, and widening the field of instruction.[27] Although the American Academy of Medicine, the Association of American Medical Colleges founded in 1890, and the Southern Medical College Association established two years later joined with the state boards of health as allies of the AMA in raising medical standards, their efforts brought only gradual improvement. The most effective action against inferior schools was taken by *The Journal of the American Medical Association* in March, 1894, with the publication of its first important article exposing fraudulent medical institutions, followed by repeated exposures in its educational issues after September, 1896.[28]

A statistical picture of the educational chaos in the healing profession near the close of the century shows the odds against which the Association and its allies fought. Schools of healing numbered 156 in 1899 and enrolled 24,119 students. Twenty-one were homeopathic with 1,833 students, seven were eclectic with 582, and three were physio-medical with 85 students. Eighty-two were separate institutions and 74 were departments of colleges and universities, while in addition to the total of 156, there were ten graduate medical schools.[29] Only 26 colleges de-

[26] AMA, *Transactions* (1867), XVIII, 363.

[27] AMA, *Transactions* (1867), XVIII, 377–84. See also p. 28 of this volume.

[28] A. Jacobi, "Medicine and Medical Men in the United States," *JAMA,* 35 (August 18, 1900), 425; *JAMA,* 37 (September 21, 1901), 775; George H. Simmons, *JAMA,* 42 (May 7, 1904), 1207; Fishbein, *History of AMA,* pp. 161, 178.

[29] Jacobi, *JAMA,* 35 (August 18, 1900), 426. The Government's Bureau of Education gave the number of such schools as 151 and the Association of American Medical Colleges set the number at 170 at the beginning of the new century. Walter A. Wells, *JAMA,* 38 (April 5, 1902), 862–63.

manded more than a total of 4,000 hours; 11 only from 2,500 to 3,000; while five required even less. Yet despite this disparity in educational requirements, as late as 1884 only three states required more than the presentation of a diploma as sufficient evidence of competency to secure a license to practice. In Indiana one applicant allegedly succeeded in substituting a Chinese napkin for a diploma.[30] The lengthy list of schools devoted to therapeutic instruction ranged from a few with high standards to some which held no sessions and others that had no graduates.[31]

Medical Journalism

While the generally low standards of education in the therapeutic arts and the rival systems of practice suggested that the healing body itself should first be healed, the caliber and quality of journalism dealing with the subjects of health and disease furnished additional evidence. Before the AMA lay the difficult task of raising the standards of medical publications. While by 1850 the scientific value of American medical literature showed some improvement, and a few journals of permanence were published,[32] there also had developed a degenerative trend that tended to overshadow the progress made. The high rate of mortality among therapeutic publications did not offset the rising volume or greatly encourage publications of superior merit. Although there were 117 professional organs which appeared between 1797 and 1850, mergers and continuations under new names reduced this number to 95. Among these publications 19 expired in less than one year, 8 in one year, 16 survived over two years, and 13 lasted from nine to fifteen years. Three years after the organization of the AMA, 24 journals were being published.[33]

The rising volume of publications on health and disease in the last half of the century was largely unrestrained either by considerations of ethics

[30] Wells, *JAMA,* 38 (April, 1902), 862; Editorial, *JAMA,* 2 (March 1, 1884) 266; Robert S., and Helen Merrell Lynd, *Middletown: A Study in American Culture* (New York: Harcourt, Brace and Company, 1929), p. 442. The three states were Ala., N.C., and Va.

[31] *American Medical Directory* (1914), 4th ed., pp. 99–109. See also *Polk's Medical Register and Directory* (1906), 9th ed., I, 152–82.

[32] Shafer, *American Medical Profession,* pp. 198–99. See also AMA, *Transactions* (1853), VI, 105–6, 118–25. The most important medical journals published in the middle of the century are among those described in AMA, *Transactions* (1868), XIX, 131–37.

[33] Shafer, *American Medical Profession,* pp. 182, 185–86.

or scientific verification. In 1866, the Committee on Medical Literature of the AMA, while asserting that the medical press was directed by "great talent," admitted that, as in most countries, "much is printed which is not worth publishing, some things positively bad and false, and a good deal that is neither good nor bad, but what is in some respects worse, indifferent. . . ."[34] As rival schools of healing became more active in the journalistic field and as pharmaceutical and promotional houses and publicity-seeking doctors advertised their cures, remedies, and inventions, the level of therapeutic journalism dropped even lower.

At least 275 periodicals on health and disease, most of them monthlies, were issued in the United States in 1898. Even when edited by physicians, these publications generally had little scientific merit, and excessive advertising often cast considerable doubt upon any claim of altruistic design. While many state societies published annual transactions and some of the medical schools and local societies had regular journals, no state medical society published a journal as late as 1899, although three had appeared by January, 1901.[35] By the time the tardy state medical societies had awakened to the generally degraded state of medical literature, exploitative agencies had already won the confidence of a great part of the credulous profession and public.

All sections contributed to the increasing volume of publications, but the East and Midwest led. New York state had 60 publications of purported therapeutic value in 1898, 54 of which came from the metropolis. Twenty-nine were published in Philadelphia, nine in Baltimore, and seven in Boston. In the Midwest, St. Louis led with 24, followed by Chicago with 22 and Detroit with seven. Among Southern cities, Richmond with five and Atlanta and Louisville with four each were ahead, while San Francisco and Denver with four each led in the West.[36]

Fortunately some journals did not succumb to the low standards of

[34] AMA, *Transactions* (1866), XVII, 442.

[35] Polk, *Medical and Surgical Register* (1898), 5 ed., pp. 156–63; George H. Simmons, *JAMA*, 52 (June 19, 1909), 2033; *JAMA*, 36 (January 12, 1901), 113. When Leartus Conner stated in 1884 that of the 509 medical journals that had been established in this country only 136 were still being published, he probably was not considering publications of pharmaceutical houses and some irregular sects. "The American Medical Journal of the Future as Indicated by the History of American Medical Journals in the Past," *JAMA*, 2 (June 14, 1884), 651. The *Journal* in 1899 set the total current number at about 230 but this figure too does not seem to include the whole field. Nathan Smith Davis and others, "Looking Backward," *JAMA*, 32 (June 3, 1899), 1245. The state societies with journals in January, 1901, were those in Penn., Ill., and N.Y.

[36] Polk, *Medical and Surgical Register* (1898), 5th ed., pp. 156–63.

the time and were experiencing a favorable reception at the end of the century. At least eight weeklies besides *The Journal of the American Medical Association* were published. These were the *Boston Medical and Surgical Register,* the *Cincinnati Lancet-Clinic,* the *Medical News* of New York, the *New York Medical Journal,* the *Medical Record* of New York, the *Maryland Medical Journal,* the *Medical Review* of St. Louis, and the *Philadelphia Medical Journal.* Among the most important monthlies were the *American Journal of Medical Sciences,* founded in 1827; the *New Orleans Medical and Surgical Register,* 1844; the *Buffalo Medical Journal,* 1845; the *American Journal of Obstetrics,* 1868; and the *Annals of Surgery,* established in 1885. While most of these were concerned with general practice, a number of specialized periodicals appeared near the end of the century.[37]

The American Medical Association protested the low levels of medical journalism long before it could enter the field with an adequate periodical of its own. Although the first volume of its annual *Transactions* appeared in 1848, not until 35 years later did it establish a publication that served effectively to elevate journalism and educate the profession. Only after enlarging the Association's membership to include physicians in good standing with their local societies who subscribed to the proposed publication and after raising pledges to defray its cost for the first year, did the newly appointed Board of Trustees dare undertake the weekly venture into the area of medical journalism. When *The Journal of the American Medical Association* first appeared on July 14, 1883, it showed promise of achieving a high place in the realm of medical literature, but its permanence was not assured in a field where not always the fittest survived.[38]

The establishment of the *Journal* did more to enhance the prestige of the Association than any other action the organization took in the nineteenth century. It afforded a medium for fighting all cults in the therapeutic realm and provided a means for disseminating knowledge about advances in medical science. Physicians throughout the United States became increasingly conscious of the AMA's activities and fell more and more within its sphere of influence. The *Journal's* circulation grew from 3,800 in 1883 to 5,450 in 1890, and to 17,446 in 1900.

[37] Davis and others, *JAMA,* 32 (June 3, 1899), 1242–45.

[38] For a fuller account of the steps that led to the establishment of the *Journal* see James Gordon Burrow, "The Political and Social Policies of the American Medical Association, 1901–1941" (unpublished Ph.D. dissertation, University of Illinois Library, 1956), pp. 19–21.

While it by no means monopolized the field of medical journalism, and as late as 1900 was received by less than one-seventh of all practitioners of healing in the United States, its growing circulation gave the Association much encouragement.[39]

The AMA also used other means to combat the degenerative trends in the field of medical journalism. Through the Association of Medical Editors, organized in 1885, it cast its influence on the side of improvement in scientific publications. At the annual meeting of the American Medical Publishers' Association, held at the same place and a day preceding the sessions of the AMA, the difficult problems associated with subscriptions and advertisements were discussed.[40] The meetings of these two organizations gave the leaders of the American Medical Association an opportunity to state their views on advancement in medical journalism and cultivate the friendship of editors of other publications.

Organizational Defects in AMA

Not only did the AMA struggle against external forces obstructing its progress but against serious internal weaknesses as well. The loose, unwieldy form of organization that the founding fathers placed on the infant Association retarded its growth for more than half a century. Division, competition, and provincialism within the profession, however, prevented the establishment of a highly centralized and efficient organization. As Nathan Davis aptly observed, the Association brought to the difficult task of overcoming the "repelling influences of sectional prejudices and the rivalry of individual institutions" no more than its own "moral weight" and the "inherent justice" of its acts.[41]

The founders of the AMA devised a complicated plan of membership and representation. At first, membership was restricted to delegates and past delegates to the annual sessions and to another group of less significance, classified as "members by invitation." Former delegates to any annual meeting became permanent members, along with any other members added to this classification by unanimous vote of the delegates.[42]

[39] *JAMA,* 40 (May 2, 1903), 1238.

[40] Charles Wood Fassett, *JAMA,* 35 (December 1, 1900), 1411.

[41] *History of AMA,* pp. 120, 119.

[42] For the constitution of 1847 in full see Davis, *Medical Education,* pp. 143–52. Membership required the payment of dues which the constitution limited to three dollars but which was later raised to five by sec. 5 of the bylaws.

Members by invitation were not classified as delegates although they represented sections of the nation that had no other representation in the assemblies.[43] Their accreditation extended only to one assembly, after which their membership terminated. While members by invitation lost the voting privilege in 1870, which the Association never granted to permanent members, both classes were allowed to participate in the discussions. Delegates to the annual meetings of the Association actually represented organizations composed of physicians who were not members themselves, except a few who had attained membership by previous service as delegates. Thus, the American Medical Association rested on a base that it refused to incorporate and from which it, in turn, received little strength.[44]

The plan of representation established by the constitution appeared about as weak as its provisions for membership. It allowed four types of organizations subscribing to the Association's Code of Ethics to send delegates to the annual sessions; these included county, district, and state medical societies; faculties of "regularly constituted" medical schools; professional staffs of larger chartered and municipal hospitals; and some other "permanently organized medical institutions" in good standing. A local society could send one delegate for every ten of its "regular resident members," with an additional delegate for a fraction of the membership above half that number. Medical schools and hospitals were allowed two delegates, and other medical institutions which the AMA wished to recognize could send one.[45] The Association made few changes in the representative character of the organization until 1874,

---

This section also provided that permanent membership would be forfeited for nonpayment of dues in three successive years. Some members learned to abuse this feature and maintained membership by paying the five dollars every three years instead of annually. AMA, *Transactions* (1879), XXX, 63–65; AMA, *Transactions* (1882), XXXIII, 36. For the extent of this abuse see letter of the treasurer, Richard J. Dunglison to J. H. Packard, cited in "Report of Committee, 1881, on Journalizing the Transactions of the American Medical Association," AMA, *Transactions* (1881), XXXII, 472–75.

[43] This provision was also abused. The framers of the constitution intended to include sections of the nation not otherwise represented but entitled to representation. This privilege came to be extended, however, to physicians residing near the location of the annual sessions even though their societies were fully represented. Davis, *History of AMA,* p. 114.

[44] Denial of membership to physicians in local societies, medical institutions, and hospitals was justified on the ground that if bestowed upon all members of such societies and institutions it would be valued too lightly and that a selective process produced a better membership. Davis, *History of AMA,* p. 116.

[45] *Ibid.,* p. 144.

when it instituted a plan basing representation almost exclusively on "permanently organized medical societies, and such other county and district medical societies as are recognized by representation in their respective state societies."[46]

Growth of medical societies, however, made the new plan of representation theoretically obsolete from the outset. Of the 38 state and territorial medical societies in the United States in 1874, 26 were established after the organization of the American Medical Association, and, of the 371 local medical societies in existence in 1873, a great part originated after the establishment of the AMA. If only the 365 societies which reported 20,800 active members in 1873 had sent their allowed representation of 2,080 voting delegates to the annual session, other changes in the plan of representation would have appeared imperative.[47] The extension of membership in 1882 to include members by application only increased the cumbersome character of the annual sessions by admitting a group that could enter into discussions but could not vote.[48]

Sectional Character of AMA

The location of the annual sessions, more than total attendance figures, reflects the regional character of the Association throughout the

[46] AMA, *Transactions* (1879), XXX, 321.

[47] Stanford E. Chaillé, "State Medicine and State Medical Societies," AMA, *Transactions* (1879), XXX, see table between 320–21. J. M. Toner, "Statistics of Regular Medical Associations and Hospitals in the United States," AMA, *Transactions* (1873), XXIV, 288–89. The statistics that Chaillé gives are used for the number of state medical societies, and those of Toner for all known medical societies generally classed as state, district, and county. Toner admitted that his statistics were not complete but derived from all the information he could secure. There are minor discrepancies in the two sets of statistics but these are not serious enough to discount the value of the information. The 38 state medical societies included the one in the District of Columbia.

[48] JAMA, 2 (June 28, 1884), 702; Davis and others, *JAMA,* 32 (June 3, 1899), 1262. It seems that a trend developed toward the end of the century of confining the participation of all except delegates to discussions in the sections but this practice apparently did not prevail in the early years after the organization of the sections. The *Journal* says that the new provision for membership "did not tend to increase the number registered" but adds that the list of permanent members began to increase. *JAMA,* 32 (June 3, 1899), 1242. Oliver Garceau infers that the problem of large attendance was not very serious before the basis of membership was enlarged to include members by application; this assumption seems to be incorrect. The date of the change in policy was 1882 and not 1862 as he states. *The Political Life of the American Medical Association* (Cambridge: Harvard University Press, 1941), pp. 14–15.

nineteenth century.[49] While the AMA reached the Pacific Coast with an annual session in 1871, it held most of its meetings in cities of the East and Midwest, areas of its principal strength. Ten years after the first annual session, the meeting in Washington, D. C. brought together 435 voting delegates. More than half of these came from five states, Massachusetts, Pennsylvania, New York, New Jersey, and Connecticut, while Mississippi, Louisiana, Florida, Arkansas, and Texas, among the Southern states, sent no delegates and Alabama only one. No delegates came from most of the Western states and territories. The five states of the East had 897 of the 2,079 permanent members of the Association in 1858, while Louisiana had but ten; Mississippi, five; Arkansas, two; and Florida and Texas none.

The same five Eastern states controlled half of the votes at the session of 1868 and, with the District of Columbia, were represented by 179 of the 281 voting delegates present. Ten years later the Buffalo session drew nearly half of the voting delegates from these five states, while representation from the Southern states was relatively insignificant at both sessions. By 1878, however, a new group of states had emerged to challenge the control of the East as Ohio, Indiana, Illinois, and Michigan sent 134 voting delegates to this session. The permanent membership of the five Eastern states, which had been the source of strength for the Association in 1858, fell to less than 700 of the 2,077 total of 20 years later, closely rivaled by the total of the four Lake states.

Until 1885 when the Association's records became inadequate for determining attendance by states, the same general pattern of control prevailed. While the New Orleans session of 1884 brought sizable delegations from several Southern states, the Association's strength remained in the East and the North Central states. The roll of over 5,100 members and permanent subscribers to the *Journal* in 1891 gave New York and Pennsylvania alone nearly 1,100 members, while Ohio, Indiana, Illinois, Minnesota, Nebraska, and Iowa claimed 1,870. The Association showed considerable strength in Kentucky and Tennessee, but had made little progress in the states farther South.[50] By 1900, 1956 of the Asso-

[49] See Appendix, p. 398 for the location of the annual sessions and for the incomplete attendance figures. The statistics used below pertaining to the attendance of voting delegates at the annual sessions and the size of the Association in different years are derived from the lengthy lists of delegates and members as reported in AMA, *Transactions* and the *Journal* for the years indicated. Chaillé, in AMA, *Transactions* (1879), XXX, 320–21 is the source for the AMA's membership in 1878.

[50] *JAMA,* 17 (December 26, 1891), 996–1013.

ciation's 8,401 members resided in the Middle Atlantic states and in Massachusetts, while the eight states of the Middle Atlantic and East North Central groups claimed 4,493 or more than half of the total (See Table I).[51] The seven West North Central states, with 1,092 members, had more than twice the membership of the eight Mountain states

TABLE I

MEMBERSHIP OF THE AMERICAN MEDICAL ASSOCIATION AND SUBSCRIBERS TO THE JOURNAL IN 1900[a]

State	*Members*	*Subscribers*[b]
New England		
Connecticut	105	6
Maine	47	10
Massachusetts	266	60
New Hampshire	47	8
Rhode Island	57	4
Vermont	43	10
Middle Atlantic		
New Jersey	172	20
New York	430	131
Pennsylvania	1088	126
South Atlantic		
Delaware	25	6
D.C.	120	43
Florida	44	4
Georgia	138	20
Maryland	142	63
North Carolina	46	26
South Carolina	50	22
Virginia	81	88
West Virginia	68	56
East South Central		
Alabama	71	15
Kentucky	167	155
Mississippi	49	21
Tennessee	152	76
West South Central		
Arkansas	66	26
Indian T.	14	14
Louisiana	52	52
Oklahoma T.	18	12
Texas	124	126
East North Central		
Illinois	885	1052
Indiana	443	211
Ohio	866	528
Michigan	323	290
Wisconsin	286	173
West North Central		
Iowa	356	225
Kansas	102	62
Minnesota	167	156
Missouri	266	176
Nebraska	144	70
North Dakota	35	24
South Dakota	22	17
Mountain		
Arizona T.	18	5
Colorado	327	32
Idaho	15	4
Montana	33	7
Nevada	5	3
New Mexico T.	19	5
Utah	37	3
Wyoming	15	7
Pacific		
California	268	54
Oregon	46	13
Washington	41	15

[a] Federal services and foreign countries not included.

[b] Subscribers to the *Journal* included those not members of the association who subscribed. Members automatically received it.

[51] Calculations are based on *JAMA*, 34 (June 16, 1900), 1555.

and the territories, and the North Central states and the Middle Atlantic together had almost two-thirds of the total membership.

Even in areas where the Association had its largest strength only a small percentage of physicians were members. If allowance is made for a large number of sectarian practitioners who were ineligible for membership, the Association still appears to have had only a weak hold on the medical profession. The ratio of members to the total number of practitioners stood at 1 to 19 in Massachusetts, 1 to 9 in Pennsylvania, and 1 to 28 in New York. Farther to the west the ratio was 1 to 10 in Ohio, 1 to 12 in Indiana, 1 to 10 in Illinois, and 1 to 8 in Wisconsin. In the South the ratio was 1 to 24 in Tennessee, 1 to 24 in South Carolina, 1 to 31 in Mississippi, 1 to 36 in Arkansas, and 1 to 40 in Texas. The ratio was 1 to 4 in Colorado, 1 to 9 in Montana, and 1 to 13 in California.[52]

After more than 50 years of painful growth, the position of the American Medical Association was still insecure. It could speak neither for the entire healing profession, nor for the practitioners of conventional medicine in any section of the nation. While stronger than any other medical organization, it had not become in reality the voice of American medicine.

Throughout the nineteenth century the Association struggled along with a constitution that discouraged the development of skilled and experienced executives to conduct its affairs. The officers included "a president, four vice-presidents, two secretaries and a treasurer" elected for one year. By 1864, the office of permanent secretary had been created.[53] The unchartered Association continued for nearly 35 years without a board of trustees, which it appointed in 1882, and had selected no city for its national headquarters. The satisfactory offer made by a Chicago firm to publish the *Journal* seems to have been an important factor in establishing headquarters in that city, but the Association occupied only rented property there throughout the century.[54]

[52] *Polk's Medical Register and Directory* (1906), 9th ed., I, 45. This ratio is determined to the nearest whole number by dividing the total number of physicians in the states as given in the register by the number of physicians in these states who were members of the AMA as given in the preceding table.

[53] Davis, *Medical Education,* p. 146; George H. Simmons, *JAMA,* 54 (June 11, 1910), 1964.

[54] AMA, *Transactions* (1882), XXXIII 54, 6–26; Fishbein *History of AMA,* pp. 144–49. The first Board of Trustees consisted of Nathan S. Davis (Ill.), Edward M. Moore (N.Y.), Joseph M. Toner (Washington, D.C.), Henry F. Campbell (Ga.), John H. Packard (Penn.), Leartus Conner (Mich.), P. O. Hooper (Ark.), Alonzo Garcelon (Me.), and Louis S. McMurtry (Ky.).

Internal Harmony and Discord

The AMA did not always offset organizational instability and insecurity with a membership united in spirit. Conflict brought on by minor issues sometimes shook the Association, but it was usually able to handle its major problems without difficulty. Unlike many religious and political organizations, the AMA did not split over the Civil War, and the Northern-controlled organization elected William O. Baldwin of Alabama president in 1868 and chose New Orleans as the location of the next session.[55] No disturbance was created by the election of the rabid and prominent former abolitionist, Henry I. Bowditch, as president in 1877, or of the Southern-born J. Marion Sims the preceding year. The session of 1870, however, was considerably disturbed over the question of admitting delegates from Negro institutions.[56] Seven years later Bowditch felt that the organization had lost strength in several parts of the nation due to disputes over matters of ethics, and because of the unjustified expectations of achievement which it could not fulfill.[57]

In 1883 and 1884 further disturbance developed when the Association cancelled the membership of a large number of physicians in the New York State Medical Society, following its repudiation of the Code of Ethics. Hardly had this trouble passed, when preparation for the Ninth International Medical Congress of 1887 touched off a controversy with several Eastern editors over the part the AMA was to play in the formation of the congress, and over the admission of sectarian practitioners to the American delegation. The session of 1888 was disturbed by the determined efforts of one group to elect its choice as the next president.[58] A tempestuous scene occurred at the session of 1895 when William Osler, then of The Johns Hopkins University School of Medicine, publicly challenged the competence of the permanent secretary and tried to secure a change. Even the customary introductory prayer did not please one delegate who sought its abolition in 1884.[59]

[55] Fishbein, *History of AMA,* pp. 67, 78. The AMA kept controversial political questions off the agenda of the sessions and the *Transactions* of 1859 leave no hint of the impending struggle. The AMA's failure to split may be partially explained by the fact that it held no sessions in 1861 and 1862 and no delegates from the Confederate States attended the session of 1864.

[56] *Ibid.,* pp. 93, 92, 80.

[57] *Ibid.,* p. 93.

[58] Nathan S. Davis, *JAMA,* 8 (June 25, 1887), 710; Fishbein, *History of AMA,* pp. 124–25; Editorial, *JAMA,* 12 (February 2, 1889), 165.

[59] Fishbein, *History of AMA,* pp. 170–71, 116.

Limits of Reform Agitation

Despite the magnitude of its own internal problems, the American Medical Association took its place among the reform movements that followed the Civil War without capturing much of their initial fervor. Agricultural unrest expressed itself in the Grange, Greenback, and Populist uprisings, while Labor sought its rights through such organizations as the Knights of Labor and the American Federation of Labor. These movements attacked the abuses of the existing order on a rather wide political and economic front. Other reform movements with more restricted objectives included the Woman's Christian Temperance Union, the Prohibition party, the Indian Rights Association, the National Divorce Reform League, the Civil Service Reform League, charity organizations, and movements for prison reform, woman suffrage, world peace, and against polygamy.[60] The scientific character of the AMA and its primary concern for problems in the sphere of medicine placed it among the reform movements with very limited objectives.

The AMA never allowed itself to be carried by the currents of reform into areas of remote connection with medical science. A close alignment with any broad political reform movement would have been disastrous to the unity it had achieved. In fact, grave problems arose on the industrial scene not far removed from the province of medicine, about which the Association showed no great concern. Oppressive child labor systems, excessive hours for women employees, hazardous and oppressive employment situations for men, and defective general educational systems did not incite the Association to vigorous protest. It took no official stand on the prohibition issue and raised only a feeble voice against wretched tenement conditions, misleading advertising, and food adulteration. In fact, President Charles A. L. Reed told the fifty-second

[60] The agricultural uprisings are treated in Solon J. Buck, *The Agrarian Crusade* (Vol. 45 of Chronicles of America Series, Allen Johnson, ed.; New Haven: Yale University Press, 1920); John D. Hicks, *The Populist Revolt* (Minneapolis: The University of Minnesota Press, 1931), see especially pp. 54–95, 404–23. For a treatment of other reform groups and agitations see Louis Filler, *Crusaders for American Liberalism* (Yellow Springs, Ohio: The Antioch Press, new ed., 1950), pp. 19–28; Arthur Meier Schlesinger, *The Rise of the City, 1878–1898* (Vol. 10 of *A History of American Life,* Arthur M. Schlesinger and Dixon Ryan Fox, eds. [New York: The Macmillan Company, 1938]), pp. 353–56, 370, 154, 402, 144–48, 45–47; Timothy Nicholson, "A Glance at the Past, A Look at the Present, A Vision of the Immediate Future," National Conference of Charities and Corrections, *Proceedings* (Boston: Geo. H. Ellis Co., 1902), XXIX, 2–8.

annual session in June, 1901, that "The American Medical Association, during the first fifty years of its existence, exerted relatively little influence on legislation, either state or national."[61] Yet several of these evils were perhaps better exemplified near the Chicago headquarters than in any other American city. There, near the end of the century, the Haymarket Riot had occurred; Jane Addams had publicized the filth and poverty of the tenement districts; the Pullman strike had been broken; the united Populists and Democrats had aired their grievances; and from there "embalmed beef" had been shipped.

American metropolises were not alone, however, in portraying the lagging character of the nation's social legislation and its meager emphasis on matters of health. Only three states in 1898 provided a per capita expenditure for state boards of health of more than two cents, while twelve provided less than two mills and six, none at all. Hospitals were generally inadequate and poorly distributed, and while often engaged extensively in charity service, met only a fraction of the nation's needs. Although physicians serving the nation's medical needs were often in plentiful supply, the physician to population ratio showed astonishing extremes. The ratio of 1 to 391 in the Pacific states was offset by a ratio of only 1 to 781 in the South Atlantic group. Between states there was even greater variations. Colorado had a ratio of 1 to 364, while that of North and South Carolina was 1 to 1,087 and 1,163 respectively. The nation's health records also varied greatly among the states and, when measured in terms of life expectancy, infant mortality, and the death tolls from major diseases, left no room for complacency.[62]

On the political front, the AMA turned its reform energies largely to the task of agitating for adequate vital statistics legislation and expanding the role of the federal government in areas of public health. The session of 1847, which established the Association, also charted its

[61] *JAMA,* 36 (June 8, 1901), 1601. Although the AMA took no stand on prohibition some of its leading members established the American Medical Temperance Union in 1891, "to advance the practice of Total Abstinence in and through the medical profession" and to study the effect of alcohol on the human system. N. S. Davis, *JAMA,* 19 (July 9, 1892), 29. Individually, some of the Association's leaders waged a vigorous attack on social abuses. For the reform crusades of Nathan S. Davis see Thomas N. Bonner, "Dr. Nathan Smith Davis and the Growth of Chicago Medicine, 1850–1900," *Bulletin of the History of Medicine,* 26 (May–June, 1952), 360–74.

[62] For an analysis of the nation's health resources about 1900 and for a comparison of its health record with other nations see Burrow, "The Political and Social Policies of the American Medical Association, 1901–1941," pp. 65–72.

policy on the question of reliable and adequate vital statistics that it consistently followed throughout the century. Reliance by the Census Bureau on state and municipal data, often nonexistent and usually inadequate, made federal health statistics only of limited value. Gradually the situation improved, but as late as the census year 1899–1900, only nine states met the requirements of the Census Bureau for classification as "registration states."[63]

The AMA also assumed leadership in the agitation for a federal department of health. In 1874 the Association's Section on State Medicine and Hygiene, created two years earlier, urged the establishment of a national sanitary bureau, but also appointed a committee to report on a proposal for a national health department at the session of 1875. The resulting Bowditch report contained plans for such a department, but discouraged the idea of its establishment until boards of health had been created in all states.[64]

To the newly formed American Public Health Association fell the principal task of pressing for a national health department until the American Medical Association took up the issue. But some of the prominent officials of both organizations were the same. In fact, Henry I. Bowditch, who helped establish the Board of Health in Massachusetts in 1869, was one of the founders of the American Public Health Association in 1872, president of the AMA in 1877, and on the federal Board of Health created two years later.[65] The National Board of Health owed its creation as much to the epidemics (especially of yellow fever) of 1878 as to the agitation of the American Public Health Association. While the board soon added to its investigatory functions control over quarantine, its establishment was but a feeble step toward federal assumption of responsibility for public health. Despite some constructive achievements, Congress abolished the board in 1883 through failure to make appropria-

[63] Richard Harrison Shryock, *The Development of Modern Medicine* (Philadelphia: University of Pennsylvania Press, 1936), p. 222; Cressy L. Wilbur, "The Registration of Vital Statistics in the United States," *JAMA,* 44 (February 25, 1905), 591. Only ninety per cent accuracy was required for admission into the classification of registration states. These states were Conn., Mass., Me., Mich., N.H., N.J., N.Y., R.I., and Vt.

[64] Robert D. Leigh, *Federal Health Administration in the United States* (In Harper's Public Health Series, Allan J. McLaughlin, ed. [New York: Harper & Brothers Publishers, 1927], p. 465.

[65] *Ibid.,* pp. 465–67; Shryock, *Development of Modern Medicine,* pp. 234–35; Vincent Y. Bowditch, *Life and Correspondence of Henry Ingersoll Bowditch* (Boston: Houghton Mifflin Company, 1902), II, 217–19, 242–43.

tions for its continuance, and part of its work passed to the Marine-Hospital Service.[66]

The Association renewed interest in a national health department in 1888, when the *Journal* urged establishment of a department powerful enough to prevent the adulteration of foods. Three years later the Association established a committee to press the health department issue on Congress. This committee composed of C. G. Comegys, N. S. Davis, and William B. Atkinson secured the introduction in the Fifty-second Congress in December, 1891, of a bill providing for a health department with cabinet status, but reported in June, 1893, that the measure had not reached the floor of either House.[67] It urged the Association to solicit President Grover Cleveland's support of the proposal and took upon itself the largely unrewarding task of circulating 8,000 appeals for assistance to state boards of health, medical societies, and the American Public Health Association. Although the committee increased its membership in 1896 to include one physician from each of the 45 states and the District of Columbia, and sometimes thereafter bore the title Committee on National Legislation, its effectiveness did not materially increase.[68]

The health department bill that the Association sought to have enacted varied in some of its features during the decade, but in its strongest form included several basic provisions. It called for a health department to collect statistics on sanitation from state and municipal authorities from which a weekly abstract would be published. It provided for a more adequate registration of vital statistics, and for the collection of information about the climatic conditions of various sections of the nation and their influence on health. The bill, as amended in 1893, authorized the Secretary of Health to investigate:

> The state of comfort of the laboring classes in respect to their lodgment, their trades, occupations, the healthfulness of their workshops and the contents of the atmosphere they habitually breathe, and the prevalence of premature degeneration of the nervous and muscular systems by the exactions of piece-work employment. He shall obtain information in regard to the soundness of their food and purity of water supply. He shall ascertain the ages at which the children of the poor are put to work, and its

[66] Leigh, *Federal Health Administration*, pp. 473–75, 478.

[67] Fishbein, *History of AMA*, p. 132; *JAMA*, 10 (January 21, 1888), 82; *JAMA*, 22 (March 31, 1894), 474; *JAMA*, 20 (June 24, 1893), 682–84.

[68] *JAMA*, 18 (June 25, 1892), 800; *JAMA*, 28 (January 16, 1897), 136; *JAMA*, 28 (June 19, 1897), 1190.

hindrance to their physical development, and their lack of common-school education.[69]

From later versions of the bill, however, this provision is strangely missing, as the committee possibly decided that its inclusion would create friction and delay passage.

When the Special Committee on the Department of Public Health gave up hope for the early establishment of a health department with cabinet status, it urged the Association to change its strategy. In 1897, it proposed that the AMA seek the expansion of the Marine-Hospital Service and its incorporation into a department of health headed by a commissioner.[70] The brief and vague reference to food adulteration in the bill would have been unobjectionable even to the corrupt food processors themselves. With minor modifications, Senator John C. Spooner and Representative Theobold Otjen (both of Wisconsin) introduced this bill into the Fifty-fifth Congress. Despite the discouraging reception given the measure by the Senate Committee on Public Health and National Quarantine, and its preference for the Caffery bill endorsed by the Marine-Hospital Service, the medical leaders did not lose interest in the proposal.[71] Yet, the war with Spain and the Philippines overshadowed all the Association's feeble attempts to secure national health legislation during the remainder of the decade.

War excitement, however, did not prevent the Association from establishing machinery for making its agitations more effective on the national level. At the Columbus session of 1899, it created a permanent three-member Committee on National Legislation to represent the organization before Congress.[72] This committee soon demonstrated its earnestness when it called upon state societies and the medical and health services of the federal government to send representatives to a conference in Washington, D. C., early in May, 1900, to consider pending legislation involving the interests of the medical profession. While the conference brought only a few delegates together, it opened the way for discussion of

[69] *JAMA,* 22 (March 31, 1894), 477.

[70] *JAMA,* 31 (July 9, 1898), 89; *JAMA,* 28 (June 19, 1897), 1190–91.

[71] *JAMA,* 31 (July 9, 1898), 90–91.

[72] *JAMA,* 32 (June 10, 1899), 1337; *JAMA,* 34 (June 16, 1900), 1547. The committee appointed consisted of H. L. E. Johnson (Washington, D.C.), William H. Welch (Baltimore), and William L. Rodman (Philadelphia). Originally the representatives had to be selected from the cities named but this restriction was later changed to include the states of Pennsylvania and Maryland rather than the cities of Philadelphia and Baltimore. *JAMA,* 34 (June 16, 1900), 1559.

important medical questions, including the establishment of a national health department and the unification of state and national medical practice acts.[73] Following the conference, the committee revived agitation for expanding the functions of the Marine-Hospital Service and urged each state society to appoint a committee to consider legislative measures within the states, and to appoint a delegate and alternate to meet with the national committee on its request.

Although the American Medical Association had little influence upon the legislative developments of the nineteenth century, it had gained from its agitations valuable political experience. Out of the frustation of ineffectiveness had come the realization that new techniques must be employed in bringing its strength to bear on political issues. It had created weak but permanent machinery through which its policies could be expressed. Yet the Association faced the public responsibilities of the new century with little more than a sense of political failure in the old.

[73] *JAMA,* 34 (June 16, 1900), 1547–51. The invitation brought no response from 22 state and territorial societies and the Navy Medical Staff and eight societies that replied could send no representatives. There were 12 present at the first session of the conference (probably including the committee) and 16 present at the second session including the committee.

Chapter 2

THE AWAKENING OF THE AMA

THE EFFECTIVENESS OF the American Medical Association in promoting political reforms in the early twentieth century depended in a large measure upon the correction of its own organizational deficiencies, the recapture of the profession's lost prestige through the improvement of medical education, and upon the expansion and activation of its membership. Affected by a spirit of reform that had begun to stir restlessly on the American scene and that had already revolutionized medical education in the leading nations of western Europe and diminished abuses of their industrial orders, the AMA prepared for a more influential role in public affairs by first dealing with its own most pressing problems. None of these appeared more urgent than the execution of broad constitutional reforms which would allow the Association to function efficiently. Inspired also by the British Medical Association's successful attempt at reorganization, the AMA was able to discard within a year a type of organization that had checked its progress for half a century.[1]

Reorganization of AMA

To the task of instituting major organizational reforms, the Atlantic City session of June, 1900, gave serious thought. It authorized the creation of a committee to co-operate with the Committee on National Legis-

[1] The reforms adopted by the British Medical Association are described in Ernest Muirhead Little, comp., *History of the British Medical Association, 1832–1932* (London: British Medical Association), pp. 79–87. The close contact of the two organizations brought to the readers of the official organs a general knowledge of the activities of both organizations.

lation and to assist in the organization of the profession throughout the United States. This committee, later known as the Committee on Organization, consisted of one member from each state and territory represented in the AMA, usually drawn from a list of retiring presidents of state associations.[2] The assembly also authorized the establishment of another committee of three members, vaguely given power to co-operate with the larger committee and to begin correspondence with the officers of state associations. To the committee of three, known as the Special Committee on Reorganization, and composed of Joseph N. McCormack of Bowling Green, Kentucky; P. Maxwell Foshay of Cleveland, Ohio; and George H. Simmons of Chicago fell most of the work in formulating plans of reorganization.[3]

The Special Committee on Reorganization found many defects in the organization and operation of the AMA when it reported to the St. Paul session in 1901. Offering no hope for correcting these weaknesses apart from a thorough constitutional revision, it presented basic proposals for reform. Urging the assembly to allow all parts of the plan to stand or fall together, it hoped to prevent the vitiation of its schemes by serious modifications. The special committee seemed highly pleased when, after a one-day discussion, the assembly enthusiastically adopted its plan.[4]

While the revised constitution did not greatly alter the conditions of membership in the Association, it changed the classifications of members. It abolished the old category of members by application and included this group in the list of permanent members which embraced all members of local societies affiliated with the state societies who applied for membership, supplied a certificate of good standing, and paid the annual fee. Members by invitation and honorary members included eminent foreign physicians that the Association accepted for membership. The amended constitution provided for a new group called associate members that included "Representative teachers and students of the allied sciences not physicians," to whom the proposed house of delegates decided to grant

[2] *JAMA,* 34 (June 16, 1900), 1558.

[3] Charles A. L. Reed, *JAMA,* 36 (June 8, 1901), 1605. While the resolution creating these committees indicated that the committee of three was somewhat subordinate to the Committee on Organization, this did not prove true. President Reed in his address to the Association in 1901 speaks of the committee of three as the Committee on Reorganization and of the larger committee as the Committee on Organization or a "supplementary committee." See also *JAMA,* 36 (June 8, 1901), 1643.

[4] *JAMA,* 36 (May 25, 1901), 1437–39, 1442–51; *JAMA,* 36 (June 8, 1901), 1642, 1643, 1648.

membership. While accreditation of members by invitation extended only to one assembly, they shared the same privileges as permanent members in attending the meetings of the assembly and voting in the sections, but the constitution denied this voting privilege to honorary and associate members.

Although many executive and administrative features of the amended constitution were very similar to the old, considerable changes appeared in the provisions for the legislative body. The revised constitution created a new legislative organ called the House of Delegates with representation based exclusively upon the state medical association instead of local bodies, except for the representation allowed the United States Army, Navy, and Marine-Hospital Service, and the sections of the Association. A ratio of one delegate to every 500 members or fraction thereof became the basis of representation from the state and territorial societies, with the provision that any state or territorial association could have one delegate regardless of its size. The membership of the House of Delegates could not exceed 150, and the constitution provided that as the membership of the state associations increased, the ratio of physicians would rise and that a general reapportionment of delegates would occur every three years. With these stipulations the Special Committee on Reorganization laid the plans for a representative body, providing adequate safeguards against cumbersomeness and inefficiency.

The revised constitution not only introduced structural reforms, but joined the AMA more closely to local societies. It preserved features of the old system which had not been enforced, prohibiting membership in the national organization to all who had not joined local societies or who had been expelled therefrom. No longer were members delinquent in the payment of dues retained for several years on the roll. Unless absent from the country, they were dropped after one year following notification of the forfeiture of membership. The framers of what was virtually a new constitution tried to guarantee that complete control of the American Medical Association would lie inside the organized medical profession.

Reorganization of Constituent Societies

The Special Committee on Reorganization had only partially completed its assignment when it had thoroughly remodeled the old constitution and secured the Association's endorsement of its work. Under the broad powers of the resolution that created the committee, it proceeded to infuse new life into weak medical organizations throughout the nation and carry through a general plan of reorganization for state and local societies. The same issue of the *Journal* that carried its sweeping plan for the revision of the AMA's constitution also contained the commitee's recommendations for the reorganization of societies on the state and local level, although the model constitution for state associations did not appear until 11 months later.

The committee stressed the necessity of strong county and state or territorial associations as component parts of the AMA, but considered most district associations a source of weakness to medical unification and raised even greater objection to most tri-state organizations. Doubting the need for organizations other than on the local, state, and national level, it emphasized the importance of unity in a trinity.[5] Over a period of several months, the *Journal* which shared the same view pointed out features of state and local organizations that prevented the development of a cohesive organizational system. It charged that "from top to bottom, there has been no system" and asserted that in several states the Associations were weaker than 20 years before.[6]

The attack on the chaotic state of medical organization centered on specific examples of weakness and disunity. Only a few of the state associations were incorporated, and some of these had virtually no power. The *Journal* found few instances of close federation between state, district, and county societies and only in the New York Medical Association and the associations in Alabama, Connecticut, Indiana, Massachusetts, New Jersey, and Pennsylvania did membership in the local society carry with it membership in the state body. Some state organizations had only an indirect and nebulous relationship with the local societies, and a great number did not recognize any subordinate organization. The same isolation that characterized societies within the state prevailed among the different state societies as well.[7] State associations, like the AMA before reorganization, relied upon the government of large, unwieldy bodies that only added to the weaknesses of isolation and disorganization. While asserting that the great movement for structural reform had to begin at the top, the *Journal* confessed that "the American Medical Association

[5] *JAMA,* 36 (May 25, 1901), 1436–51.

[6] *JAMA,* 38 (February 1, 1902), 325; *JAMA,* 38 (February 8, 1902), 400. The *Journal* played an indispensable role in the reorganizational process and George H. Simmons, the editor, also served on the special committee.

[7] *JAMA,* 38 (February 22, 1902), 514.

has gone as far as it can and now calls on the state and territorial societies to do their part. . . ."[8]

Under the pressure of criticism from the central body, leaders of several state associations appealed to the national headquarters for aid in unifying and strengthening their state societies. The president of the AMA made belated appointments to a committee that had been provided for by the St. Paul session and assigned the task of assisting the state societies in drafting new constitutions. This committee was identical with the Special Committee on Reorganization created the preceding year.[9] Early in 1902, the *Journal* pushed the movement along with a serial account of the disorganized condition of state and local societies. After allowing the matter to rest for about ten weeks, it reintroduced the problem in the issue of May 3 and submitted a model constitution that the drafting committee had prepared.[10]

The constitution proposed for the state societies followed roughly the plan that the central organization had just previously adopted. While expecting slight variations in details, the committee urged close adherence to the general features of the model plan. The constitution restricted membership in the state associations to physicians in good standing with county societies, although guests could attend the annual sessions at the request of the association or its council. The model plan allowed one representative in the proposed house of delegates of the state association to every county society with 100 members or major fraction thereof, if the society held a charter from the state association and paid the annual assessment. The new instrument allowed counties in sparsely settled sections to combine, provided the name that the counties adopted as the name of the society was hyphenated to distinguish it from other types of district medical organizations.

Novel features of the model constitution demonstrated the drafting committee's intentions of carrying through a complete program of reorganization. The plan proposed a division of each state into ten councilor districts, each under a councilor who would be "organizer, peacemaker and censor for his district." The councilors' work consisted of visiting each county within their jurisdiction at least once a year and of organizing component societies where none existed. The constitution called for

[8] *JAMA,* 38 (February 15, 1902), 460.

[9] *JAMA,* 38 (June 25, 1902), 1642.

[10] The following analysis of the model constitution is based on the final draft appearing in the *JAMA,* 38 (May 3, 1902), 1156–61.

the submission of an annual report to the state associations on conditions within the councilors' jurisdictions. Collectively, the councilors constituted the Board of Censors of the association. This board had power to consider questions on the standing of members and their relation to the county or state association, and constituted a court of appeal on all questions that involved the discipline of a member or county society when the decision of a local councilor was challenged.

Although all power in determing major policies resided in the house of delegates, the model constitution called for an adequate executive staff. It followed the plan of the American Medical Association in providing for a president, vice-presidents (although an unspecified number), a treasurer, and a secretary. Anticipating heavy duties for the secretary, the framers of the constitution suggested remuneration for his services at a sum determined by the House of Delegates, and for the employment of assistants if considered advisable.

Incorporation Issue

Before the Association had carried through its plan for the reorganization of societies on the state level, however, it faced the problem of incorporating nationally. When the advising attorney, Jesse A. Baldwin, stated his view on March 13, 1903, that the constitution of 1901 was invalid since adopted at a session outside the state of Illinois which had chartered the Association, the whole organizational program seemed jeopardized.[11] In response to a resolution for national incorporation adopted by the Atlantic City session in 1904, the Committee on Reorganization appealed to Congress for a national charter, but the bill as amended prevented the transaction of business outside the District of Columbia, retaining the very type of restriction that the Association sought to escape.[12]

The AMA continued to press Congress for a national charter which would allow the transaction of business anywhere in the United States, but the Judiciary Committee of the House, doubting its constitutionality, refused to approve it. A further check to the movement for national incorporation appeared in the trustees' report to the Portland session of 1905 which seemed unsympathetic toward the idea.[13] The House of

[11] *JAMA,* 40 (May 9, 1903), 1316.
[12] *JAMA,* 42 (June 18, 1904), 1634; *JAMA,* 45 (July 22, 1905), 269.
[13] Charles A. L. Reed, *JAMA,* 46 (January 20, 1906), 212.

Delegates refused to allow an official investigation of the validity of the new constitution and voted down a resolution proposing the appointment of a committee for this purpose. The legality of the Association's conduct in transacting business outside the state of Illinois lay in doubt until 1916, when the Supreme Court of the state decided that nonprofit corporations, with which the AMA was classed, had this privilege.[14]

Raising Educational Standards

The enthusiasm that the Association brought to the task of reorganization characterized its efforts to improve medical education as well. Finding it unnecessary to make more than minor modifications in its Code of Ethics, which became the "Principles of Medical Ethics of the American Medical Association" in 1903, the AMA turned to medical education as the area in greatest need of reform.[15] Leaders of the Association saw little hope of advancing either professional ethics or political reforms on health and medical fronts as long as the profession made no effort to raise the generally low levels of medical training. In January, 1904, the editor of the *Journal* called attention to the backward state of medical education, its inferiority to that of many nations, and to the flood of graduates that annually took their place in the profession. He noted that medical schools, numbering 90 in 1880, had increased to 154, which would supply the nation with twice as many physicians as would be required to maintain the already "absurdly crowded conditions."[16]

[14] *JAMA,* 45 (July 22, 1905), 285; *JAMA,* 70 (June 15, 1918), 1835–36; Fishbein, *History of AMA,* p. 305. The case that culminated in the state Supreme Court decision grew out of the unsuccessful effort of G. Frank Lydston to remove the trustees because they were elected at a meeting held outside the state of Illinois.

[15] The Committee on Reorganization proposed no revisions to the Code of Ethics but a few changes suggested by the New York State Medical Association were endorsed by the AMA's Committee on Medical Ethics and accepted by the House of Delegates. The AMA left state societies with the power to draw up their own rules of professional conduct as long as their standards harmonized with its own. *JAMA,* 36 (June 8, 1901), 1642; *JAMA,* 38 (June 21, 1902), 1649; *JAMA,* 40 (May 16, 1903), 1379.

[16] George H. Simmons "Medical Education and Preliminary Requirements," *JAMA,* 45 (May 7, 1904), 1205. This article was an address Simmons gave at Drake University, Des Moines, Iowa, January 29, 1904, at the dedication of a new building of the medical department. An editorial of August, 1904, reported 157 medical schools which included 133 regular, 19 homeopathic, ten eclectic, three physiomedical, and one offering various forms of sectarian instruction. *JAMA,* 43 (August 13, 1904), 466.

Several months later a *Journal* editorial attacked the superficial character of most internship training, charging that "the staff of some hospitals is encumbered with men who are incapable of teaching internes . . ." and added that probably more than half of all graduates took no internship work whatever.[17]

The *Journal's* exposure of the worsening crisis in medical education was only a part of the Association's effort to bring about reform. With the creation of a Council on Medical Education in 1904, which supplanted the Committee on Medical Education, it made its greatest contribution to the advancement of medical standards. Establishment of the council rested on the Association's belief that the American form of government made federal control "improbable if not impossible" and placed upon the organization much of the responsibility for improving conditions. The AMA authorized the council to make annual reports to the House of Delegates on medical education, to suggest methods of improving standards, and to serve as an agency for advancing the Association's reform policies.[18] A few months later the *Journal* sketched the dimensions of the committee's task. It noted the lack of co-operation among most agencies dealing with medical standards and referred to the inadequacy of state requirements for licensure. It cited the low admission requirements for medical training in most institutions and weaknesses in their educational programs. It also noted the limited access medical schools had to the clinical materials of hospitals and referred to the frequency with which the performance of medical institutions fell short of announcement claims.[19]

The Council on Medical Education approached its arduous task with considerable vigor, but reconciled to the process of gradual reform. In April, 1905, it held a conference in Chicago, attended largely by delegates from most state and territorial licensing bodies and committees of the Association of American Medical Colleges and the Southern Medical College Association to discuss the advancement of medical education. About three weeks later it submitted an "ideal standard" to the House of Delegates meeting in Portland, Oregon, as well as a statement of

[17] *JAMA*, 43 (August 13, 1904), 469–70.

[18] *JAMA*, 42 (June 11, 1904), 1576, 1582. A temporary Committee on Medical Education made the recommendation for the creation of a permanent committee. First appointees to the five-member permanent committee were V. C. Vaughan, Charles H. Frazier, A. D. Bevan, John A. Witherspoon, and W. T. Councilman. *JAMA*, 43 (August 13, 1904), see frontispiece.

[19] Editorial, *JAMA*, 43 (August 13, 1904), 468–69.

goals that could be more readily reached. This standards set a high school education and a year's training in several basic science courses as a prerequisite for admission to medical schools and called for a four-year medical program and a year's internship. Recommendations that the council felt might be adopted earlier included requirements of a high school education for medical training without a year of basic science work, a four-year medical course of not less than seven months each year, and passage of an examination given by the state board.[20]

Despite formidable obstructions to the council's work, it had reversed the degenerating trends in medical education by the end of the decade and could report substantial gains. After two tours of medical institutions, the council announced in 1910 that the current rate of medical progress would soon place standards of American medical education among the highest in the world. Yet it found no reason for complacency and proceeded to challenge medical schools with an appeal for greater improvement. As a guide for establishing higher standards it proposed a 25-point program which it called "Essentials of An Acceptable Medical College." This program greatly enlarged on the council's earlier recommendations and left no area of medical education untouched. In addition, the council had assisted in drafting a model bill for state adoption, regulating admission to the practice of medicine.[21]

Among the most important contributions that the Association made to the improvement of medical education, however, was the assistance it gave to Abraham Flexner in his investigation of American medical schools. The editor of the *Journal* advised Flexner on problems related to his difficult assignment, and N. P. Colwell, secretary of the Council on Medical Education, made available its many reports and accompanied him during some of his investigations. The fearless exposure of deficiencies in medical education appearing in 1910 in what soon became widely known as the "Flexner Report" rested in some measure on the contributions of the American Medical Association. It ably supplemented the Association's own limited exposures and jarred medical schools as no earlier criticisms had done.[22]

[20] *JAMA*, 54 (July 22, 1905), 269–70.

[21] *JAMA*, 54 (June 11, 1910), 1974, see also p. 1970.

[22] Abraham Flexner, *I Remember: The Autobiography of Abraham Flexner* (New York: Simon and Schuster, 1940), pp. 114–15, 121, 130–31. Flexner, whose life was threatened after the publication of this study, later wrote that he did not have to proceed as tactfully in his investigations as did Colwell, who was dealing with fellow physicians, and added, "The medical profession and the

Improvement in medical education that continued during the Progressive Era did not stop when the international issues raised by World War I largely turned the nation's attention from most areas of domestic reform. A number of the older medical schools moved forward with impressive strides, while The Johns Hopkins University School of Medicine, of the newer group, lived up to its international renown. Forces that brought about the strengthening of some medical schools, closed the doors of others and left the nation with 86 at the end of the decade. The demise of 76 institutions between 1906 and 1920, however, gave the Council on Medical Education no cause for regret and inspired its fight for even higher standards. In 1918, it raised its prerequisites for medical training to two years of college work and reported in 1920 that 78 of the 86 schools required this. It also reported substantial improvements in the equipment of medical institutions and the requirement of an internship before licensure of physicians in ten states.[23]

The Association added to its successful struggle for higher standards in medical education a vigorous program to expand and activate its membership. Following its own reorganization and the drafting of the model state constitution, it launched a drive to start medical societies where physicians were not organized and to strengthen existing bodies. For an organization still partially paralyzed from the inactivity of more than 50 years, the task seemed all but overwhelming.

McCormack's Organizational Crusade

The organizational work of the Association in the first decade of the twentieth century fell largely on Joseph N. McCormack, who deserves much of the credit for its rapid growth. In taking up the duties of official organizer, McCormack left behind an impressive record in Kentucky, his native state, where the success of his agitation for supplanting the state's archaic health laws with more adequate statutes commended

faculties of the medical schools, as well as the state boards of examiners, were absolutely flabbergasted by the pitiless exposure. We were threatened with libel suits, and in one instance actually sued for $150,000." The Carnegie Foundation for the Advancement of Teaching sponsored this investigation which appeared in published form as *Medical Education in the United States and Canada.*

[23] *JAMA,* 74 (May 1, 1920), 1243, 1244, 1245, 1246; Bertram M. Bernheim, *The Story of the Johns Hopkins* (New York: Whittlesey House, 1948), see esp. pp. 7–17, 118–21.

him to the public and profession alike. Endowed with personal charm and bountless enthusiasm, this indefatigable organizer overcame almost insuperable obstacles to the Association's growth.

McCormack never allowed promotional responsibilities, however, to dull his sensitivity to the gravity of great national problems and abuses. Although stressing the need of medical organization for combating imposture, investigating lodge and contract practice, and protecting physicians against unjustified lawsuits,[24] he seemed keenly aware of the great social obligations of the profession as expressed in an article for state councilors in 1905:

> No great reform is possible without high ideals, and our ideal was a society in every county, in every state, containing as many as three or four medical men, embracing in its membership every reputable physician in the country and existing solely for improvement and helpfulness in everything related to the prosperity and well-being, not only of every member of the profession as a whole, but of every citizen of this jurisdiction.[25]

In the same article he suggested a plan of meetings for physicians either weekly or more often. He proposed a course of study "after some well-modeled postgraduate or university extension plan" which would bring to physicians of even the most isolated areas an acquaintance with the latest and best medical literature. Aware of the inadequacies of medical service, he concluded: "I am firmly convinced that there are not enough doctors in the United States to do the practice if every sick person received the careful, intelligent, scientific examination to which he is entitled."[26]

Nine months after the model constitution for state societies had been framed, McCormack entered the field urging state associations to adopt it and assisting them in the process of unifying and strengthening their own organizations. For sometime he entertained hopes of combining the different state associations into seven strong branches of the AMA, but opposition within the Association defeated this idea. The work of reviv-

[24] The Medical Historical Research Project of the Work Projects Administration of the Commonwealth of Kentucky, *Medicine and Its Development in Kentucky* (Louisville: The Standard Printing Company, Incorporated, 1940), pp. 263–64, 282–83; *JAMA,* 78 (May 13, 1922), 1475; Irvin Abell, "A Retrospect of Surgery in Kentucky and The Heritage of Kentucky Medicine" (1926), 63.

[25] *Councilor's Bulletin* (Chicago: American Medical Association, 1906), 1 (January 15, 1906), 34.

[26] *Ibid.*

ing dormant state societies often proved very discouraging. Writing in 1906, he stated that although the AMA entirely financed his work, "it is not well known that I have had almost literally to beg my way into most states and that I am still kept out of others where the need for everybody to do something to arouse and help the profession is even more evident."[27] He added, however, that the opposition of many physicians stemmed not from resentment to him or the association, but from the "delusion that their organizations are already so advanced that only the element of time is needed to make them complete." McCormack not only met opposition within the profession, but hostility from outside sources as well. This opposition he described as the proprietary medicine interests:

> . . . a powerful, alert and implacable foe to organization . . . with its agencies and tentacles reaching into and utilizing every distracting and disaffected element in every section. Resourceful, untruthful and unscrupulous, with unlimited funds, and backed by a powerful element of both the professional and lay press, its literature, multiplied, distorted and misleading, has been showered on the profession like the leaves of Vallombrosa.[28]

His brief work in North Carolina in 1903 illustrates both the opposition of the profession to his plans and the immediate success that frequently crowned his efforts. Meeting with the society assembled at Hot Springs, North Carolina, at its annual session in June, he found the organization proud of its accomplishments in the field of health legislation and at first impervious to the novel idea of reorganization. After two days of extensive discussion, however, he convinced his strongest opposition of the value of the proposed new constitution that the assembly unanimously accepted before the session closed. At his insistence, the society divided the state into ten councilor districts and appointed councilors in each. As the plan put into operation followed the pattern of the model constitution and illustrates that adopted by several other societies, it appears below.[29]

The reports of McCormack's work reveal the extent of his travels, the nature of his audiences, and the rigor of his schedule. In 1905 his activi-

[27] *Ibid.*, p. 52. For the plan of branch organizations see *JAMA*, 42 (June 11, 1904), 1580. McCormack entered the field as organizer in February, 1903. *JAMA*, 42 (June 18, 1904), 1639.

[28] *JAMA*, 46 (June 16, 1906), 1870.

[29] J. N. McCormack, *JAMA*, 40 (June 20, 1903), 1740. For the list of councilors in other states see the *Councilor's Bulletin*, 1 (November 1, 1905), 30–32, and 1 (May 15, 1906), 162–64.

COUNCILOR PLAN ADOPTED IN NORTH CAROLINA

First District	Oscar G. B. McMullan	Elizabeth City
Second District	David T. Tayloe	Washington
Third District	Frank H. Russell	Wilmington
Fourth District	Albert Anderson	Wilson
Fifth District	Jacob F. Highsmith	Fayetteville
Sixth District	Hubert A. Royster	Raleigh
Seventh District	Edward C. Register	Charlotte
Eighth District	Henry S. Lott	Winston
Ninth District	Thomas E. Anderson	Statesville
Tenth District	James A. Burroughs	Asheville

ties covered the Northern and Western states and ended in the Southwest. Between the annual sessions of 1906 and 1907, his organizational work extended to 13 states of the South, East, and Midwest, in addition to addresses delivered before the legislatures of Alabama, Tennessee, and Arkansas. In the fall of 1907, besides extensive organizational work in West Virginia, Indiana, Maryland, and Delaware, he spoke before the American Pharmaceutical Association in New York; addressed the general meeting of the national Woman's Christian Temperance Union at Nashville; spoke before the faculty and Civic Federation of Connecticut at Yale University; addressed the American Health League of New York; and the legislatures of Virginia and Kentucky.[30]

In 1908 favorable comments of his work appeared in the newspapers of Louisiana, Mississippi, Pennsylvania, South Dakota, and Ohio, and yet these states did not exhaust the list of those visited in the interest of the Association. Between the annual sessions of 1908 and 1909, his work, which often involved four speeches a day, was highlighted by addresses before the legislature of North Carolina, Minnesota, Indiana, Missouri, and Kansas. A little later he carried on widely publicized work in New England and the Northwest. Between the sessions of 1910 and 1911, he delivered addresses in 97 cities in 11 states. The South was the scene of much of this work where he spoke in ten cities of North Carolina, held 14 meetings in Georgia, and ten in South Carolina that attracted many laymen as well as physicians. In the fall of 1911, he worked again in the Western states and spent one week for the Association in Honolulu. While not neglecting matters of organization, his emphasis gradually shifted to the problems of educating the public on

[30] *Councilor's Bulletin,* 1 (November 1, 1905), 8; *JAMA,* 48 (June 15, 1907), 2043; *JAMA,* 50 (June 6, 1908), 1925–26.

national health topics and bringing the public and the profession closer together.[31] The crowded speaking schedule of his Texas trip in 1905 shows the extent of his organizational and publicity work there and illustrates the extent of his activities in other states as well.[32]

McCormack's Speaking Schedule in Texas, 1905

El Paso	October 30-31	Greenville	November 14-15
San Antonio	November 1-3	Tyler	November 15-16
Austin	November 3	Pillsbury	November 16-17
Beaumont	November 4-5	Texarkana	November 17-18
Galveston	November 5-7	Paris	November 18-20
Houston	November 7-8	Bonham	November 20
Waco	November 8-9	Sherman	November 20-21
Cleburne	November 9	Denison	November 21-22
Fort Worth	November 9-11	Gainesville	November 22-23
Mineral Wells	November 11-13	Amarillo	November 24
Dallas	November 13-14		

The *Councilor's Bulletin,* first published by the Association in November, 1905, provided McCormack with a means of reaching localities he could not visit in person. This publication, addressed primarily to state councilors and state and county secretaries, confined its interest largely to the work of organization.[33] In the *Bulletin* McCormack gave detailed instructions to state councilors about the process of organizing county societies and prepared them in advance for the problems that they would likely meet. Gradually the AMA broadened the functions of this organ and its successor, the *American Medical Association Bulletin,* to cover other matters of concern to state medical leaders, including abstracts of state medical practice laws and discussions of medical education.[34] While these publications appeared only bimonthly from September to

[31] *JAMA,* 50 (April 11, 1908), 1213–14; *JAMA,* 50 (May 2, 1908), 1446–47; *JAMA,* 50 (May 30, 1908), 1833–35; *JAMA,* 51 (September 19, 1908), 1025–26; *JAMA,* 51 (November 14, 1908), 1714–15; *JAMA,* 52 (January 30, 1909), 402; *JAMA,* 52 (June 19, 1909), 2056; *JAMA,* 54 (June 18, 1910), 2063; *JAMA,* 57 (July 1, 1911), 63; *JAMA,* 58 (June 8, 1912), 1803; George H. Simmons, *JAMA,* 49 (November 23, 1907), 1739.

[32] *Councilor's Bulletin,* 1 (November 1, 1905), 8; Pat Ireland Nixon with a foreword by Merton M. Minter, *A History of the Texas Medical Association, 1853–1953* (Austin: University of Texas Press, 1953), p. 251.

[33] *Councilor's Bulletin,* 1 (November, 1905), 1.

[34] *American Medical Association Bulletin,* 3 (November 15, 1907), 34; *JAMA,* 40 (May 23, 1908), 1732. The first issue of the *Bulletin* is cited in this footnote.

May for many years, they served as invaluable aids in the work of organization and reorganization.

The services of McCormack as organizer and field representative of the Association lasted until December, 1911, despite his desire much earlier to terminate personal connection with this work. Hoping that the session of 1908 would relieve him of these duties, he reminded it that "For eight years I have been almost a stranger to my home and my family that I might serve you."[35] The Board of Trustees, mindful of the heavy expenses involved in this activity, recommended abolishing the office of organizer at the same session, but suggested that the services of McCormack be retained in educating the public on food matters, arousing the legislatures to the need for uniform medical statutes, and informing the public on medical topics.[36] Although persuaded to continue with the Association in a somewhat different role, it does not appear that the quantity of work appreciably diminished.

McCormack's Success

The immediate success of the Association's scheme for the organization and reorganization of state and local medical societies exceeded all expectations. While the constitutions of the state association in Alabama, Connecticut, Massachusetts, and Pennsylvania so closely resembled the model that revision appeared unnecessary, McCormack informed the Portland session of 1905 that all the states except Virginia and Maine had accepted "practically" the plan of the Association and that almost 1,800 of the 2,830 counties of the United States had some form of organization.[37] The medical societies of Hawaii and Puerto Rico had also adopted the basic features of the plan before the Portland meeting.[38] The reports that state associations made of their rapid progress following reorganization encouraged the AMA. The membership of the Kentucky Medical Society jumped from 400 to 1,600 two years after reorganization, and that of the Michigan society rose from 500 to 1,800 in about

[35] *JAMA,* 50 (June 6, 1908), 1927. He dates these eight years from the time of his appointment to the Committee on Reorganization.

[36] *JAMA,* 50 (May 23, 1908), 1738.

[37] *JAMA,* 43 (December 17, 1904), 1875; *JAMA,* 45 (July 22, 1905), 274. Virginia adopted the reorganizational plan shortly before the New Orleans session of 1920. *JAMA,* 74 (May 1, 1920), 1233.

[38] J. N. McCormack, "An Epitome of the History of Medical Organization in the United States," *JAMA,* 44 (April 15, 1905), 1213.

the same period. In the spring of 1905, the Tennessee society reported a growth of from 400 to 1,200 following reorganization; the Indiana society showed a 25 per cent increase; the membership of the Illinois society multiplied fourfold, and the societies of many other states showed great gains.[39]

While the state societies experienced phenomenal growth following reorganization, statistics at the beginning of 1907 showed that the work was far from complete. The societies in Alabama, Delaware, Iowa, Maryland, Massachusetts, Michigan, New Hampshire, New Jersey, Ohio, Rhode Island, and South Carolina had completed or almost finished the county organizational work, but a number of societies especially in the South and West lagged far behind. The following table indicates the progress of organizational work at that time and the magnitude of the task ahead.[40]

The progress of local societies continued unchecked throughout the rest of the decade and many appear to have established their growth on a sound basis. The membership of all local medical societies that numbered not more than 35,000 in 1901 rose to over 70,000 in 1908, and by the following year at least 200 had established postgraduate training courses. These courses were intended to supply the practicing physicians with a thorough knowledge of a wide variety of practical medical subjects, and to aid local societies in starting them, the *Councilor's Bulletin* published in 1907 a schedule of courses that John H. Blackburn of Bowling Green, Kentucky, had prepared.[41]

Besides the growth of local societies, the appearance of many new state association medical journals indicated an awakening within the profession. While no state societies published official journals in 1899, 19 appeared in the following decade. In addition, eight other state societies had recognized certain publications as their "official organs."[42] The pub-

[39] F. W. McRae, *JAMA,* 44 (April 8, 1905), 1138–39.

[40] *Councilor's Bulletin,* 2 (January 15, 1907), 96. Compare membership figures with Table I, p. 18. The discrepancies do not obscure the trend.

[41] *AMA Bulletin,* 4 (November 15, 1908), 74, and 5 (November 15, 1909), 187–92; *Councilor's Bulletin,* 3 (September 15, 1907), 9–32. The original plan was for a schedule of courses that would cover four years after which the cycle with some variation would be repeated. *JAMA,* 57 (July 1, 1911), 70.

[42] *JAMA,* 52 (June 19, 1909), 2033. The nineteen state societies were those in Ark., Cal., Colo., Ill., Ind., Kan., Ky., Md., Mich., Mo., N.J., N.M. T., N.Y., Ohio, Okla., Tenn., Tex., S.C., and W. Va. The Medical Society of the State of Pennsylvania with a journal not actually its own is classed here with the associations in La., Minn., Miss., Neb., S.D., Va., and Wis. as the eight state societies with "official organs."

TABLE II

Progress of Organizational Work: January, 1907

State or Territorial Medical Society in	*No. of Counties*	*No. of County Societies*	*No. of Councilor Districts*	*No. of Physicians*	*No. Members of State Societies*
Alabama	66	66		2,022	137
Arizona	14	5	3	185	104
Arkansas	75	65	10	2,080	766
California	57	37	9	3,935	1,783
Colorado	57	20	5	1,469	716
Connecticut	8	8		1,288	780
Delaware	3	3		195	104
District of Columbia				985	484
Florida	45	22	8	605	281
Georgia	137	81	11	2,699	1,020
Hawaii					63
Idaho	21	4[a]		259	149
Illinois	102	105[b]	9	7,863	4,087
Indiana	92	86	13	4,763	2,109
Iowa	99	98	11	3,594	1,719
Kansas	105	64	8	2,458	1,202
Kentucky	119	99	11	3,238	1,602
Louisiana	59	46	7	1,395	746
Maine	16			1,167	486
Maryland	24	24	11	1,682	929
Massachusetts	14	18[a]		5,066	3,044
Michigan	83	80	12	4,100	1,966
Minnesota	83	71	8	1,920	1,105
Mississippi	75	59	10	1,631	930
Missouri	115	96	26	5,811	2,235
Montana	27	15	7	340	175
Nebraska	90	60	12	1,651	714
Nevada	14			80	53
New Hampshire	10	13[a]		671	403
New Jersey	21	21	5	2,245	1,228
New Mexico	21	8		177	123
New York	61	59	5	1,995	6,378
North Carolina	97	89	10	1,414	1,242
North Dakota	39		10	311	207
Ohio	88	87	10	7,950	3,482
Oklahoma		25	5	988	676
Oregon	33	24	10	659	332
Pennsylvania	67	61	9	9,379	4,574
Philippine Islands				170	57
Rhode Island	5	6[a]		690	322
South Carolina	41	41	7	1,050	659
South Dakota	69	54	9	510	245
Tennessee	96	61		3,169	1,055
Texas	243	159	15	4,826	2,690
Utah				278	130
Vermont	14	11		680	416
Virginia	100			1,825	1,413
Washington	36	19		808	507
West Virginia	55	22	5	1,319	597
Wisconsin	71	66	12	2,393	1,395
Wyoming	14		1	124	62

[a] Is organized by districts. [b] Apparently a misprint.

lication of these journals provided a needed contact with local physicians and facilitated the work of organization.

Broadening Public Relations Work

With the second decade of the new century, the Association's activities for the unification of the profession and instruction of the public entered a broader phase. These aspects of its work no longer centered around the activities of one individual, as an increasing number of new bureaus and councils performing more varied tasks largely overshadowed personalities. While the plan of the Association for pushing the interests of organized medicine and enlightening the public on medical questions remained the same, changing conditions justified changes in strategy.

The creation of the Council on Health and Public Instruction in 1910, similar to a board proposed at the Boston session four years earlier, indicated the desire of the House of Delegates to unify the activities of agencies in charge of this work. The governing body gave this new council authority over the work of the Committee on Medical Legislation, the Board of Public Instruction on Medical Subjects, the Council on Defense of Medical Research, and the Committee on Organization. The council was also given charge of the work of several subordinate committees, including the Committee of Public Health Education, better known as the Committee on Public Health Education Among Women. It consolidated the work of these agencies into five new bureaus, with one member of the council in charge of each. W. C. Woodward headed the Bureau of Medical Legislation; J. N. McCormack, Organization; Henry B. Favill, Public Instruction; W. B. Cannon, Protection of Medical Research; and H. M. Bracken directed the work of the Bureau of Public Health.[43]

The Bureaus of Organization and Public Instruction became immediately active in executing their functions. McCormick's work of organization and publicity in widely scattered states was now supplemented by the activities of the Bureau of Public Instruction. This bureau began the publication and circulation of regular bulletins on health topics that it sent to 4,818 newspapers and journals in less than a year after its

[43] *AMA Bulletin,* 7 (January 15, 1912), 3, 96; House of Delegates of the American Medical Association, *Proceedings* (62 Annual Session, June, 1911), p. 7. The House of Delegates, *Proceedings* are hereafter referred to as HD, *Proceedings,* with session and year.

creation.[44] Topics discussed in these bulletins included occupational diseases, white phosphorus, lead poisoning in Illinois, different aspects of the pure food problem, and other subjects of national interest.

After the Los Angeles session of 1911, the Council on Health and Public Instruction inaugurated a wider program of work. Stating as its principal mission "the development of public confidence in the purposes and work of the American Medical Association and of the profession," it planned for the extension of the work of the Press Bureau, as the Bureau of Public Instruction was sometimes called, the organization of a speaker's bureau, the compilation of a handbook for speakers, and the organization and development of a bureau of literature.[45] While the Press Bureau temporarily increased its production, its circulation later included only about 2,200 newspapers showing interest in its releases, and the pressure of other work led to its discontinuance in January, 1916.[46]

The Speaker's Bureau, established January 1, 1911, to provide a list of physicians throughout the nation capable of speaking at public meetings that the profession sponsored, proved unusually successful. The Association selected physicians whom their state societies recommended and requested them to fill speaking appointments not farther away than in adjacent states, receiving from the Council on Health and Public Instruction $25.00 for each engagement. Seventeen months after the establishment of the bureau, 64 speakers had accepted appointment to the panel.[47]

With the establishment of the Speaker's Bureau, the need for materials on public health topics became more urgent. The Council on Health and Public Instruction soon prepared a speaker's handbook that devoted a chapter to most of the common diseases and other health topics.[48] This book enabled busy physicians on the speaker's panel to prepare for speaking engagements with the least expenditure of time and effort.

Between the annual sessions of 1913 and 1914, the bureau, with an expanding panel, sponsored 133 meetings in all parts of the nation and deserved credit for the arrangement of many more. At the San Fran-

[44] HD, *Proceedings* (62 Annual Session, June, 1911), p. 8.

[45] *Ibid.* (63 Annual Session, June, 1912), p. 31.

[46] *Ibid.* (65 Annual Session, June, 1914), p. 27; *ibid.* (66 Annual Session, June, 1915), p. 31; *JAMA*, 66 (June 17, 1916), 1948.

[47] HD, *Proceedings* (63 Annual Session, June, 1912), p. 33. Although 64 physicians had agreed to serve on the panel the council's published record lists only 57.

[48] *Ibid.* (64 Annual Session, June, 1913), p. 16.

cisco session of 1915, it reported a total of 151 meetings and announced that 49 calls for speakers had come from 23 states after the funds allotted for this work had been exhausted. The list of speakers registered with the bureau had increased to 255 by June, 1917, but the expense fund provided by the Association had been discontinued the preceding year, and each society requesting a speaker then assumed responsibility for paying traveling expenses.[49]

The time required in the organization and work of the Speaker's Bureau retarded the development of the Bureau of Literature. The first literature circulated by this agency consisted mostly of materials against nostrums and quackery, as well as a few other timely articles reprinted from the *Journal.*[50] But the work of the bureau gradually expanded and by the time of the Minneapolis session of the Association in 1913, it had issued a wide variety of important pamphlets on public health. The following year it succeeded in securing co-operation from the secretaries of the state boards of health in preparing a standard series of twelve pamphlets on major diseases, written by eminent American physicians.[51] The extent of its work is indicated by the printing and circulating of 285,400 health pamphlets on 49 subjects between June 1, 1914, and May 15, 1915.[52] The Council on Health and Public Instruction reported to the New York session of 1917 that it had printed and distributed 1,133,500 pamphlets from June 1, 1915 to May 16, 1917, and the Bureau of Literature probably performed most of this task.[53]

Another agency, the Committee on Public Health Education Among Women, created in 1909, played an important part in the publicity work of the Association. It appears to have absorbed the functions originally planned for the public health bureau, and was organized to make use of the talents of women physicians in the AMA in disseminating public health information on the prevention of disease through women's clubs and other women's organizations. Three years after its creation, it had established organizations for this purpose in all but three states, and

[49] *Ibid.* (65 Annual Session, June, 1914), pp. 27–29; *ibid.* (66 Annual Session, June, 1915), pp. 31–33; *JAMA,* 68 (June 9, 1917), 1719.

[50] HD, *Proceedings* (63 Annual Session, June, 1912), p. 34.

[51] *Ibid.* (64 Annual Session, June, 1913), p. 17; *ibid.* (65 Annual Session, June, 1914), pp. 27, 30. Eight of the 12 manuscripts for the health series were completed when the Council on Health and Public Instruction reported to the session of 1914.

[52] *Ibid.* (66 Annual Session, June, 1915), p. 33.

[53] *JAMA,* 68 (June 9, 1917), 1719.

in one nine months' interval in 1911 and 1912 these affiliates gave 3,342 lectures to audiences representing the general public and 935 to groups of school children.[54] Along with the attempt to secure representatives of the committee in as many local societies as possible and "to connect the work of the American Medical Association with the women's clubs of the country," the committee encouraged a variety of successful projects that state branches initiated.[55]

Among these was the baby health contest movement started by the Iowa committee, under the chairmanship of Lenna L. Meanes, that soon developed into a national movement under the direction of the central committee. The Iowa committee's record in working with mothers for the proper growth and health of infants became so impressive that the Iowa legislature appropriated $75,000 for a woman's building at the state fair. The national committee changed its name in 1914 to the Committee on Women's and Children's Welfare. About the same time it began circulating a score card prepared by the AMA to determine the health and fitness of babies that local branches had the opportunity to examine.[56] Although a reduced budget and the war soon interfered with the work of the committee, it continued to emphasize the importance of proper baby care, working in conjunction with the federal Children's Bureau. It also expanded its activities to include agitation for adequate vital statistics laws in all states.[57]

While the Association's publicity and public instruction activities constituted a large part of the work of the Council on Health and Public Instruction, the council did not ignore the organizational work in which McCormack had been so successful. When state societies approved of the idea, the AMA paid organizers to work in building up the membership, giving the state organizations a percentage of the income received from "new business." However, it required the state societies to bear a part of the expense, asking that they turn over to the central organization one half or less of the first year's assessment of each new member. Although the immediate return did not make the work financially profit-

[54] HD, *Proceedings* (63 Annual Session, June, 1912), p. 41; *ibid.* (64 Annual Session, June, 1913), pp. 28–29.

[55] *Ibid.* (65 Annual Session, June, 1914), p. 36.

[56] *Ibid.* (64 Annual Session, June, 1913), p. 29; and (65 Annual Session, June, 1914), pp. 36–37; and (66 Annual Session, June, 1915), p. 36. Meanes soon became chairman of the national committee and was a prime mover in the work.

[57] *JAMA*, 70 (June 15, 1918), 1843; *JAMA*, 72 (June 14, 1919), 1751.

able to the AMA, both national and state organizations eventually derived strength from this co-operative endeavor.[58]

Aside from the work of the different bureaus and committees, the Council on Health and Public Instruction also engaged in several activities that did not fall exclusively within the sphere of any particular department. The council announced its intention in 1914 of making a study of the health activities of the federal, state, and municipal governments, and voluntary public health societies. It commissioned Charles V. Chapin, Commissioner of Health of Providence, Rhode Island, to conduct this study, part of which was completed in a few months. It sponsored a meeting in New York City, April 12, 1913, of representatives of 39 health agencies in order to bring about a better co-ordination of their work which led to a survey of the activities of voluntary public health organizations.[59] It did not conduct the proposed survey of municipal and federal health activities, although the Association joined with state health officials in securing the introduction of a resolution in Congress later in the decade providing for a survey of federal health work.[60]

On November 11, 1920, the council announced its intention of beginning other phases of work. It planned to urge the adoption of state legislation requiring compulsory courses on health subjects for all public school students and for all prospective teachers in state-supported institutions. It also urged the establishment of sections on public health and sanitation in all local societies that would prove particularly interesting to laymen. In addition it referred to the Board of Trustees the matter of establishing a journal on sanitation and epidemiology.[61]

The council manifested considerable interest in the question of social insurance at home and abroad and initiated an elaborate study of the subject. H. B. Favill, chairman of the council, persuaded Alexander Lambert, chairman of the Judicial Council, to join him in a committee to get this study under way.[62] They secured the services of the well-known

[58] *JAMA,* 66 (June 17, 1916), 1941–42. Surprisingly little is said of this phase of the work, which may indicate that little along this line was done.

[59] HD, *Proceedings* (65 Annual Session, June, 1914), pp. 25–26; *ibid.* (66 Annual Session, June, 1915), pp. 30–31.

[60] *JAMA,* 74 (May 1, 1920), 1239–40.

[61] Victor C. Vaughan, *JAMA,* 75 (December 4, 1920), 1574.

[62] *AMA Bulletin,* 11 (March 15, 1916), 250. Frederic J. Cotton of Boston, who had been chairman of the Committee on Compensation of the Massachusetts State Medical Society, became the third member of the committee.

expert, Isaac M. Rubinow, whose thorough survey was presented by the Social Insurance Committee to the Detroit session of 1916. At the next annual session the committee reported on other aspects of the subject and recommended that its work on developments in this field be continued.[63]

While the entrance of the United States into World War I checked the normal growth of the health and public relations work of the AMA, the postwar period brought about a change in the type of health and publicity work that the Association conducted. With the return of peace, the Association faced the problem of determining the nature and extent of further work in these fields. It did not revive the Press Bureau when the Council on Health and Public Instruction reported to the Atlantic City session of 1919 that many national and state health organizations had begun to supply health information and press bulletins and that "the propaganda period in public health is past."[64] The same report rejected the idea of reviving an active speaker's bureau, but suggested the maintenance of a list of speakers available to medical societies on request. It announced that the program for the distribution of pamphlets had become largely self-supporting, but indicated no plans for greatly expanding this activity. By the end of the decade, the Association had completed another stage of its public health work.

Growth of AMA

The supremacy that the Association had achieved over the medical profession after two decades of struggle contrasted strikingly with its precarious position at the beginning of the century. By enlarging the basis of membership in 1913 to include all members in good standing with state and local societies, the total membership had jumped from 8,401 in 1900 to 70,146 in 1910 and reached 83,338 in 1920. More indicative of actual growth, however, was the number of "fellows" in the Association in 1920, a term adopted in 1913 to indicate all physicians in good standing with a local society who applied for membership, subscribed to the *Journal,* and paid the annual fee. This number, that

[63] *JAMA,* 66 (June 17, 1916), 1951; *JAMA,* 68 (June 9, 1917), 1721–55.
[64] *JAMA,* 72 (June 14, 1919), 1747.

reached 47,045 in 1920, exceeded by more than five and one-half times the total membership in 1900.[65]

The ratio of fellows in the AMA to the total number of physicians within the states in 1920 showed a great advancement over the ratio of members to the number of practitioners 20 years earlier. The ratio in Massachusetts that stood at 1 to 19 in 1900 was 1 to 2.6 in 1920, while Pennsylvania's ratio climbed from 1 to 9 to 1 to 2.6 in the same period and New York's from 1 to 28 to 1 to 3. States farther to the west showed a similar increase. Ohio's ratio rose from 1 to 10 to 1 to 3; Indiana's from 1 to 12 to 1 to 3.6; Illinois' from 1 to 10 to 1 to 2.4; and Wisconsin's from 1 to 8 to 1 to 2.5. In the South, the ratio changed from 1 to 24 to 1 to 5.3 in Tennessee; from 1 to 24 to 1 to 4 in South Carolina; from 1 to 31 to 1 to 7 in Mississippi; from 1 to 36 to 1 to 6.6 in Arkansas; and from 1 to 40 to 1 to 4.5 in Texas. The ratio in California jumped from 1 to 13 to 1 to 2.8; in Montana from 1 to 9 to 1 to 3.5; and in Colorado from 1 to 4 to 1 to 2.9.[66] While the South Atlantic and the East and West South Central states showed the lowest average percentage of fellowships in the Association, the higher averages in other sections raised the general level and reflected clearly the Association's growth. (See Appendix, pp. 399–400).

Despite the Association's rapid growth from 1900 to 1920 and its ascendancy over all other medical organizations, a great part of the medical profession did not have membership in the AMA. The percentage of the entire profession that held membership in 1920 varied from 51.5 in the West South Central states to 64.2 in New England. Fellowships in the Association, a far better indication of the organization's strength, varied from 18 per cent in the East South Central states to 35.8 in the Middle Atlantic group. Even in the section with the highest percentage of fellowships the ratio stood at only 1 to 2.8.[67]

The membership figure for local societies of state associations that reached 82,894 in 1920 appears less impressive when other phases of the development of local societies is considered. Although some experi-

[65] *JAMA,* 57 (July 1, 1911), 58; *JAMA,* 74 (May 1, 1920), 1233. For the constitutional changes adopted providing for "fellows" in the Association see HD, *Proceedings* (64 Annual Session, June, 1913), pp. 10–12, 50. The figures for the Association's growth include the members and fellows in the territories and government services as well as the states. The membership of the local societies of the states in 1920 was 82,894, and the number of fellows was 44,992.

[66] The ratios for 1920 are calculated from statistics in *JAMA,* 74 (May 1, 1920), 1233, and those for 1900 from statistics in *JAMA,* 34 (June 16, 1900), 1555, and *Polk's Medical Register and Directory* (1906), 9th ed., I, 45.

[67] Calculations are based on figures in Appendix, pp. 399–400, 401–2.

enced rapid growth between 1911 and 1920, others showed a decline. Thirteen state societies reported fewer counties organized in 1920 than in 1911, and the total drop in the nation was 123. The membership of the local societies in Indiana, Mississippi, Nevada, New Hampshire, New Mexico, South Carolina, Vermont, and Wyoming decreased while the societies in Delaware, Georgia, Maryland, South Dakota, and Texas showed very little growth. The increase in the total number of counties not organized and the decline in the membership of some component societies (Appendix, pp. 401–2) indicate that in some cases enthusiasm created by McCormack's crusade soon waned, and that many district councilors became less interested in organizational activities.[68]

Success of the Journal

Perhaps the growing circulation of the *Journal* serves as the best barometer for reflecting the Association's rise in influence and prestige. Under the long editorship of the energetic George H. Simmons, who assumed this position in March, 1899, the *Journal* became a most effective instrument for advancing the organization's interest, while improving as a scientific publication as well.[69] Table III shows this growth over two decades.[70]

The 74,372 widely-scattered fellows and subscribers who received the *Journal* in 1920 stood out as convincing proof that this publication was more than a regional organ. In five of the nation's nine geographical divisions at least 50 per cent of all physicians received the *Journal,* and the West North Central states barely missed this mark. The East South Central states had the lowest percentage, not far surpassed by the West South Central group, while the South Atlantic states with 41.5 per cent led in the South by a wide margin. Within many states the percentage of physicians receiving the *Journal* increased remarkably during the second decade, and only in six states, Florida, Kentucky, Louisiana,

[68] The impact of World War I may have obstructed the progress of the organizational work in some states.

[69] Fishbein, *History of AMA,* pp. 191–92. Simmons was both secretary of the Association and editor of the *Journal* until 1911 when the two offices were separated. He continued in the position as editor. *JAMA,* 57 (July 8, 1911), 142.

[70] *JAMA,* 74 (May 1, 1920), 1237. The figures here vary somewhat from those cited above in giving the numerical strength of the Association but not enough to be significant. The different reports may have cited the Association's statistics as they appeared at different times during the year.

TABLE III

CIRCULATION OF THE JOURNAL: 1900-1920[a]

	Fellows[b]	*Subscribers*
January 1, 1900	8,445	4,633
" 1901	9,841	8,339
" 1902	11,107	10,795
" 1903	12,553	12,378
" 1904	13,899	14,674
" 1905	17,570	15,698
" 1906	20,826	17,669
" 1907	26,255	20,166
" 1908	29,382	20,880
" 1909	31,999	18,983
" 1910	33,032	19,832
" 1911	33,540	20,504
" 1912	33,250	21,620
" 1913	36,082	19,863
" 1914	39,518	19,751
" 1915	41,254	20,430
" 1916	41,938	22,921
" 1917	42,744	22,156
" 1918	43,420	23,117
" 1919	42,366	24,687
" 1920	44,340	30,032

[a] This does not include copies sent to libraries, colleges, advertisers, exchanges, etc.

[b] Before the constitutional changes of 1913 there was no class entitled "fellows" and before that time these were actually the members of the Association who met the same requirements as "fellows" after 1913 and are actually predecessors of this group.

Iowa, Montana, and New Mexico did it show an actual decline. (See Appendix, pp. 403–4).

Figures for the *Journal's* circulation in any given year, however, do not accurately indicate its influence. It reached many more than those on the mailing list, although the exact number cannot be known. The Association made several efforts to determine the actual percentage of physicians who had access to the *Journal.* In 1916, when the mailing list included 45.3 per cent of the physicians in the United States, the Board of Trustees concluded that it was available to 75 per cent of the medical profession.[71] On this basis of calculation, it probably reached at least 80 per cent in 1920 when the mailing list included 48 per cent. The formulation of plans for the publication of a semi-monthly edition in the Spanish language in 1918 assured the Association of a wider circulation beyond the nation's borders. Published with the aid of the Rockefeller Foundation, the Spanish edition appeared the next year. Before the year had ended, the Association received subscriptions from 2,908 persons in 21 countries where Spanish was the predominant language or widely spoken.[72]

The first two decades of the twentieth century spread the power and influence of the Association at home and abroad and firmly entrenched the organization in Chicago as well. Three lots at Indiana Avenue (now Grand) and North Dearborn Street, which the Association purchased in 1902 and 1903, became the site on which it erected its first office building in the former year. The addition of a new story and the extension of the building back 50 feet in 1905 reflected the growth and prosperity of the organization. Although it erected an adjacent building in 1911, it needed even more room eight years later. The Board of Trustees were considering the construction of an impressive building of six stories and a basement near the close of the second decade.[73]

[71] *JAMA,* 66 (June 17, 1916), 1941.

[72] Editorial, *JAMA,* 71 (December 7, 1918), 1914; *JAMA,* 74 (May 1, 1920), 1234.

[73] *JAMA,* 72 (June 14, 1919), 1742. No mention is made of these plans in the report of the trustees to the New Orleans session of 1920. This may be partially explained by the fact that the *Journal* was in financial difficulty; a special session of the House of Delegates raised the rates from $5.00 to $6.00 later in the year. *JAMA,* 75 (November 20, 1920), 1425, 1432.

Chapter 3 THE POLITICAL MACHINERY OF THE AMA, 1901–1921

As the American Medical Association pressed its organizational crusade in the early twentieth century, it also recognized the urgent need for making its growing membership politically influential. Lamenting the Association's political ineptitude in the nineteenth century, the *Journal* challenged physicians to recapture the spirit of public service that had moved the profession in earlier years. It contrasted the impressive public record made by outstanding physicians in the early years of the Republic with the political obscurity into which the profession had passed.

Political Heritage

The *Journal* had reason to point with pride to the influence of many politically prominent physicians. Three practitioners, Benjamin Rush of Pennsylvania and Josiah Bartlett and Matthew Thornton of New Hampshire, signed the Declaration of Independence and, along with 27 others, constituted the list of physicians that 12 of the 13 states sent to the Continental Congress.[1] Although this list included a number who achieved no particular distinction, it also contained the names of David Ramsay of South Carolina, who was president pro tempore of the last session that he attended, and Hugh Williamson of North Carolina, who later became a delegate to the Constitutional Convention. Other physicians achieving some political prominence were John Archer, a representative from Maryland in the early nineteenth century, who received the first medical degree awarded in colonial America, and Nathaniel

[1] See Appendix, p. 405.

Peabody, who shared the travail of giving to the nation its first birth of freedom, only to have his own taken away by 20 years of confinement in a debtor's prison.[2]

The Association was also justified in deploring the dwindling influence of the profession in national politics. Only 161 physician members served in Congress in the last half of the nineteenth century and none appears to have achieved any great distinction in either House.[3] On November 3, 1900, the *Journal* stated that only two men in Congress identified themselves as physicians and added:

> It seems strange that a profession so close to the people and representing such an aggregate of culture should furnish hardly the half of one per cent. of our lawmakers, while the other learned secular profession, the law, furnishes over nine-tenths of the total number. . . . No other country with legislative government, so far as known, so practically excludes the medical profession from its law-making bodies, and it has not always been the case with us.[4]

Seven years later, Charles A. L. Reed, chairman of the Committee on Medical Legislation, observed that while 92 physicians then served in the central legislative body of France, only four appeared on the register of the Fifty-ninth Congress that ended in March, 1907, and considered that so small a representation of the medical profession hindered the enactment of legislation bearing on national health.[5]

[2] Clifford P. Reynolds, Chief Compiler, *Biographical Directory of the American Congress, 1774–1961* (U.S. Government Printing Office, 1961) pp 1494, 1826, 486, 1436.

[3] Figures are derived from typewritten list [in AMA library] entitled "Physicians Serving in Congress, 1774–1961," prepared by the AMA's Division of Scientific Publications and based on material in *ibid*. The list includes a few members of Congress who were only students of medicine.

[4] *JAMA,* 35 (November 3, 1900), 1161. Actually there were ten members of Congress in 1900 who had either taken or completed medical training. Those who appear to have been at sometime practicing physicians were, in the Senate, Jacob H. Gallinger (Rep., N.H.), and in the House of Representatives, Henry D. Allen (Dem., Ky.), William J. Deboe (Rep., Ky.), James A. Norton (Dem., Ohio), Joseph B. Showalter (Rep., Pa.), and Frank E. Wilson (Dem., N.Y.). In the House, those who had studied medicine were John F. Fitzgerald (Dem., Mass.), Joseph W. Gaines (Dem., Tenn.), Joseph C. Sibley (Dem., Pa.), and James W. Stokes (Dem., S.C.). Rep. Henry R. Gibson (Rep., Tenn.) served as a professor of medical jurisprudence at the Tennessee Medical College but apparently never studied medicine. See Reynolds, *Biographical Directory of the American Congress.*

[5] "Medical Legislators of Two Republics," *JAMA,* 48 (May 25, 1907), 1733. Actually there were four who apparently had experience in medical practice and all were Republicans. These were Reps. Andrew J. Barchfeld (Pa.), Harold

Establishment of Political Machinery

In urging doctors to seek positions in legislative bodies, the Association did not rest the fate of reform legislation upon their acceptance of its advice. Instead, the AMA placed greater emphasis on the establishment of effective machinery through which it could put its potential strength to political use. During the early years of the century it not only carried through a program of organizational expansion, but attempted to make of the profession an important pressure group as well.

The creation of the Committee on National Legislation in 1899 was the Association's first step in the establishment of permanent machinery for the advancement of its political goals.[6] This committee moved swiftly to strengthen contacts of the Association with state societies and encourage their interest in political affairs. Only six weeks after convening the conference in Washington, D. C. in May, 1900,[7] it urged state societies to appoint legislative committees for reviewing all medical bills proposed in their states and in Congress. It also urged the appointment of one delegate and an alternate from each state society to a proposed committee, later called the State Auxiliary Legislative Committee, which it could call into session to consider urgent political issues.[8]

The Committee on National Legislation and the auxiliary committee often bore the title "Committee on Medical Legislation" and both secured legal status in the Bylaws of the revised constitution of 1901. The constitution authorized the president of the AMA to secure recommendations for membership on the state auxiliary committee from the presidents of state societies, and at the next annual session, President John Allen Wyeth reported that he had complied with this requirement.[9] The Association, moving with considerable speed to create most of its political

---

R. Burton (Del.), Edmund W. Samuels (Pa.), and Gallinger, who remained in the Senate until 1917. Gaines, who had studied medicine, was still in Congress. The two physicians entering Congress in December, 1907, were Reps. Martin D. Foster (Dem., Ill.) and Addison D. James (Rep., Ky.).

[6] The AMA had created committees with specific political objectives at different times which functioned for a few years. One committee of this type was the Committee on the Department of Public Health. The Committee on National Legislation was established as a permanent committee for promoting all of the Association's political objectives. See pp. 24–25.

[7] See pp. 25–26 above.

[8] *JAMA,* 34 (June 16, 1900), 1548, 1552.

[9] *JAMA,* 38 (June 14, 1902), 1553. While chap. vii, sec. 3 of the bylaws was specific with reference to the representatives from each state composing the Committee on Medical Legislation, it was very indefinite with regard to the status of the Committee on National Legislation, vaguely referred to as the

machinery, soon found that it would be more difficult to operate than to establish.

Glaring defects in the Association's political apparatus appeared from the outset. State committees charged with responsibility of surveying medical bills found their membership too small to function satisfactorily. The Committee on National Legislation, hoping to increase the effectiveness of state machinery and co-ordinate that of all state associations, proposed the organization of a new committee at its meeting in New York City, June 7, 1903, which would include official correspondents in almost all counties of the United States.[10] It called upon presidents of state societies to name capable representatives of the profession from all the counties of their states to serve on the newly created National Auxiliary Congressional Committee. Although two did not co-operate and two others were not able to make nominations immediately, by June, 1904, the Committee on National Legislation had secured a list of about 1,940 names, most of which it had obtained by the preceding December.[11] On February 11, 1904, the Committee on Medical Legislation (consisting of the State Auxiliary Legislative Committee and the Committee on National Legislation) met in Washington, D. C. and further complicated the picture by adopting the title "National Legislative Council" as another name for the two combined committees.[12]

"Committee on Legislation." See *JAMA,* 36 (June 8, 1901), 1646. Not until an amendment to the constitution was adopted in 1902 does the structure of the Committee on Medical Legislation become clear. This amendment shows that the committee was composed of "three members appointed by the president," being actually a continuation of the Committee on National Legislation, and "an auxiliary committee to be composed of one member from each state and territorial society represented in this association" and also one member from the Army, Navy, and Marine-Hospital Service. See *JAMA,* 38 (June 21, 1902), 1657–59.

[10] *JAMA,* 40 (May 16, 1903), 1375; *JAMA,* 42 (June 11, 1904), 1577. The Committee on National Legislation proposed that this large committee be called the National Auxiliary Legislative Committee but as incorporated into the by-laws of the Association it was known as the National Auxiliary Congressional Committee. *JAMA,* 50 (May 23, 1908), 1742.

[11] *JAMA,* 42 (June 11, 1904), 1577. The president of the Association in Alabama declined stating that he had no authority to perform this function while the president of the Massachusetts society refused on the ground that such an action would imply an affiliation between the state society and the AMA which he believed did not exist. In Alabama, however, the Committee on Medical Legislation secured the appointment of a representative for the state society through another channel. *JAMA,* 42 (June 11, 1904), 1579.

[12] *JAMA,* 42 (March 5, 1904), 670. As the name "Committee on Medical Legislation" remained the title generally used in referring to the combined committees it is usually employed in this chapter instead of the title "National Legislative Council."

The committees that functioned as the Association's political apparatus operated along rather clearly defined lines. The Committee on National Legislation, which in 1904 consisted of Reed, William H. Welch, and William L. Rodman, held occasional meetings for considering political developments on the national scene and plotting the Association's strategy. Besides assuming the routine work of correspondence, this committee called for conferences that brought representatives of the entire National Legislative Council together. While the committee had a large measure of freedom in dealing with procedural matters, it followed policies on pending and proposed legislation that the whole council established.[13] With decisions on political policy resting with the entire council, the Association hoped to add greater credibility to the position that it spoke for organized medicine.

Since the National Auxiliary Congressional Committee consisted of a large group of widely scattered physicians, its functions made possible fairly close contact with the Committee on Medical Legislation. All physicians of the auxiliary committee were originally authorized to call the attention of doctors and laymen within their respective counties to matters referred to them by the legislative committees of their own state societies or by the Committee on Medical Legislation of the AMA. They had instructions to press the interests of the profession on either the state legislative bodies or the national Congress "by every honorable means, personal and political, individual and professional, private and public, direct and indirect. . . ." and report their efforts on the state level to the chairman of the state society's legislative committee, and on the federal level to the chairman of the Committee on Medical Legislation.[14] As much of the work assigned to members of the National Auxiliary Congressional Committee duplicated that which the legislative committees of state societies sometimes performed, the auxiliary committee members were later relieved of this assignment.[15]

The early success experienced by the Committee on Medical Legislation in perfecting and strengthening the legislative machinery of the Association gave promise of making the AMA an effective political force. The committee multiplied its contacts and reported to the annual session of June, 1904, that the chairman's office had issued 30,000 communications and received over 13,000. The volume of correspondence of

[13] *JAMA,* 45 (July 22, 1905), 262, 259.

[14] *Ibid.,* p. 259; quotation, *JAMA,* 42 (June 11, 1904), 1577.

[15] Charles A. L. Reed, *JAMA,* 43 (July 9, 1904), 143.

the central office grew by 17,000 pieces before the Portland session convened in July, 1905, and additions to the list of local physicians serving on the National Auxiliary Congressional Committee increased by 860, reaching a total of 2,800.[16] In order to protect the Association's interests, the committee refused to publish this list which probably never got much larger. Table IV shows the decline in the membership of the National Auxiliary Congressional Committee by December, 1907.[17]

TABLE IV

STRENGTH OF THE NATIONAL AUXILIARY CONGRESSIONAL COMMITTEE: DECEMBER, 1907

State	*No. of Counties*	*Aux. Members*	*State*	*No. of Counties*	*Aux. Members*
Alabama	66	50	Nebraska	99	60
Arizona	14	12	Nevada	14	
Arkansas	75	51	New Hampshire	10	9
California	57	21	New Jersey	21	14
Colorado	59	53	New Mexico	25	14
Connecticut	8	8	New York	61	24
Delaware	3	3	North Carolina	97	13
Dist. of Col.			North Dakota	45	26
Florida	45	27	Ohio	88	61
Georgia	145	62	Oklahoma	54	13
Idaho	21	5	Oregon	33	15
Illinois	102	57	Pennsylvania	67	31
Indiana	92	60	Rhode Island	5	5
Iowa	99	57	South Carolina	41	22
Kansas	105	42	South Dakota	69	31
Kentucky	119	98	Tennessee	96	25
Louisiana	59	35	Texas	243	46
Maine	16	12	Utah	27	14
Maryland	24	19	Vermont	14	13
Massachusetts	14	13	Virginia	100	
Michigan	83	53	Washington	36	13
Minnesota	83	25	West Virginia	55	12
Mississippi	76	44	Wisconsin	71	61
Missouri	115	72	Wyoming	14	11
Montana	27	6	Total	2,882	1,420

[16] *JAMA,* 42 (June 11, 1904), 1578; *JAMA,* 45 (July 22, 1905), 261, 259.

[17] Charles A. L. Reed, *JAMA,* 43 (July 9, 1904), 143; Frederick R. Green, *AMA Bulletin,* 3 (January 15, 1908), 126.

The immediate success that the Committee on Medical Legislation experienced in the recruitment of membership on the large auxiliary committee inspired the conception of another scheme for increasing the local effectiveness of the AMA. It prepared a register of local political leaders in all recognized and organized political parties which, by the middle of 1905, included the names of over 11,000 political figures from about 900 counties, as well as information on the political climate of these counties.[18] The committee attempted to promote the development of friendly relations between members of the national auxiliary committee and local political leaders by urging each to consult the other about pending political issues.

The Committee on Medical Legislation reported in 1905 that the few attempts made to use this plan had been successful, and that the list of local political figures would be frequently revised.[19] A year later it noted that many physicians had already made use of the Association's political machinery. The committee found that they had learned to present their views for consideration at medical meetings, and to refer them through established channels to legislative bodies instead of appealing directly to their congressmen.[20]

The difficulty that the AMA experienced in building up and maintaining its political machinery in a profession that remained largely unorganized clearly demonstrated the need for a national directory of physicians. Preparation for this directory, which the Association published in 1907, involved contact with the 70 licensing boards and 161 medical schools and the creation of a staff of local correspondents that numbered about 5,000.[21] Through these correspondents, who probably represented in many instances the personnel of the National Auxiliary Congressional Committee, and by direct contact with physicians, the Association compiled a register far more complete and accurate than any ever published in the United States. The new directory provided a convenient source of information on all licensed practitioners, but a more detailed account appeared in the card index that the Association compiled while prepar-

[18] *JAMA,* 45 (July 22, 1905), 259.

[19] *Ibid.*

[20] *JAMA,* 46 (June 16, 1906), 1859. The committee noted only one exception to the willingness of members to use the legislative machinery. This instance occurred in the hearings on the pure food and drugs legislation.

[21] George H. Simmons, *JAMA,* 49 (November 23, 1907), 1737; *JAMA,* 48 (June 8, 1907), 1963; *JAMA,* 50 (May 23, 1908), 1737.

ing the register. Not only did the directory enhance the prestige of the Association, but it also gave the AMA an effective medium for damaging the position of unlicensed practitioners, all of whom it refused to list.[22]

Machinery Improved

Having established its political apparatus on the state and federal levels, the AMA attempted to make it function efficiently. The State Auxiliary Legislative Committee and the National Auxiliary Congressional Committee found that their functions often duplicated those assigned to committees established by state organizations. At the Chicago session of 1908, the House of Delegates adopted a resolution urging all state societies that had not perfected a legislative organization to do so. It also recommended the inclusion of the chairmen of the state legislative committees on the AMA's State Auxiliary Legislative Committee, and the inclusion of members of the state societies' auxiliary committees on the National Auxiliary Congressional Committee of the AMA. It also authorized that the name of the National Auxiliary Congressional Committee be changed to National Auxiliary Legislative Committee, indicating that the committee's interest included both state and federal legislation.[23]

Growth in the responsibilities of the Committee on Medical Legislation required a further enlargement of the AMA's political machinery. In 1905, the committee insisted on the establishment of a bureau of medical legislation at the Chicago headquarters that would place the political functions of the Association on a more orderly basis, expedite the handling of correspondence, and provide for efficient co-operation with the *Journal* offices. Although the House of Delegates adopted the committee's recommendation, the Bureau of Medical Legislation was not established until January 1, 1907, and not until eight months later did the energetic Frederick R. Green become its secretary.[24]

[22] *JAMA,* 50 (May 23, 1908), 1737; Editorial, *JAMA,* 47 (September 29, 1906), 1024–26.

[23] *JAMA,* 50 (May 23, 1908), 1742; *JAMA,* 50 (June 6, 1908), 1925; *AMA Bulletin,* 4 (September 15, 1908), 3–4.

[24] *JAMA,* 45 (July 22, 1905), 261, 277; Frederick R. Green, *AMA Bulletin,* 3 (January 15, 1908), 127.

Machinery in Operation

With the assistance of the Bureau of Medical Legislation, the Committee on Medical Legislation undertook work that it had contemplated for some time. The bureau aided in the collection of information on medical practice acts, the compilation and analysis of federal and state supreme court decisions on these acts, the framing of a model vital statistics bill, and the accumulation of material on the pure food and drugs legislation and other state health laws.[25] The committee hoped that this material would prove valuable in the formulation of model laws on health and other medical subjects. While the collection of this data placed heavy burdens on the bureau and required the co-operation of state boards of health and state boards of medical examiners, it created a reservoir of information available to the AMA and to the state health and medical agencies as well.

Starting with what material the Committee on Medical Legislation had accumulated, the bureau made rapid progress in carrying out its difficult assignment. On November 15, 1907, it published a preliminary study of the medical practice acts of the states and territories in the *American Medical Association Bulletin,* with the assurance that this study would be kept up-to-date.[26] The compilation and analysis of decisions of state and federal courts on medical practice laws required a longer time. While this study progressed, the Committee on Medical Legislation urged no major changes in these acts until after a model practice bill had been prepared. Although the bureau generally found the state records on court decisions and the opinions of attorney generals in a chaotic condition, by the time of the St. Louis session of 1910, it had completed this work and had classified and indexed 200 Supreme Court decisions.[27] Nor did this include the material it had collected on the decisions of lower courts.

Although the bureau appears to have taken little part in framing the model vital statistics bill, it was probably responsible for getting this measure before state boards of health and the registrars of vital statistics in all the principal cities before June, 1908. The Committee on Medical

[25] *JAMA,* 50 (May 23, 1908), 1740–41; Frederick R. Green, *AMA Bulletin,* 3 (January 15, 1908), 127–29.

[26] Frederick R. Green, *AMA Bulletin,* 3 (January 15, 1908), 127; *JAMA,* 50 (May 23, 1908), 1741.

[27] *JAMA,* 50 (May 23, 1908), 1741; Frederick R. Green, *AMA Bulletin,* 3 (January 15, 1908), 127; *JAMA,* 54 (June 11, 1910), 1970–72.

Legislation reported to the House of Delegates in 1909 that a new vital statistics bill had been framed and that the committee and the bureau would continue to work for its adoption in all non-registration states. It believed that the model bill was suitable for adoption in all states without any major alterations.[28]

The Committee on Medical Legislation sought to implement the national Pure Food and Drugs Act with corresponding state laws. While reluctant to draft a model bill because of the difficulty of establishing uniformity, it upheld the laws of Kentucky and Tennessee as among the best. At the annual conference of the committee in Chicago in January, 1909, however, it endorsed a model bill that had been prepared for the Association of National and State Food and Dairy Departments by an assistant to the Attorney General of the United States, R. M. Allen, who had drafted the Kentucky law. Following the conference, the bureau printed the model bill and gave it wide circulation.[29] It also began the compilation of state health laws with the expectation of later publishing a volume that included these measures, and by June, 1910, had collected over 300 health laws from 43 states. The Committee on Medical Legislation decided against publication, however, since the volume would meet no great demand and entailed excessive publication costs.[30]

As the Committee on Medical Legislation came to the close of the decade, its work afforded grounds for both pride and disappointment. While not successful in all of its political activities on the national level, it rejoiced over the passage of the federal Pure Food and Drugs Act. It looked with pride at the vast and valuable materials it had acquired on matters related to the profession's interest. It also found that its own prestige had risen in the Association. In 1909, the House of Delegates agreed to leave "to the discretion of the Committee on Medical Legislation" matters pertaining to "policy and procedure relative to legislation not specifically covered by resolutions passed at the present session....[31] While this affirmation of confidence appears to have endorsed a policy that had existed for several years, it can be taken as a complimentary gesture on the part of the House of Delegates.

[28] *JAMA,* 54 (June 11, 1910), 1972; *JAMA,* 52 (June 19, 1909), 2042. The model vital statistics bill was framed by representatives of the Committee on Medical Legislation after consultation with leading authorities on the subject.

[29] *JAMA,* 50 (May 23, 1908), 1741; *JAMA,* 52 (June 19, 1909), 2042.

[30] *JAMA,* 54 (June 11, 1910), 1970. A new building at the headquarters that was soon to be completed necessitated the efforts for economy.

[31] *JAMA,* 52 (June 19, 1909), 2081.

The committee, however, had less reason for pride when it assessed the strength of the legislative machinery established throughout the Nation. The State Auxiliary Legislative Committee and the larger National Auxiliary Legislative Committee did not maintain a high degree of interest in the discharge of their activities. As already indicated, the list of members of the National Auxiliary Legislative Committee that increased to 2,800 by July, 1905, dropped to a little over half that number by the end of 1907. The Committee on Medical Legislation complained to the Boston session of 1906 that at the last meeting with the State Auxiliary Legislative Committee many of the state and territorial societies sent no representatives, either due to a failure to make appointments or to provide for the expense of the trip.[32] Although the roll of the National Legislative Council in 1906 included 50 names, only 15 members attended the January conference at the nation's capital, and attendance at later conferences was hardly more encouraging.[33]

The legislative work of the Association, like its organizational activities, entered a somewhat broader phase at the beginning of the second decade of the new century. Indications appeared early in 1910 that a movement was under way for the consolidation of many of the Association's bureaus when the Council on Medical Education and the Committee on Medical Legislation began holding their conferences together. In the same year the Association's attempt to merge some of its scattered bureaus and agencies with related functions brought the legislative work of the organization under the direction of the Council on Health and Public Instruction. The House of Delegates established a Bureau of Legislation within the council, headed by William C. Woodward, and the Board of Trustees appointed Frederick R. Green, formerly the secretary of the old Bureau of Medical Legislation, as secretary of the newly created council.[34]

Under Woodward's leadership, the new bureau retained and used the Association's state and local machinery and worked toward the completion of several projects that the Bureau of Medical Legislation left unfinished.[35] It continued collecting state health laws and abstracting

[32] *JAMA,* 46 (June 16, 1906), 1859.

[33] Charles A. L. Reed, *JAMA,* 46 (January 20, 1906), 210. While this roll was not altogether up-to-date it was the latest information the AMA had on the members of this committee. For attendance at some later meetings see *JAMA,* 48 (January 12, 1907), 152, and *JAMA,* 52 (February 27, 1909), 722.

[34] *JAMA,* 54 (March 5, 1910), 813; HD, *Proceedings* (62 Annual Session, June, 1911), p. 7.

[35] HD, *Proceedings* (62 Annual Session, June, 1911), p. 8.

Supreme Court decisions on medical practice acts, but not until the creation of the Medicolegal Bureau within the council, January 1, 1913, did the work get well under way.[36]

Under the capable direction of John Hubbard, the bureau rapidly completed the work of collecting laws on public health matters, revised the model vital statistics bill, and undertook the task of preparing a series of model health laws. It also prepared a mailing list of about 1,000 names which included many governors, chief justices, noted members of the American Bar Association, and other prominent figures and asked for their opinions as to the ten most important topics for further state legislation. By the June session of 1914, it had established contact with legislative reference bureaus in many states and had begun to exchange information with them on public health topics.[37] Before another session of the House of Delegates opened, it had published *The Digest of Supreme Court Decisions on Medical Practice Acts.* It had also begun the compilation of Supreme Court decisions on malpractice, "medicolegal relations of physicians," and "the powers and duties of state boards of health."[38]

Decline of Operations

The problems that confronted the nation during World War I not only checked the organizational and publicity work of the AMA, but arrested its work along legislative lines as well. The Council on Health and Public Instruction that ordinarily informed the annual sessions about these matters had little to report toward the close of the decade. The national crisis checked the growing work of the Bureau of Medical Legislation and the Medicolegal Bureau, contact with state and local committee members seems to have been largely lost. The political functions of the Association were in need of revival by the end of the second decade.

The Association, however, could look in retrospect over 20 years of political agitation with some degree of pleasure. Both the federal and state governments had yielded to the enlightened pressure of progres-

[36] *Ibid.,* p. 8; HD *Proceedings* (63 Annual Session, June, 1912), p. 35 and (64 Annual Session, June, 1913), p. 19.

[37] *Ibid.* (64 Annual Session, June, 1913), p. 19 and (65 Annual Session, June, 1914), p. 31.

[38] *Ibid.* (66 Annual Session, June, 1915), p. 34; *JAMA,* 66 (June 17, 1916), 1949.

sive groups by enacting better laws on health and medical matters.[39] The Association believed that some of its hardest battles had been fought. Its efforts were not very successful, however, in drawing members of the profession into legislative bodies. If representation in Congress is an indication of their influence in state legislatures, the profession made no real gains. Only 27 physicians served in Congress during these two decades, and none appears to have achieved an unusual degree of prominence.[40]

[39] In most areas of agitation for public health reforms significant results were achieved. By 1920 all but five states had adopted the model vital statistics bill and forward steps in the development of preventive medicine had been taken. See *JAMA,* 74 (May 1, 1920), 1241.

[40] See Appendix, pp. 406–7 for physicians serving in the twentieth century. Reed, in 1907, gave a list of physicians in 25 states known to be serving in state legislatures. The highest numbers were 14 for Pennsylvania and 11 for Missouri. Only one physician is listed for a number of states. *JAMA,* 48 (May 25, 1907), 1736.

Chapter 4

THE STRUGGLE FOR THE ENACTMENT AND ENFORCEMENT OF THE PURE FOOD AND DRUGS ACT, 1901–1921

As THE OLD CENTURY BEQUEATHED its bewildering problems to the new, it also transmitted a protest spirit that soon publicized the great liabilities that the new century had assumed. Out of the turbulence of the nineties, and from the agrarian revolts and agitations of minor reform elements sprang vigorous critics of the American scene, whose stirring exposures of corruption accelerated the momentum of reform and shaped considerably the direction of the Progressive Movement. About the time that the American Medical Association resolved on a more aggressive role in public affairs, and before it had perfected its machinery for political action, the alarming indictments of a few daring prophets had already offended the pride of a victorious nation still exulting over recent territorial conquests. While the AMA was at first too preoccupied with its own internal problems to give their agitation much support, it later joined the forces that contributed so mightily to the reform efforts of the Progressive Era.

Agitation for Reform

The rise of reform agitation among a group commonly known as "muckrakers,"[1] is largely explained in terms of the abuses created and

[1] Theodore Roosevelt "popularized the term 'muckraking'" in 1906 when he compared the man with the muckrate in John Bunyan's *Pilgrim's Progress* with

perpetuated by the industrial order and the ineptitude of the state and national governments in taking remedial action. Even the imperialistic impulse could not permanently obscure the gravity of domestic problems, as the passage of the frontier slowly removed the mirage of opportunities in the West and as social injustices and inequalities multiplied.[2] The muckraking movement, long overdue, capitalized on the dissent of earlier groups, but captured the support of a larger portion of the population than any earlier revolt. Whereas the agrarian and proletarian elements were moved by the agitations of the nineteenth century, the work of the muckrakers appealed to the middle class citizens in general and brought the support of popular magazines to their cause. Their severe exposures of specific businesses and individuals attracted the notice of a public largely unmoved by the more general indictments of critics in earlier years.[3]

While several articles uncomplimentary of the industrial order were published in the popular magazines of 1900 and 1901, not until the fall of the next year did the muckraking movement get well under way. Frank Norris pioneered in the crusade with his exposure in *Everybody's* of the ruinous speculation in the wheat market and the dismal life of coal miners in periods of strikes. A greater sensation came, however, with the publication of an article in *McClure's* by Claude H. Wetmore and Lincoln Steffens on "Tweed Days in St. Louis," followed immediately by the installment publication of Ida M. Tarbell's "History of the Standard Oil Company." The widespread popularity of the articles reveal-

---

those who exposed the corruption in American economic life, and according to his view, saw little else. C. C. Regier, *The Era of the Muckrakers* (Chapel Hill: The University of North Carolina Press, 1932), p. 1. Regier, while referring to earlier literature of exposure, says that "The years 1900, 1901, and 1902 witnessed the real beginnings of the muckraking movement" but considers Lincoln Steffens whose work got under may in the latter year "in some respects the real founder of the movement." *Ibid.*, pp. 49, 59. Louis Filler regards Henry Demarest Lloyd's *Wealth against Commonwealth,* published in 1894, as really the first muckraking book and hardly accepts Regier's estimate of Steffens. See his *Crusaders for American Liberalism,* pp. 26, 55–57.

[2] Regier, *Era of Muckrakers,* pp. 2–9; Walter Lippmann, *Drift and Mastery* (New York: Mitchell Kennerley, 1914), p. 5, attributes the success of this movement in part to the passage of the frontier. For evidence that the frontier was little more than a false hope throughout most of the nineteenth century see Murray Kane, "Some Considerations on the Safety Valve Doctrine," *The Mississippi Valley Historical Review,* 23 (September, 1936), 169–88, and Fred. A. Shannon, "The Homestead Act and the Labor Surplus," *The American Historical Review,* 41 (July, 1936), 637–51.

[3] Filler, *Crusaders for Liberalism,* p. 13; Regier, *Era of Muckrakers,* pp. 49–50.

ing the sordid state of business and politics plunged *McClure's* into a campaign of exposure that initiated a rivalry with other publications.[4]

Everybody's startled the nation with the publication of Thomas W. Lawson's "Frenzied Finance" in 1904, a picture of Wall Street corruption. The next year the *Independent* published John Spargo's vivid portrayal of the plight of children in industrial employment, and *Cosmopolitan* published Edwin Markham's account during the next two years. David Graham Phillips's "Treason in the Senate," published by *Cosmopolitan* in 1906, shook popular confidence in the higher legislative body, just as Burton J. Hendrick's exposure of the corruption in the insurance business, published by *McClure's* in the same year, further discredited business practice. When Gustavus Myers published *The History of Great American Fortunes* in 1910, most readers were satisfied that the prevailing corruption in business methods was no departure from past standards of conduct.[5]

While these exposures were of vital concern to the nation, other aspects of the muckraking movement were more closely identified with the interests of the AMA. Of increasing concern to the Association was Harvey W. Wiley's work that extended into the new century and received widespread publicity with the organization of the "Poison Squad" in 1902. This group consisted of young men upon whom he tested the effects of various chemicals frequently used in the manufacture of foods. When the Bureau of Chemistry published parts of its famous *Bulletin No. 84,* revealing the harmful effects of many food preservatives, it supplied valuable material in the fight for food and drugs legislation. Nor did the official phase of Wiley's courageous fight for the protection of the nation's health end until he resigned as chief of the bureau in 1912.[6]

Additional evidence damaging to food processors was supplied by Charles Edward Russell, writing in *Everybody's* in 1905. He showed that while cattle prices declined considerably in the three years before

[4] Regier, *Era of Muckrakers,* pp. 50–58.

[5] *Ibid.,* pp. 126–31, 151–52, 110–14, 139–40; Filler, *Crusaders for Liberalism,* pp. 118–19.

[6] Harvey W. Wiley, *An Autobiography* (Indianapolis: The Bobbs-Merrill Company, 1930), pp. 215–20; Oscar E. Anderson, *The Health of a Nation* (Chicago: University of Chicago Press, 1958), pp. 149–52; Harvey W. Wiley, *The History of a Crime against the Food Law* (Washington, D.C.: Harvey W. Wiley, publisher, 1929). Anderson's excellent study provides a needed balance in weighing the evidence offered by all sides in the struggle for pure food and drugs. See especially pp. 197–279.

January 1, 1905, the retail price of meat steadily advanced, and his exposure better prepared the public for the revolting picture of the meat packers' menace to national health that appeared the following year. Based on seven-weeks' observation inside Chicago packinghouses and numerous interviews with plant workers, Upton Sinclair's *The Jungle* revealed the incredible filth and corruption associated with the processing of meat, and the total disregard of the managements for the health of the consumer or the welfare of the workers in the industry. His stinging disclosures, never successfully denied, showed that these firms preserved rotten hams and slaughtered for human consumption horses, animals dying in transit, and diseased and boil-covered cattle.[7] The American people, generally tolerant of business corruption, became more indignant.

Still more closely linked with the interests of the AMA were the contributions of its allies in the battle against patent medicine frauds. Although Mark Sullivan and Edward W. Bok made significant exposures, the attacks of Samuel Hopkins Adams were the most destructive.[8] In 1900, the number of patent medicine establishments reached 2,026, with a production valued at $59,611,335, that had quadrupled in twenty years. Fortunes rolled in to firms whose extensive and extravagant advertisements baited a gullible public. Under such alliterative titles as Pink Pills for Pale People, Pierce's Pleasant Pellets, Radway's Ready Relief, and Swifts' Syphilitic Specific, crafty medicine promoters for years had exploited human ignorance and disease.[9] During 1905 and 1906, with 12 articles in *Collier's* entitled "The Great American Fraud," Adams attacked the nostrum racket, revealing the generally high alcoholic content of the mixtures, as well as the pretentious claims and enormous profits of the makers. His work did not end with these exposures, for six years later he began another attack when many of the conditions against which he fought passed uncorrected.[10]

[7] Regier, *Era of Muckrakers,* pp. 132–33; Upton Sinclair, *The Jungle* (New York: The Viking Press, 1946), see especially pp. 96–98, 134. For an account of the dubious methods used in an unsuccessful attempt to answer Sinclair see his *The Brass Check: A Study of American Journalism* (9th ed.; Long Beach, California: published by the author, 1928), pp. 28, 33–34, 37, 54. The first edition was published in 1920.

[8] Regier, *Era of Muckrakers,* pp. 181–82.

[9] David Livingstone, Dykstra, "Patent and Proprietary Medicines: Regulation Control Prior to 1906" (unpublished Ph.D. dissertation, University of Wisconsin, 1951), pp. 36, 45, 67, 85. For a careful study of the nostrum menace largely devoted to the years before 1906, see James Harvey Young, *The Toadstool Millionaires* (Princeton: Princeton University Press, 1961).

[10] Regier, *Era of Muckrakers,* pp. 181–82.

While several magazines and individual writers waged a determined battle against corrupt food processors and nostrum manufacturers, a number of organizations were aligned with the AMA in the same fight. As early as 1883, the national Woman's Christian Temperance Union established a Department of Non-Alcoholic Medication, and before the century closed the National Temperance Society also enlisted in the war against nostrums. The interest of several other organizations in the growing menace of adulterated food and drugs was reflected in the organization of the National Pure Food and Drug Congress which held its first meeting in March, 1898. Mrs. Walter McNab Miller encouraged the General Federation of Women's Clubs to enter the fight, and in 1904 this organization established a Pure Food Committee.[11] Largely through the efforts of Miss Alice Lakey, the Consumers' League began agitation for remedial legislation and became an important ally in the crusade. Other organizations that made significant contributions to the movement were the American Public Health Association, the Patrons of Husbandry, and the federated labor organization.[12] While these interests operated without the aid of effective press facilities for carrying their appeals to the public, they played vital roles in the agitation for reform.

Abortive Attack on Nostrums

When Congress was unwilling to extend federal control over the manufacture of food and drugs at the close of the nineteenth century, the American Medical Association embarked on a program of its own in exposing the nostrum evil. Showing some concern over the reports of unsanitary food processing that occasionally leaked out, the Association began its fight against the corrupt proprietary medicine interests, whose expanding business provided a growing threat to the nation's welfare. Long before the end of the old century, the *Journal* occasionally warned its readers of the evils associated with this business, but not until 1900 did it begin a feeble crusade against the nostrum menace. Under the heading "Relations of Pharmacy to the Medical Profession," the *Journal* published a series of eight articles between April 21 and July 14, 1900, that started its campaign of exposure.

[11] Dykstra, "Patent and Proprietary Medicines," pp. 180–84; Wiley, *Crime against the Food Law,* p. 52.

[12] Wiley, *Crime against the Food Law,* p. 52; Mark Sullivan, *Our Times* (New York: Charles Scribner's Sons, 1929), II, 521–52.

The leaders of the Association recognized the magnitude of the task before them. An editorial of June 2 announced that:

> The field is so large that nothing short of the most thorough consideration of the entire subject, in all its phases, will be adequate to furnish a basis for such conclusions as may be necessary in determining the status of the various medical agents and compounds which the enterprise and genius of foreign and domestic manufacturers are constantly evolving and offering to the medical profession.[13]

The second installment of the series, appearing in the issue of April 28, outlined ten phases of the proprietary medicine business that the Association planned to investigate and proposed a study of the medical instrument and surgical equipment business as well. The AMA promised to examine "patent medicines" of secret composition, in which the proprietary right was maintained through a "copyrighted label and in an arbitrary trade-mark or title," as well as "patent medicines" actually protected by patents.[14] Other aspects of the proposed work included an investigation of proprietary pharmaceuticals, pharmaceutical specialties, dietetic preparations, chemical products, and external antiseptics which included disinfectants and deodorants.

This broad offensive planned against the proprietary interests necessitated the announcement of another policy that, while threatening the foundations of proprietary medicine, was a serious economic threat to medical journalism as well. The *Journal* began agitation for the removal of secret nostrum and cure-all advertisements from the pages of medical publications, and, while admitting that its own pages contained such advertisements, promised that these would be removed when current contracts expired. Despite the *Journal's* contempt for medical prepara-

[13] Editorial, *JAMA,* 34 (June 2, 1900), 1420.

[14] "Relations of Pharmacy and Chemistry to the Medical Profession," *JAMA,* 34 (April 28, 1900), 1049. This installment also tells why almost all "patent medicines" sold to the public were a misnomer. "It should be remembered that the so-called 'patent medicines' are not patented for this all sufficient reason that, in order to comply with the requirements of the patent laws, the composition would have to be divulged, to which the originator or rather 'appropriator' would never consent, since it would disclose the fact that there was neither originality nor virtue in the alleged discovery. On the contrary, secrecy of composition is the *vis medicatrix* of all 'patent medicines,' since this admits of the most mendacious representation to bolster up their alleged virtues and puff them to the credulous public." For a fuller account of the distaste of the proprietary medicine business for patents, see Dykstra, "Patent and Proprietary Medicines," pp. 5, 24. Harvey Wiley saw one reason for using the term "patent medicine" saying that "patent means to lie open, and the literature of these nostrums lied openly." Wiley, *Autobiography,* p. 205.

tions of secret composition, it explained that preparations intended for external use need not necessarily be accompanied by the formula unless "active or toxic agents" were present.[15] It hoped that as medical journals removed false and misleading advertisements from their pages, lay periodicals and newspapers would also cut the life line of nostrum manufacturers.

Unfortunately, the Association defaulted on its promise to carry through an immediate and complete exposure of corruption in the manufacture of proprietary medicines and failed to live up to its pledge of purging its own publication of unfit advertisements. The issue of the *Journal* of July 14, 1900, carried the last installment of the article on proprietary medicines, and the work outlined in an earlier issue was left incomplete without any explanation. Renewed interest in the nostrum menace appeared in 1903 when the *Journal* announced that a committee had been appointed to consider the establishment of a National Bureau of Medicines and Foods, sponsored by the AMA and the American Pharmaceutical Association.

The original plan contemplated an association of reputable manufacturers and pharmacists who were in agreement with the officials of the proposed bureau "on standards of identity, purity, quality, and strength to which their products shall comply. . . ."[16] The bureau was to "secure adherence to prescribed formulas of all drugs, chemicals, foodstuffs, and of all articles intended for use in the arts and sciences or for human consumption . . ." and could make inspections and analyses of the products of affiliated firms that were taken from the open market.[17] The expense of the bureau was to be borne by the firms connected with it. The House of Delegates at the Atlantic City session of 1904 rejected

[15] Editorial, *JAMA,* 34 (June 2, 1900), 1420. For earlier, unsuccessful efforts of the Association to cleanse the pages of the *Journal* of nostrum advertisements see Fishbein, *History of AMA,* pp. 109, 152, 168–69.

[16] *JAMA,* 40 (April 11, 1903), 1002–3. While the amount spent annually in advertising patent medicines is not known, Wiley's estimate that the figure reached about $100,000,000 at the beginning of the twentieth century was only an extravagant guess, since patent medicine production in 1900 was valued at $59,611,335. See Wiley, *Autobiography,* p. 208 and p. 70 of this chapter. The fact that the acceptance of nostrum advertisements seemed necessary for the survival of many struggling publications made this phase of the Association's work even more difficult.

[17] *JAMA,* 40 (April 11, 1903), 1002–3. See also *JAMA,* 42 (June 18, 1904), 1640, for the final report as presented to the House of Delegates. The proposed bureau's supervision over firms connected with it seemed complete when it was empowered to examine all articles manufactured by them that were used "in the arts or sciences or for human consumption. . . ."

a proposal embodying most of these ideas.[18] The Association was not yet ready to begin a persistent campaign of exposure against the nostrum evil or to adopt constructive policies aimed at driving fraudulent proprietary interests from the scene. The work of exposure passed largely into the hands of laymen, as the AMA temporarily surrendered the enviable position of leadership in the battle against the nostrum menace.[19]

Having discontinued a tentatively aggressive fight against corruption in the manufacture and promotion of proprietary medicines, the Association actually abetted the growth of the business by retaining the advertisements of questionable and fraudulent compounds in the *Journal.* In complying with the *Journal's* requirements, proprietary concerns supplied formulas for the products advertised, but these were often untrue and the *Journal* exerted no sustained effort to enforce honesty among its advertisers. A study of proprietary advertisements in five medical journals in 1905 indicated that the *Journal* accepted fewer than the others, but none of the periodicals had a commendable record.[20] The *Journal* had placed itself in a poor position to lead the movement for establishing higher standards in advertising.

Revived Attack on Nostrums

Although the Association had done little to check the advance of the nostrum evil up to 1905, that year marked the beginning of a campaign that gradually gave the AMA leadership of the forces attacking the corrupt proprietary interests. The Association took an encouraging step at the Portland session in July, when the House of Delegates endorsed a resolution closing the pages of the *Journal* to all nostrum advertisements.[21] More important, however, was the organization of the Council on Pharmacy and Chemistry at Pittsburgh on February 11, providing the Association with an agency capable of testing the claims and contents of proprietary medicines. While planned originally as a council through which the claims of "ethical" proprietary medicines (those sold or prescribed through physicians) could be tested, its functions were later

[18] *JAMA,* 42 (June 18, 1904), 1644.
[19] *JAMA,* 45 (July 22, 1905), 264–65.
[20] Robert Hessler, "A Study of Proprietary Advertisements," *JAMA,* 44 (June 24, 1905), 1983.
[21] *JAMA,* 45 (July 22, 1905), 276–77.

expanded to include the examination of "patent medicines" sold to the public directly.[22] The organization of this council profoundly impressed the Portland session. The reference committee, of which Frank Billings was chairman, told the assembly that "The Report of the Board of Trustees on the creation of the Council on Pharmacy and Chemistry is, in the opinion of your committee, the most important and effective measure ever undertaken by this Association to rid the profession of the abuse of the nostrum evil."[23] The extensive influence of the council was soon indicated when in September the Medical Society of California asked it to check the last issue of the *California State Journal of Medicine* and give advice about any advertisement that should be discontinued.[24]

At the Pittsburgh meeting of 1905 the council framed a code of ten rules, as a guide for determining what articles manufactured by pharmaceutical and proprietary concerns could be accepted and listed in the first issue of *New and Nonofficial Remedies,* published in 1907. It sought the co-operation of these firms and invited their representatives to attend its next meeting at Cleveland in September, 1905. The rules were thoroughly discussed at Pittsburgh, and several concerns showed interest in the work. Especially encouraging was the pledge of co-operation received the same month from James Wilson, the United States Secretary of Agriculture, and the willingness of his associates, Wiley and L. F. Kebler, to serve on the council.[25]

Struggle for Federal Regulation

Even before the organization of the council, however, the AMA had joined forces pressing for the passage of food and drugs legislation in Congress. Through the vigilance of the Committee on National Legisla-

[22] *JAMA,* 45 (July 22, 1905), 265–66; Lewis S. McMurtry, *JAMA,* 46 (June 16, 1906), 1851.

[23] *JAMA,* 45 (July 22, 1905), 276.

[24] Austin Smith, "The Council on Pharmacy and Chemistry and the Chemical Laboratory," in Fishbein, *History of AMA,* p. 877.

[25] *JAMA,* 45 (July 22, 1905), 265; *JAMA,* 46 (June 16, 1906), 1866; Smith, in Fishbein, *History of AMA,* pp. 871, 875–77; George H. Simmons to Wiley, Feb. 18, 1905; C. S. N. Hallberg to L. F. Kebler, Dec. 27, 1905 (Records of the Bureau of Agricultural and Industrial Chemistry, National Archives, referred to hereafter as BCR). Kebler had headed the Chemical Laboratory of the Department of Agriculture since March, 1903. Anderson, *Health of a Nation,* p. 103.

tion, the *Journal* kept its readers informed of the general character of the struggle and the forces opposing effective legislation. The committee took great interest in the Hepburn bill, passed by the House on January 20, 1904, and worked for its passage by the Senate. The National Legislative Council, meeting on February 11, recommended that every auxiliary committeeman in the United States write Senator Weldon B. Heyburn, chairman of the Senate Committee on Manufacturers, and the representative and United States senators from his district and state, expressing interest in the passage of the Hepburn measure. In addition, the council proposed that auxiliary members urge their county medical societies to pass resolutions favoring the measure and to send them, as well as any favorable newspaper clippings, to Senator Heyburn. When the Senate substituted its own measure (basically the McCumber bill), which the Committee on National Legislation considered superior to that passed by the House, the council ordered local committeemen to exert pressure for its passage. Reed, still chairman of the Committee on National Legislation, secured from Senator Heyburn the names of all physicians answering these appeals and announced that the response was encouraging.[26]

Failure of the second session of the Fifty-eighth Congress to enact food and drugs legislation only increased the determination of the AMA's Committee on National Legislation to secure its passage. Reed kept the Association's machinery in readiness for further political activity when Congress reconvened in December, 1904. On August 30, his secretary informed Wiley that the Association planned to renew its efforts to secure passage of food and drugs legislation. Late in November Reed inquired if additional letters from members of the Council on National Legislation to each of their senators would be helpful. He assured Wiley that "This office is at your disposal and we will do anything that we can to help the good cause along."[27]

The third session of the Fifty-eighth Congress had just assembled when the Committee on National Legislation renewed its agitation. On December 6, Reed urged Senator Heyburn to support the bill which the Senate Committee on Manufacturers had favorably reported on in March, contending that it was the only measure "that can in any effec-

[26] *JAMA,* 42 (June 11, 1904), 1577–78; Reed to Wiley, March 8, 1904, BCR; Anderson, *Health of a Nation,* pp. 160–62; Charles A. L. Reed, *JAMA,* 42 (June 11, 1904), 1578.

[27] Georgia A. H. Scanniger to Wiley, Aug. 30, 1904; Reed to Wiley, Nov. 24, BCR. Reed was in Europe at the time his secretary wrote.

tual way, secure the purity of food now notoriously vended in adulterated forms and the equal purity of drugs that are now all too frequently sophisticated." He also requested that the Senator bring to the attention of the upper house the many petitions that he had received from physicians and medical organizations and assured Heyburn that further petitions could be presented to the Senate within ten days. On the same day Reed addressed a communication to members of the National Legislative Council, urging them to ask their senators again to support the measure.[28]

Against the formidable opposition which the bill aroused in the Senate, the AMA and its allies fought a futile battle. The Proprietary Association, the National Wholesale Liquor Dealers Association, and many food processors found influential senators to champion their cause and prevent the measure from coming to a vote. This group included Henry Cabot Lodge, Joseph B. Foraker, Shelby M. Cullom, Arthur P. Gorman, Hernando D. Money, Orville H. Platt, and Thomas C. Platt who proved particularly sensitive to the interests of powerful home-state pressure groups opposing the measure. Although Heyburn succeeded twice in getting the bill briefly before the Senate, obstructionists denied the measure adequate consideration and turned the attention of the body to matters fraught with fewer political perils.[29]

Mounting public interest in the adulteration problem, however, forced the Fifty-ninth Congress that met in December, 1905, to deal with the troublesome issue that its predecessors had brushed aside. Exposures of nostrums and quackery, made by Adams and Sullivan during the year, awakened a large part of the public to the seriousness of the problem and aroused prominent lay organizations to action. President Theodore Roosevelt, who had shown little interest in the matter during his first administration, began to sense growing public interest. In November at a meeting with a committee advocating corrective legislation (which included Reed), the President promised to place a food and drugs law among recommendations for legislative reform in his message to Congress the next month.[30]

Into the renewed struggle for adequate legislation that lasted for many months, the American Medical Association brought the strength of its growing membership. In September, the *Journal* warned that "we shall

[28] Reed to Heyburn, Dec. 6, 1904; enclosure in Reed to Wiley, Dec. 6, 1904, BCR.

[29] Anderson, *Health of a Nation,* pp. 167–70.

[30] *Ibid.,* pp. 172–73; Mark Sullivan, *Our Times,* II, 530.

be compelled to put in sleepless nights to be sure that the measure is not passed in emasculated and deformed shape," but declared the following month that if the profession did its duty, the passage of a pure food law could not be prevented. Tempering confidence with caution, the AMA moved to the front lines of attack against forces that had strengthened their defenses against the passage of effective food and drugs legislation.[31]

The Association strongly supported the bill that Senator Heyburn introduced on December 6, basically the same measure that his colleagues had considered at the last session. On December 18, Reed inquired about further Senate hearings on the measure (which never occurred) to which he might send the entire National Legislative Council that would meet in the capital city in January.[32] When the council convened, January 9-11, Chairman Reed told the group that no further appeal for pressure from the profession at large was probably advisable, but asked that it reaffirm its position and convey to Senator Heyburn and Representative William P. Hepburn an expression of appreciation for their contribution to the fight. On January 10, the group visited Heyburn and discussed opposition to the measure. Before the adjournment of the council, the Committee on the Pure Food and Drugs Bill (composed of three members of the council) reported favorably on the Heyburn and Hepburn bills, and its chairman suggested that the report of the council and Reed's speech to that body be sent to the appropriate congressional committee.[33]

Early in February the editor of the *Journal* hoped to promote the passage of the legislation by building up even greater support within and without the profession. He urged Wiley to accept an invitation to speak on the issue before the Chicago Medical Society, promising to publish the address and to circulate at least 25,000 reprints. Senate debate on the measure that started on the nineteenth, however, left the AMA with little time to do more than apply pressure directly upon that body. Following Wiley's instructions, Reed prepared a petition to send

[31] *JAMA,* 45 (September 16, 1905), 858; *JAMA,* 45 (October 7, 1905), 1090.

[32] Reed to Wiley, December 18, 1905; Simmons to Wiley, Feb. 5, 1906, BCR.

[33] *JAMA,* 46 (January 20, 1906), 210, [Charles A. L. Reed] 211; *JAMA,* 46 (January 20, 1906), 213, 215. The recommendation of A. S. Von Mansfelde follows this report. The Committee on the Pure Food and Drugs Bill apparently served no other purpose than to keep the council informed on the nature of the food bills proposed in Congress and the time of its creation is uncertain. The committee was composed of A. S. Von Mansfelde, chairman, Silas B. Presbrey, and John S. Fulton.

to each senator, urging passage of the bill which would reach their desks at the opening of the session on the twenty-first, the day when Wiley expected the vote.[34]

The Association's petition, perfectly timed, stressed the urgency of the legislation. It informed the senators that the AMA's appeal rested on the "unanimous petition of the medical profession from each of over 2,000 counties. . . ." and an enclosure gave Reed's description of the opponents of the measure as they appeared in the last Congress:

> . . . the antagonism was derived from the manufacturers of blended and otherwise adulterated liquors, from the fabricators of foodless foods, from importers of foods and medicines so worthless as to be denied a market in Europe where they are made, from the makers and purveyors of worthless, dangerous, and enslaving drugs—interest in which, in the aggregate, and judged by the character of their business, cannot go clean-handed into any court of justice or command an honest footing before any legislative committee or legislative body in the country.[35]

Probably feeling more the political pressure of the AMA than the strength of its arguments, the Senate, reacting to agitation for remedial legislation coming from many sources, passed the bill by a comfortable majority.[36]

As organized opposition now turned to the House of Representatives for a last stand against the enactment of effective food and drugs legislation, the AMA also turned to that body to defeat their efforts. The *Journal* warned the profession that "All the influences that have been at work heretofore will now be more active than ever to prevent the passage of the bill or to emasculate it by amendments," and urged physicians to write their congressmen expressing approval of the Hepburn bill. On February 28, Reed wrote Wiley to determine whether the House would consider the Heyburn or the Hepburn bill, stating that his committee would petition each member of that body on the day of the vote, just as it had petitioned the Senate. On March 3, the editor of the *Journal* informed Wiley of his fear that if manufacturers succeeded in writing into the final measure provision for a "board of experts" to which decisions of government officials could be appealed, the measure would be vitiated. A week later he wired for an exact copy of the amended bill which James R. Mann, chairman of the Committee

[34] Simmons to Wiley, Feb. 5, 1906; telegram, Reed to Wiley, Feb. 17 [1906], BCR.

[35] Reed to Wiley, Feb. 19, 1906, BCR.

[36] Anderson, *Health of a Nation,* p. 180.

on Interstate and Foreign Commerce, had reported on three days earlier.[37]

The Committee on National Legislation waited anxiously for the House to open debate on the pure food and drugs issue. On March 14, Reed wired Wiley inquiring about the date of the vote assuring him that the AMA was ready to set its political machinery in motion. Less than a week later he forwarded a copy of a form letter that he had prepared to send to all members of the House. Instead of supporting the amended Hepburn bill, however, Reed's letter called upon the House to enact the Heyburn bill which the Senate had passed. Impressed by the Senate bill which made no provision for a board of experts, Reed favored the measure over the amended Hepburn bill, although the latter alone held promise of checking the worse abuses of proprietary firms. Reasserting the Association's readiness to act, he assured Wiley that "The letters to the House are ready to be mailed when we receive intimation from you to do so."[38]

The AMA had hardly prepared its ranks for battle, however, when internal dissension threw its leadership into confusion. The *Journal's* attack on the Committee of Experts deeply offended Victor C. Vaughan, Dean of the University of Michigan School of Medicine, member of the AMA's House of Delegates and Council on Medical Education, who, while connected with some food manufacturers, had recommended inclusion of a provision for such a committee in the Hepburn bill before a congressional hearing. This influential physician entered into a sharp controversy with the editor that broke into the *Journal* and reduced the effectiveness of the AMA's agitation. On March 28, Simmons wrote Wiley of a decision to drop temporarily discussion of "the Pure Food Bill" and added: "The Vaughan matter has complicated things frightfully, and I think it is best not to get Vaughan's open opposition just at this time."[39]

Although public interest in the enactment of food and drugs legislation mounted in the spring of 1906, the AMA watched the turn of battle

[37] *JAMA,* 46 (March 3, 1906), 660; Reed to Wiley, Feb. 28, 1906; Simmons to Wiley, Mar. 3, 1906; Simmons to Wiley, Mar. 10, 1906, BCR. Anderson, *Health of a Nation,* pp. 185–86.

[38] Telegram, Reed to Wiley, Mar. 14, 1906; Reed to Wiley, March 19, 1906, BCR. Anderson, *Health of a Nation,* pp. 180, 186–87.

[39] Vaughan to Simmons, Mar. 19, 1906; telegram, Simmons to Vaughan, Mar. 20, 1906; telegram, Vaughan to Simmons, Mar. 20, 1906; BCR; Fishbein, *History of AMA,* p. 728; V. C. Vaughan, *JAMA,* 46 (March 24, 1906), 901, see also editor's comment, p. 901; Simmons to Wiley, Mar. 28, 1906, BCR.

with keen disappointment. The editor of the *Journal* quickly reversed his decision to remain out of the fight and renewed his attack on forces trying to weaken proposed legislation. Early in April he bitterly protested the provision for a committee of experts in the amended Hepburn bill, which, he contended, could become a board established purely through political procedures and warned of the enormous power it could exercise. Just as strongly did he denounce another provision appearing in both the amended Hepburn bill and a measure proposed in Massachusetts, which allowed manufacturers to conceal the names and quantities of several potentially dangerous drugs which might be present in minimal quantities in their products. He declared that:

> The mere proposition that these drugs, such as opium, morphin, heroin, chloral hydrate and other narcotics are to be exempted because they occur in a certain apparently small proportion is as vicious as it is stupid. To enact such a law would be virtually to grant a license for the unlimited sale of enslaving drugs in a state of dilution.[40]

A little later he contended that "It is in the insidious small dose, gradually increased, either in time or in size, that the danger lurks," and added:

> There should be no compromise with the crime. Better let matters go as they are until the public is awakened a little more rather than adopt such a law as is now proposed in Massachusetts and in the amendments to the Pure Food Bill.[41]

Although the *Journal* found temporary defeat preferable to compromise on the food and drugs issue, it demonstrated no knowledge of strategy that a spokesman for the measure in the House had employed to secure passage of an effective law. Just as the AMA seemed unaware of the deficiencies of the bill which the Senate passed for controlling proprietary enterprises, it did not know that Representative Mann had weakened the Hepburn bill to discomfit proprietary interests fighting the measure, expecting to introduce stronger controls too late for the opposition to rally.[42] Believing that proponents of the original bill had sacrificed public welfare for private interest, the *Journal* seemed about ready to desert the fight.

[40] *JAMA,* 46 (April 7, 1906), 1036, quotation, p. 1037.

[41] *JAMA,* 46 (April 21, 1906), 1209.

[42] See Anderson, *Health of a Nation,* pp. 189–90 for Mann's strategy and how opponents of effective legislation learned of it.

Legislative Victory

Probably discounting the impact of Sinclair's *Jungle,* published in February, on the American public and the growing interest of many groups and organizations in the food and drugs issue, the *Journal* remained despondent even as late as the month of victory. On June 2, it demonstrated an unjustifiable spirit of loneliness in stating that while many organizations opposed the enactment of pure food and drugs legislation, only the AMA represented the people. Two days later at the Boston session, Reed showed no greater optimism in announcing that "At this moment [the bill] lies between the subcommittee having it in charge, the Committee on Rules, and the Speaker—if, indeed, the order ought not to be reversed."[43]

The House of Delegates at Boston restored a sense of direction to the Association's leadership that had been groping somewhat aimlessly.[44] On June 4 it passed resolutions that referred to the revolting meat scandals and the frauds of proprietary medicines and urged the House of Representatives to pass the pending Hepburn bill. These resolutions were telegraphed to Representative Hepburn with the request that they be submitted to the House, to the Speaker, and to the Committee on Rules. A short time later the Association made its appeal more direct and telegraphed the Speaker of the House and the Chairman of the Committee on Rules asking that consideration of the Hepburn bill be delayed no longer. The Association's decision to work for the passage of the Hepburn measure allowed it to participate significantly in the closing moments of the struggle. Within 24 hours after the telegrams were sent, the House on June 21 had reviewed and passed the bill.[45] By the twenty-ninth a conference committee had worked out differences between the House and Senate bills and submitted proposals that both bodies readily adopted. The following day President Roosevelt signed the Pure Food and Drugs bill, as well as the Agricultural Appropriation bill that carried the meat inspection rider. After the President's signature cli-

[43] *Ibid.*, p. 188; *JAMA,* 46 (June 2, 1906), 1701; *JAMA,* 46 (June 16, 1906), 1860.

[44] Leaders of the AMA supporting the Heyburn over the Hepburn bill appear not to have been well acquainted with the former and its limitations. It seems that they were thrown off tract by business interests opposing the Hepburn bill who began agitating for the passage of the Heyburn bill. They objected, of course, to the provision for a board of experts in the Hepburn bill. See Anderson, *Health of a Nation,* p. 192.

[45] *JAMA,* 46 (June 16, 1906), 1860–61; *JAMA,* 48 (June 8, 1907), 1966.

maxed the victory, Senator Heyburn paid fitting tribute to the American Medical Association, asserting that without its aid the pure food and drugs bills would not have been passed.[46]

AMA's Appraisal

The AMA enthusiastically endorsed the new measures and looked upon their enactment as a step toward safeguarding the health of the population. A week after the President signed the bills, the *Journal* referred to the passage of the food and drugs measure as "too good to be true," and the following issue referring to the same matter said:

> The law is far better in every respect than its most ardent supporters could reasonably have expected. When we consider the determined and able efforts which have been continuously made by the opponents of this legislation, and when we think of the wealth of expert testimony which has been advanced against it, we must confess to a feeling of grateful surprise that the measure is as strong as it is.[47]

The Association found absent in the Pure Food and Drugs Act some of the weaknesses which it had strongly denounced in the Hepburn bill as once amended. The new law called for no committee of experts and required that the presence of several potentially dangerous drugs appear on the labels of products offered for human consumption. While rejoicing over the enactment of the Pure Food and Drugs Act, the *Journal* also observed that its effectiveness was enhanced by the passage of the meat inspection amendment.[48]

[46] *Ibid.*, 1966; C. C. Regier, "The Struggle for Federal Food and Drug Legislation," *Law and Contemporary Problems,* 1 (December, 1933), 14–15. Wiley apparently did not place quite this high a value on the work of the AMA. He considered the work of the Federated Women's Clubs of America and the Consumers' League more important. Wiley, *Crime against the Food Law,* p. 52. The AMA was not disposed to minimize its own part in the fight. The *Journal* stated on July 14 that "undoubtedly, the strongest and most effective of these [forces working for the act] was the medical profession . . . and the American Medical Association, acting for the medical profession, through its Committee on Medical Legislation, with its far-reaching state and county auxiliaries, made it possible for physicians all over the country to act in unison, and consequently with effect." Editorial, *JAMA,* 47 (July 14, 1906), 117.

[47] Editorial, *JAMA,* 47 (July 7, 1906), 41; *JAMA,* 47 (July 14, 1906), 116.

[48] Anderson, *Health of a Nation,* pp. 192–94, 197; Young, *Toadstool Millionaires,* pp. 243–44; Editorial, *JAMA,* 47 (August 4, 1906), 365.

Enthusiasm over the passage of the legislation, however, did not blind the Association to the limited control it gave the federal government over the food processing industries or to the more glaring weaknesses in the measures themselves. While the AMA believed that fairly effective safeguards had been provided against the shipment of corrupted foods in interstate commerce, it recognized that the food laws of most states were extremely weak. The *Journal* observed that the exclusive application of these federal laws to the territories, the District of Columbia, and interstate and foreign commerce left the consumer unprotected who resided in the state where the product was manufactured. It contended that:

> . . . while foreigners and residents of other states and territories have the assurance of protection against fraudulent, adulterated, unwholesome and misbranded meat products of the Chicago packing houses, the residents of Chicago and Illinois are left unprotected except as they may be protected by the laws of Illinois.[49]

It also showed with reference to "patent medicines" that the Hartman firm could still "humbug the temperate people" of Ohio with Peruna, and that the manufacturers of Kopp's Baby Friend were left unchecked in killing the babies of Pennsylvania. While the contents of Bromo-Seltzer must be revealed in shipments outside of Maryland, the people of that state were left uninformed that acetanilid remained the principal ingredient.[50]

Besides the impossibility of regulating intrastate commerce through federal legislation, the AMA felt that certain features of the new measures were also detrimental to the most effective control of commerce that crossed state lines. The *Journal* was displeased that the new food and drugs measure, which gave the people some safeguards against preparations containing habit-forming or poisonous drugs, offered no protection against compounds that contained useless drugs. It contended that if people prescribed for themselves, the label should reveal fully the contents of the prescription.[51] The misunderstandings resulting from the guarantee provisions of the act made this feature also objectionable. The measure exempted any dealers from prosecution who could produce a signed guarantee from the manufacturer, jobber, or wholesaler residing in the United States, asserting that the article was not misbranded or

[49] *Ibid.*
[50] *Ibid.*, pp. 365–66.
[51] *Ibid.*

adulterated according to the meaning of the act. The public and a portion of the medical profession were led to believe that the government had already inspected and approved products carrying these guarantees. The *Journal* observed that while some manufacturers were making full use of this provision as a means of deception, the guarantee did not mean that a product was pure or had been inspected or approved by federal authorities.[52]

Leaders of the AMA also complained of the omission of the date of inspection on labels attached to meat examined under the meat inspection amendment. Henry L. E. Johnson, president of the Committee on the Department of Public Health, observed that:

> . . . and immense quantity of meat and meat products, prepared under presumably careless and objectionable methods, now in cold storage or warehouse, [is placed] on an equality with, and indistinguishable from, recent products prepared under careful government inspection.[53]

He also charged that the failure to place a label on examined meat, showing the date of inspection, allowed unwholesome meat labeled and preserved in cold storage for five or ten years to pass as meat recently inspected and approved. As these new measures were not effective until January 1, 1907, Johnson also criticized this seeming neglect of public welfare. Believing that the meat inspection amendment was generally too lax in dealing with the "adulterating, embalming, misbranding, and counterfeiting processes" of many firms, he concluded that the people who provided $3,000,000 to enforce this measure should have "insisted on . . . adequate inspection, dating certificates or labels, and severe penalties for violations."[54]

Unfinished Struggle

The failure of Congress to deal adequately with the problem of adulterated food and drugs in 1906 provided the AMA with an opportunity for leadership in the battle for effective governmental regulation. The Association saw the need not only for strengthening this legislation and the agencies charged with its enforcement, but for defeating the efforts of that part of the manufacturing and processing fraternity, which, having

[52] *JAMA,* 48 (January 5, 1907), 55.
[53] *JAMA,* 47 (October 27, 1906), 1372.
[54] *Ibid.,* pp. 1371–72.

been checked by Congress, hoped by subtle evasion, lax enforcement, and favorable judicial interpretations to render the new law innocuous. In championing the cause of reform, the Association's activities consisted largely of working for effective enforcement, agitating for more adequate legislation, and calling for certain structural changes among governmental agencies concerned with public health.[55]

The AMA strengthened its power by co-operating with other organizations striving for the same objectives. Even before the passage of the food and drugs legislation, the House of Delegates in early June adopted a resolution favoring the creation of a national society devoted to the preservation of public health. Another resolution that the House of Delegates endorsed authorized the Association to send a delegate to a meeting of laymen in New York, November 15, 1906, to consider ways of combating "the dangerous attacks now being made . . . on public health . . . and morals."[56] From this meeting there came the Public Health Defense League, which merged about a year later with the American Health League. The AMA also maintained contact with other lay groups, including the Committee of One Hundred, composed of many eminent lawyers, professors, and scientists organized by Professor Irving Fisher of Yale University.[57]

Encouraged by the increasing popular interest in health problems, the Association pressed the political aspects of its crusade by aiding in the defeat in 1908 of powerful candidates who had opposed the food and drugs legislation two years before. Reed, still chairman of the Committee on Medical Legislation and supported by the AMA, became a candidate for the United States Senate from Ohio. Although his candidacy was not successful, the legislature chose Theodore E. Burton to succeed the vigorous opponent of this legislation, Joseph B. Foraker. An alert medical profession also contributed to the defeat of Representative James H. Southard of the same state and Senator James A. Hemenway of Indiana, who were backed by powerful proprietary medicine interests.[58] While the outcome of the elections was in many ways dis-

[55] The following two chapters discuss the Association's efforts to secure a reorganization of governmental health services and to assist in the effective enforcement of the drug provisions of the Pure Food and Drugs Act.

[56] *JAMA,* 46 (June 16, 1906), 1861.

[57] Charles A. L. Reed, *JAMA,* 48 (January 12, 1907), 154; *JAMA,* 48 (June 8, 1907), 1968. For Fisher's account of the organization of this committee and for its membership see *JAMA,* 48 (January 19, 1907), 251.

[58] *JAMA,* (May 2, 1908), 1428; Lewis S. McMurtry, *JAMA,* 50 (June 13, 1908), 2008. The *Journal* was mistaken in 1909 in reporting that Hernando D.

couraging, the Association was aware that these victories were but a minor phase of a larger battle.

The Association quickly found that interpreting and enforcing the food and drugs legislation would be as difficult as its enactment. The drafting of regulations under the law was a task resulting in inevitable frictions among government officials and affected firms. Industries chaffing somewhat under the pressure of federal restraints increasingly looked upon Wiley as the principal source of their woes. In the bitter controversy over the effect of benzoate of soda as a preservative, the enforcement problem attracted national attention.[59] While siding with Wiley from the first, the AMA did not object when President Roosevelt on February 20, 1908, appointed a Referee Board of Consulting Scientific Experts to give advice on the issue, headed by the chemist Ira Remsen, president of The Johns Hopkins University.[60] The AMA did answer the charge of a representative of the Pacific Coast Borax Company and numerous trade journals, however, that this action was a repudiation of Wiley.

The Association was disappointed when the referee board failed to support Wiley's contention that the addition of benzoate of soda to canned foods constituted an adulteration and was unlawful. It was fully aware that corrupt food processors and proprietary medicine concerns would cite this incident to discredit Wiley's entire work. The *Journal,* presenting its own view, declared, like Wiley, that the only two reasons for the use of benzoate of soda were "to take the place of cleanliness and care in preparing or to permit the use of inferior products." The same article expressed appreciation of Wiley's work:

Money, who remained in the Senate until 1911, had retired. His fight against effective food and drugs legislation, however, did arouse much opposition among physicians in Mississippi, but he was not a candidate for re-election in 1908. Editorial, *JAMA,* 52 (January 9, 1909), 139; Reynolds, *Biographical Directory of the American Congress, 1774–1961,* p. 1344.

[59] Anderson, *Health of a Nation,* pp. 209–11, 216–18.

[60] Editorial, *JAMA,* 50 (April 4, 1908), 1126. Others on this board were "Russell H. Chittenden, Director of the Sheffield Scientific School, Yale University; Alonzo E. Taylor, University of California; C. A. Herter, College of Physicians and Surgeons, New York; and John H. Long, Northwestern University, Chicago, all of whom were eminent chemists." Gustavus A. Weber, *The Food, Drug, and Insecticide Administration: Its History, Activities and Organization* (Institute of Government Research, Special Monographs of the United States Government, No. 50 [Baltimore: The Johns Hopkins University Press, 1928]), p. 18.

Possibly Dr. Wiley may have overstated or overemphasized the toxicity of some of the preservatives that have been used in foods, but if he erred he did so in the interest of the public's health instead of to the benefit of the dishonest manufacturer's pocket-book.[61]

As the attack on Wiley showed no signs of abatement, the AMA followed the developments and continued to support his position. The House of Delegates in June, 1909, passed a resolution calling for adequate federal inspection of all food-processing plants engaged in interstate commerce and urged Congress "To prohibit, absolutely and unqualified, the use of benzoate of soda and similar preservatives in the preparation and preservation of foods destined for interstate commerce."[62] Late in 1911 the AMA indicated its abiding concern over the government's policy of allowing the use of sodium benzoate by citing a decision against its use rendered by the Royal Scientific Deputation for Medical Affairs of Berlin. Attempting to show the contradictory position of the government, the *Journal* asked:

Why should a catsup-maker, for instance, be forced by the government to state the presence and quantity of an ingredient of his product which the same government has officially pronounced harmless and which it permits to be used in any quantity? It is altogether unjust to rule that a manufacturer shall declare the presence and proportion of one ingredient of his product—an ingredient which the government claims to be wholesome—while the presence of any other wholesome ingredients may remain a secret.[63]

The *Journal* also charged that high government officials were actually aligned with the food-processing interests in blocking Wiley's efforts at enforcement. It leveled its criticism at Attorney General George W. Wickersham for allegedly passing over his own subordinates, and entrusting the opinion on the legality of the creation of the referee board to the Solicitor of the Department of Agriculture.[64] It hurled charges of

[61] Editorial, *JAMA,* 52 (February 13, 1909), 562. The referee board later considered the use in food of saccharin, alum, sulphur dioxide, sulphate of copper, and other substances. While only an advisory board it was continued until June 30, 1915. The *Journal* observed that the board supported Wiley's position on several points, nevertheless Wiley considered that its creation constituted a virtual repeal of the Pure Food and Drugs Act by "executive edict." Weber, *Food, Drug, and Insecticide Administration,* p. 19; Editorial, *JAMA,* 57 (July 22, 1911), 295; Wiley, *Autobiography,* p. 241.

[62] *JAMA,* 52 (June 19, 1909), 2076.

[63] Editorial, *JAMA,* 57 (November 4, 1911), 1541–42; quotation, *JAMA,* 57 (November 11, 1911), 1620. The government required that the quantity of benzoate of soda used must be specified on the label of the product.

[64] *JAMA,* 57 (July 22, 1911), 297–98. For arguments of the Attorney General justifying the referee board see Charles Wesley Dunn, ed., *Dunn's Food and*

collusion and obstruction at George P. McCabe, the Solicitor, and Frederick L. Dunlap, who, with Wiley, constituted the Food and Drugs Inspection Board. But coming in for perhaps the severest indictment was Secretary of Agriculture James Wilson, under whose aegis the *Journal* believed the whole plot to obstruct the enforcement of the law started.[65] The *Journal* accused him not only of a failure at enforcement, but of using the prestige of his department for "jamming through" the Denver Convention of the Association of State and National Food and Dairy Departments in 1909, resolutions supporting the decision of the referee board on the sodium benzoate question. It pointed to the great difficulty Indiana authorities encountered in securing data on Wiley's experiments from the Department of Agriculture, when the catsup manufacturers fought for the invalidation of the state pure food law prohibiting the use of benzoate of soda.[66]

Particularly grievous to the *Journal* in 1911 was the conspiracy of the Attorney General and Wiley's opponents in the Department of Agriculture to procure his dismissal for an alleged violation of a statutory regulation of the per diem pay of temporary advisory specialists. It saw the real fight as one between Wiley and his associates, Willard D. Bigelow and Kebler representing the public, and Wilson, McCabe, and Dunlap aligned with private interests. When the special congressional committee investigating friction over the enforcement of the law declared the contract invalid, but weighted its report generally in favor of Wiley, the *Journal* considered the chief chemist exonerated and launched another attack on his opponents.[67]

The Wiley controversy was still raging when the Association broadened its attack to include the United States Supreme Court. On May 29, 1911, a divided court decided in the case of United States *vs.* O. A. Johnson that Johnson's sale in interstate commerce of an alleged cancer

---

Drug Laws: Vol. I, *Federal* (New York: United States Corporation Company, 1st ed., 1927–1928), pp. 181–84.

[65] McCabe appears to have been a capable official. Dunlap was a young chemist from the University of Michigan but the elderly Wilson was neither a lawyer nor a scientist. Oscar E. Anderson, Jr., "The Pure-Food Issue: A Republican Dilemma, 1906–1912," *The American Historical Review,* 61 (April, 1956), 553.

[66] *JAMA,* 57 (July 22, 1911), 297–98; Editorial, *JAMA,* 57 (July 22, 1911), 295; Editorial, *JAMA,* 57 (September 16, 1911), 982.

[67] Editorial, *JAMA,* 57 (July 22, 1911), 295; *JAMA,* 57 (August 26, 1911), 747; Editorial, *JAMA,* 58 (February 3, 1912), 347. This dispute arose over Wiley's employment of H. H. Rusby, a noted pharmacologist. Wiley's opponents charged that Rusby's services were secured with a private agreement to pay more than the law allowed. See Anderson, *Health of a Nation,* pp. 244–51.

cure did not violate the Pure Food and Drugs Act. While the claims for Johnson's compound were admittedly misleading if not completely false, the court decided that Section 8, which prohibited interstate commerce in drugs and articles of food bearing statements on labels or packages "false or misleading in any particular," referred to the contents of the drug or food and not to claims about their therapeutic effect.[68] The *Journal* considered this decision an intolerable emasculation of the law. The court had interpreted the phrase "false or misleading in any particular" as " 'false or misleading' in *certain* particulars. . . ." The *Journal* charged that the interests benefiting from this decision were "as cruel a gang of swindlers as ever operated under the protection of the law" and that "cancer fakers . . . who have been driven out of business under the law as previously interpreted, will now be free to resume their damnable trade unmolested."[69]

Less than a month after the Supreme Court's decision, the Los Angeles session of the AMA registered its protest. It adopted a resolution petitioning Congress to amend the Pure Food and Drugs Act, making unlawful any false statements on the labels and circulars of food and drugs and commended President Taft for urging action on this matter in his special message to Congress. It authorized the secretary of the Association to telegraph the resolution to the President, the Vice President, and the Speaker of the House and to send printed copies to all members of Congress.[70] Congress was not long in responding to the agitation for amendment along lines that the AMA suggested. On August 23, 1912, it enacted the Sherley Amendment that corrected this weakness in the legislation passed six years earlier. The enforcement of this measure improved the standards of advertising displayed on the labels and circulars of food and drugs, and the AMA praised the Supreme Court in 1916 when it upheld the constitutionality of the amendment.[71]

A painful awareness, however, of the persistence of food-and-drug adulteration and the continued prosperity of the nostrum business dulled

[68] *JAMA,* 56 (June 17, 1911), 1832–1835. For early developments in the judicial interpretation of food and drug statutes see John G. Kuniholm, "Constitutional Limitations on the Regulation of Therapeutic Claims under 1938 Federal Food, Drug, and Cosmetic Act," *Food, Drug Cosmetic Law Journal,* 9 (November, 1954), 636–41.

[69] Editorial, *JAMA,* 56 (June 17, 1911), 1819; *JAMA,* 56 (June 3, 1911), 1660.

[70] *JAMA,* 57 (July 8, 1911), 133.

[71] Weber, *The Food, Drug, and Insecticide Administration,* p. 21; *JAMA,* 66 (January 15, 1916), 198.

the Association's satisfaction over the gradual improvement of remedial legislation. Wiley's resignation on March 15, 1912, which the Association deeply regretted, appeared to offset any advantages gained.[72] Only about a year before the enactment of the Sherley Amendment, the AMA had wired President Taft that according to reliable estimates about 2,000,000 cases of sickness and 500,000 deaths resulted annually from impure food and drugs. Soon after its passage, the *Journal* pointed to specific cases in which long litigation and small fines had rendered the Food and Drugs Act virtually ineffective.[73] It cited the work of the Connecticut Experimental Station that found 372 of 757 samples of goods offered to the public in 1912 "adulterated, misbranded, or below standard," as proof of the inadequacy of legislation and enforcement at that time.[74] It supported a bill introduced by Representative Burton L. French of Idaho, requiring all bottles shipped in interstate commerce containing poison to be so labeled, with at least one antidote given. Among objectionable practices later noted was the use of aniline dyes, by which some food processors deceived the public with inferior products. Despite the accomplishments of the food and drugs legislation, the AMA in 1915 endorsed the view of J. P. Street of the Connecticut Agricultural Experiment Station that the nation was in an "era of legal food, rather than pure food."[75]

The Association, now placing greater emphasis on the revision of drug legislation, did not allow the war in Europe to stop its political agitation. It appealed directly to President Wilson for a federal investigation of the proprietary medicine industry. Acting at the request of the House of Delegates, three representatives of the Association arranged for a conference with the chief executive on March 9, 1916. They pointed out to the President that even after the passage of the Pure Food and Drugs

[72] Congress passed another amendment to the Pure Food and Drugs Act on March 3, 1913, known as the Net Weights Act which regulated the way in which food and drugs entering interstate commerce were to be labeled as to measure, weight, or numerical count, but the AMA showed little interest in the measure. See Weber, *The Food, Drug, and Insecticide Administration,* p. 22 for this law. J. N. McCormack considered Wiley's resignation a "calamity" to the nation and believed that it justified "grave and wide-spread alarm for the welfare of our people." Telegram, McCormack to Wiley, March 16, 1912 (Wiley Papers, Manuscript Division, Library of Congress). For the resignation see Anderson, *Health of a Nation,* pp. 250–52; and Wiley, *Crime against the Food Law,* p. 92.

[73] *JAMA,* 57 (July 8, 1911), 139; *JAMA,* 59 (November 16, 1912), 1802.

[74] Editorial, *JAMA,* 60 (January 11, 1913), 132.

[75] *JAMA,* 60 (May 17, 1913), 1547; *JAMA,* 67 (July 29, 1916), 364–65; quotation, Editorial, *JAMA,* 65 (July 24, 1915), 335.

Act, the Australian Government had debarred as unsafe certain medical preparations of American origin, and that a committee appointed by the British Parliament to study the sale of patent and proprietary medicines was also critical of some American brands. They urged the appointment of a special commission, whose findings would be published for the benefit of Congress and the public, to investigate the products and advertising methods of the proprietary industry. Although the President seemed interested in their request, he failed to arrange for this investigation.[76] As the United States drew closer to war, it became less concerned about ideas of domestic reform.

By 1920, the Association's attitude about the strength of federal drug legislation had matured through close acquaintance with the corrupt and evasive practices of a number of proprietary establishments. It had seen the enemies of public health find the gaps in drug legislation and pour their products through on an unsuspecting public. It was prepared to remind a nation triumphant in war of its less impressive record in defense of public health.

On March 26, 1919, Arthur J. Cramp, Director of the Propaganda for Reform Department of the AMA, summed up the factors contributing to the weaknesses of federal drug legislation before the Chicago Medical Society. He observed that fraudulent firms could thrive in the shadow of federal legislation by avoiding interstate traffic in their products. In evading the Sherley Amendment, they had resorted to false advertisements in newspapers and handbills, uncontrolled by federal statutes. He cited the difficulty of enforcing this amendment which required not only proof of false claims, but of a deliberate intention to defraud. Federal legislation that required the revelation (only on the container or package) of certain poisons found in drugs made no provision for the disclosure of others equally dangerous. Cramp considered that the long attempt of the government to regulate the proprietary and patent medicine business had brought the public only limited protection.[77]

[76] *JAMA,* 66 (March 25, 1916), 974: *JAMA,* 66 (June 17, 1916), 1942. The representatives appointed by the Board of Trustees to visit the President were William L. Rodman, president of the AMA; W. T. Councilman, chairman of the Board of Trustees; George H. Simmons; Hiram Woods, Baltimore; and Alexander Marcy, Jr., Riverton, New Jersey. As Rodman died the day before the conference and Woods was ill, only three met with the President.

[77] Arthur J. Cramp, "The Nostrum and the Public Health," *JAMA,* 72 (May 24, 1919), 1531.

Chapter 5

STRUGGLE FOR A FEDERAL HEALTH DEPARTMENT

THE AMERICAN MEDICAL ASSOCIATION'S struggle to protect the nation's health included more than its efforts to secure the enactment, improvement, and enforcement of food and drugs legislation. Attributing much of the ineffectiveness of the government's public health activities to the disintegration and duplication of federal health agencies, it insisted on structural changes among organizations responsible for federal health functions. Although the AMA waivered somewhat in its advocacy of a national health department with cabinet status, it never abandoned the idea as an ultimate goal.[1]

Changing Strategy

The first decade of the new century well illustrates the Association's changing strategy in its efforts to secure reforms in public health administration. In 1902, President John Allen Wyeth urged the AMA to support the Perkins-Hepburn bill, which enlarged the functions and changed the name of the Marine-Hospital Service to United States Public Health and Marine-Hospital Service. He believed that the passage of this measure would hasten the establishment of a national health department.[2]

[1] The strategy of the AMA in its work for a department of health is well summarized in *JAMA,* 60 (May 3, 1913), 1366.

[2] *JAMA,* 38 (June 14, 1902), 1553; Marguerite F. Hall, *Public Health Statistics* (New York: Paul B. Hoeber, Inc., 1942), pp. 4–6, traces briefly the history of the Marine-Hospital Service which became the United States Public Health and Marine-Hospital Service in 1902, and the United States Public Health Service ten years later. At the beginning of the twentieth century the AMA's Committee on Department of Public Health supported the "Spooner-Ray Bill" that provided

When the principal features of this bill were enacted, the Association's agitation for more far-reaching changes largely subsided until developments about 1906 revised its enthusiasm. By this time the fight against disease in the Caribbean area, the victory over the bubonic plague in California, and the more recent suppression of the yellow fever epidemic in New Orleans had kindled the interest of a nation largely unconcerned with public health problems.[3] Especially encouraging to the AMA was the passage of the long-delayed food and drugs legislation, and the commencement of a crusade for a national health department by Irving Fisher's militant Committee of One Hundred and other lay organizations.[4] Supported by growing popular interest, the leadership of the Association believed that the opposition to a department of health could be rapidly overcome.

When the National Legislative Council of the AMA met in Washington early in January, 1906, the question of a federal health department was a major topic for consideration. Charles Reed pressed the viewpoint of the Association that the public health work of the nation should convey "executive authority, subordinate only to that of the chief executive to control and determine results."[5] This position, of course, demanded a place in "the supreme executive council of the country" for a director of public health functions, and Reed, as chairman of the Committee on Medical Legislation, felt that the Association should not relax its efforts until a department of health had been established.[6]

Evidently moved by Reed's appeal for immediate action, the council endorsed a resolution asking the trustees to appropriate $1,000 for securing competent legal aid.[7] The following June the House of Delegates also adopted this resolution and approved of a rough plan for a national health department that Congressman Andrew J. Barchfield, a physician

---

only for a bureau of health and not a department. U. O. B. Wingate, chairman, reported on March 10, 1900, that there was no prospect of securing a department of health soon. *JAMA*, 34 (March 10, 1900), 1591. See pp. 24–25 for AMA's early agitation for a health department.

[3] Editorial, *JAMA*, 50 (July 18, 1908), 227; Charles A. L. Reed, *JAMA*, 46 (January 20, 1906), 213.

[4] Irving Fisher, *JAMA*, 48 (January 19, 1907), 251.

[5] *JAMA*, 46 (January 20, 1906), 213.

[6] *Ibid.*

[7] *JAMA*, 46 (January 20, 1906), 215. The Committee on Department of Public Health submitted this resolution and also another, which was adopted, that called for the presentation of a health department bill to Congress "at the earliest practicable date, if possible during the present session."

from Pennsylvania, had prepared. The trustees, however, refused to authorize this expenditure and checked the movement that would have presented to Congress a bill framed under the careful direction of the Association. The perplexed Committee on Medical Legislation told the annual session of 1907 that it had followed the only reasonable alternative of turning over the responsibility of drafting the bill to the Committee of One Hundred.[8]

The refusal of the trustees to comply with the resolution indicates a sharp division within the Association's leadership over the revival of the health department issue. Although the need of such a department was not disputed, the leaders divided over the urgency of the matter. The National Legislative Council and a majority of the House of Delegates favored immediate agitation for the direct establishment of the department, but the trustees, the Section on Hygiene and Sanitary Science, and the editorial writers of the *Journal* supported a more evolutionary plan.

Less than five weeks after the House of Delegates, in June, 1908, rejected the proposal of the Section on Hygiene and Sanitary Science for the expansion of the Public Health and Marine-Hospital Service and reaffirmed its favorable position on the question of a national department of health, the *Journal* flatly contradicted the stand of the legislative body. It contended that the real issue concerned the conservation of public health, and that the manner of accomplishment, whether through the immediate creation of a health department or through the gradual expansion of existing bureaus, was immaterial. It even added that no bill for a national health department should be drafted until more study had been given to the functions of the present health agencies both in the United States and abroad.[9] While affirming that a separate department of health was the ideal, the *Journal* in October favored Roosevelt's plan for the concentration of health functions within some existing department, seeing no hope for the immediate establishment of a department of health.[10]

[8] *JAMA,* 48 (June 8, 1907), 1968. Reed had accepted membership on the Committee of One Hundred and was told by Fisher that legal talent on the committee would be employed to draft a federal health department bill.

[9] *JAMA,* 50 (June 13, 1908), 2011; Editorial, *JAMA,* 51 (July 18, 1908), 227–28.

[10] Editorial, *JAMA,* 51 (October 17, 1908), 1338–39. The *Journal* cited the announcement of Roosevelt's plan by the International Congress on Tuberculosis that had met at Washington.

Since the Committee of One Hundred had also relaxed its agitation for the immediate creation of a health department and had even helped the President draft his plan of reorganization, the Committee on Medical Legislation recognized the futility of the fight. When, along with several members of the National Legislative Council, it appeared before the subcommittee of the House Committee on Interstate and Foreign Commerce, on January 19, 1909, there was little choice but to endorse the "effect aimed at" by the President's plan. It explained its action to the House of Delegates meeting at Atlantic City in June, and this body also agreed to support the plan for an expanded federal health bureau and applauded Taft's interest in the proposal.[11]

Support of First Owen Bill

It seemed at last that the Association had committed itself to a settled policy regarding the co-ordination of federal health activities and had abandoned the plan for the immediate creation of a national health department. Yet a year had not passed before developments on the political scene revived the Association's interest in the early establishment of a department. On February 10, 1910, Senator Robert L. Owen of Oklahoma introduced Senate bill 6049, which provided for the creation of a national health department with cabinet status.[12] A few days later Reed wrote Owen apparently informing him of the Association's position on the health department issue. In a prompt reply, Owen, while welcoming criticism of his bill, expressed the view that satisfaction with less than a department of public health with cabinet status resulted from a failure to appreciate the magnitude of the public health problem.[13]

[11] *JAMA,* 52 (June 19, 1909), 2039, 2075. Roosevelt's plan, which would have given the chief executive power to move various health agencies from one department to another at his discretion, was unacceptable to some congressional committeemen. When Joseph N. McCormack observed the obstructive tactics employed to prevent Congress from considering the bill, he left Washington in disgust to continue his work as national organizer for the AMA. *JAMA,* 52 (June 19, 1909), 2056.

[12] *JAMA,* 60 (May 3, 1913), 1384. The AMA disclaimed any credit for the introduction of the Owen bill and attributed Senator Owen's interest in public health largely to the influence of his brother, Major W. O. Owen, a retired naval medical officer. *JAMA,* 58 (January 13, 1912), 134; *JAMA,* 54 (June 18, 1910), 2064.

[13] Owen to Reed, February 23, 1910, *JAMA,* 54 (March 19, 1910), 985. Reed's first letter to Owen was dated February 18, 1910. Unfortunately this letter is not published but its contents can be fairly well established by the nature of Owen's reply.

Reed, who had abandoned hope for the immediate establishment of a national department of health, quickly threw his influence behind the Owen bill. When the conference of the Council on Medical Education and the Committee on Medical Legislation met at Chicago from February 28 to March 2, a resolution favoring its creation was adopted. The *Journal* showed its approval by carrying the full text of the bill, and, while expressing doubt that the measure would pass, was gratified over the renewed interest in the subject.[14]

Although Reed highly regarded the bill, he nevertheless accepted Owen's invitation to offer criticism. Just one month after it was introduced in the Senate, Reed wrote Owen again, outlining in great detail the Association's idea of the structure and work of a national health department. While the Owen bill called for the transfer to the proposed department of all agencies concerned with public health, Reed's proposed the establishment of six bureaus within the department that would assume all scattered federal health activities. These bureaus were to be the bureau of hygiene and preventive medicine, the bureau of foods and drugs, the bureau of marine hospitals, the bureau of quarantine, the bureau of institutions and reservations, and the bureau of publication and publicity. Reed also suggested that a medical unit be attached to the department, called the United States health service, consisting of the United States Marine-Hospital Corps and a special medical corps including all other physicians and medical officers employed by the government. In addition, he proposed that the president be empowered to appoint an advisory board of health of six members to confer with the secretary of health on all public health policies, and to give other advice on request. Hoping that these suggestions would be embodied in the final bill, Reed urged that the hearings on the measure be arranged as soon as possible, and that Owen impress upon his colleagues the gravity of the health problem when "There are nearly 5,000,000 needlessly ill every year."[15]

The Association's support of the bill, however, was not dependent on Owen's acceptance of Reed's criticisms. The Committee on Medical Legislation immediately applied to Representative James R. Mann of the House Committee on Interstate and Foreign Commerce for a hearing

[14] *JAMA,* 54 (March 19, 1910), 992, 985; *JAMA,* 54 (February 26, 1910), 725.

[15] Reed to Owen, *JAMA,* 54 (March 19, 1910), 985–86. Earlier in this letter Reed stated that there were 600,000 deaths, 3,000,000 cases of sickness, and an economic loss of over $1.5 billion resulting annually from preventable causes.

on the health department bill whenever it was introduced in the House. In April, J. N. McCormack interrupted his organizational work long enough to establish contacts in Washington and petition Congress on behalf of the AMA for the passage of the Owen bill.[16] As a clear and logical plea for the creation of such a department, this petition was unexcelled. It cited the duplication of health functions and the illogical location of many health agencies as justification for the co-ordination of these agencies and functions in one department. In June, the Sixty-second session of the House of Delegates gave some attention to the health department issue. But while endorsing the principles of the Owen bill, it authorized the president of the Association to appoint a committee on national health organization responsible for framing a national health department bill for presentation to the next session of Congress in December.[17] This action indicated that while the Association liked the Owen bill, it preferred a measure of its own making and was now willing to assume the initiative in the fight.

Once again, however, the Association lost an opportunity to get its own bill before Congress. The leaders at the headquarters of the AMA actually repudiated the action of the Sixty-second session as early as November, when the entire issue of the *Bulletin* stressed the need for a department, emphasizing particularly the Owen bill. Not until March 25, 1911, did the committee appointed by the president of the AMA hold its first meeting, and this was four months after the December session of Congress convened. Although the committee assembled again a week later, it prepared no more than an outline of a national health bill and then largely shifted the responsibility by turning its suggestions over to Senator Owen. In the meantime the Council on Health and Public Instruction had already established contacts with the family physicians of the members of Congress, asking them to urge their representatives to support the Owen bill.[18]

When the first Owen bill never emerged from the Senate Committee on Public Health and National Quarantine and died with the expiration

[16] Editorial, *JAMA,* 54 (March 19, 1910), 972; J. N. McCormack, *JAMA,* 54 (May 14, 1910), 1642–44.

[17] *JAMA,* 54 (June 18, 1910), 2068.

[18] HD, *Proceedings* (62 Annual Session, June, 1911), p. 35. The Committee on National Health Organization consisted of Hermann M. Biggs, New York City; W. A. Evans, Chicago; S. G. Dixon, Harrisburg, Pa.; J. N. Hurty, Indianapolis; J. N. McCormack, Bowling Green, Ky; H. P. Walcott, Cambridge, Mass.; and William C. Woodward, Washington, D.C. See *ibid.,* p. 8 for criticism of this committee by the Council on Health and Public Instruction.

of the Sixty-first Congress, the determined senator from Oklahoma reintroduced his department of health bill on April 6, 1911. Any suggestions from the Committee on National Health Organization probably came too late to be incorporated into the new Owen bill. But the bitter hostility of some private interests to the first measure, as well as the earlier helpful criticism of the AMA, led the senator to make the second bill considerably different from the first. While the new Owen bill provided for a department of public health, it made no reference to cabinet status and referred to the administrative head as director rather than secretary. Apparently Owen had come to believe that the immediate creation of a department with cabinet rank was impossible. The second bill provided for eight bureaus in the proposed department, and, while exceeding the six recommended by the AMA, appears to have called for no superabundance.[19]

Since opponents of a national health department charged that the first bill displayed favoritism toward standard medical practitioners against a great variety of unconventional healing groups and allowed also an infringement on state rights, the new bill guarded against these alleged weaknesses. Section 3 stipulated that the proposed department "shall recognize no so-called school or system of medicine," and that the department of health could exercise no function belonging solely to a state without the consent of the proper authorities within a state, nor send its officials into any premise within a state without the owner's permission.[20] The *Journal* soon expressed general satisfaction with the Owen bill, but added that the safeguards of Section 3 would not silence the opposition of "mercenary interests arrayed against further health legislation."[21]

Support of Second Owen Bill

The Association's most effective work for a department of public health did not get well under way until after the introduction of the

[19] The eight bureaus constituting the proposed department as outlined in the new Owen bill had charge of the following matters: sanitary research, child hygiene, vital statistics and publications, food and drugs, quarantine, sanitary engineering, government hospitals, and personnel and accounts. While Owen seems to have accepted some of the suggestions of the AMA, the second bill varied considerably from its recommendations. For the text of the second Owen bill see *JAMA,* 56 (April 22, 1911), 1208.

[20] *Ibid.*

[21] Editorial, *JAMA,* 56 (April 22, 1911), 1202.

second Owen bill. Not until then did it bring into service its nation-wide legislative machinery with a direct appeal for immediate action. On April 29, the Council on Health and Public Instruction sent circular letters to the approximately 2,000 members of the National Auxiliary Legislative Committee appealing for their participation in the crusade. The council urged the local committee members to wire their senators, requesting their support of the Owen bill and to prevail on local physicians to do likewise. In addition, it asked them to secure and forward to the senators favorable resolutions from local medical societies and to urge commercial and civic organizations, women's clubs, health organizations, and newspapers to support the measure. During the first quarter of 1911, the council circulated about 20,000 copies of the *Bulletin* of the past November that were devoted exclusively to the campaign for a national department of health.[22] The political work of the Association moved steadily forward, but not without some moments of discouragement. At a medical club meeting in Philadelphia in May, Reed deplored the lack of interest most congressmen manifested in the subject and the constitutional objections that some offered. He charged that "These wiseacres seem to think it constitutional for the government to educate the people to protect swine but not to educate them how to protect themselves against disease."[23]

Attack on Enemies of the Bill

As the crusade for a national health department continued, the Association became increasingly aware of the tactics employed by forces resisting the movement. Under the name of the National League for Medical Freedom (established in 1910), opponents of the AMA frantically fought the health department bills. Asserting that advocates of a national health department would make the government "an immense anthropomorphic allopathic physician," the league charged that "The legislation that we are combating would, if successful, mark another long stride in the march of centralization and the establishment of a Russian bureaucratic system in the place of the democracy of the fathers . . ." and would place upon the taxpayers an "enormous and ever-increasing

[22] HD, *Proceedings* (63 Annual Session, June, 1912), p. 35.
[23] *JAMA*, 56 (May 13, 1911), 1402.

burden of expense. . . ."[24] It warned that the "generous" nature of constitutional interpretation in Washington and the vague powers conferred by the proposed legislation would lead to federal domination of medical care. Asserting that all of the 7,000 physicians which the federal government employed were "regular" practitioners, it called upon physicians of other systems to combat the AMA's monopolistic designs.[25]

Although this agitation appeared to come primarily from unconventional healing sects, the AMA traced its source largely to proprietary medicine interests. Simmons contended that the league had been established by proprietary firms to fight the AMA and stop its attacks on quackery and nostrums. He identified the movements as consisting of "faddists, including the antivivisectionists, the anti-vaccinationists, the Eddyites, the patent medicine fakers and quacks, the pure food adulterators and the Lord knows what else."[26] Early in 1912, the *Journal* accused this organization, boasting a membership of 200,000, of duping the eclectics, homeopaths, osteopaths, and Christian Scientists into opposing the second Owen bill by convincing them that it promoted medical favoritism. Attempting to show that no legitimate interest could be adversely affected by its passage, the *Journal* announced what it considered to be the real reason for the violent opposition. The Owen bill called for the transfer of the Bureau of Chemistry from the Department of Agriculture to the proposed department of health. The *Journal* remarked:

> That is the bureau that is headed by Dr. Wiley, who enforces the food and Drugs Act (when he gets a chance). . . . As long as Dr. Wiley is a part of the Agricultural Department he can be annoyed and hampered. But suppose he were transferred to a new department which was run for

[24] *JAMA,* 58 (February 3, 1912), 350; "The Facts about 'Collier's' Attack on the National League for Medical Freedom," (New York: The National League for Medical Freedom); "The National League for Medical Freedom: Organization and Purposes" (New York: The National League for Medical Freedom), p. 7. The National League for Medical Freedom File, Department of Investigation, American Medical Association, referred to hereafter as AMA, DI.

[25] "First Report of the National League for Medical Freedom," (New York City: National League for Medical Freedom), p. 11. (League for Medical Freedom File, AMA, DI.)

[26] Simmons to Mark Sullivan, Jan. 21, 1911; Simmons to J. E. Tuckerman, Jan. 23, 1911. (League for Medical Freedom File, AMA, DI.) The president of the League in 1911 was B. O. Flowers, editor of *Twentieth Century Magazine.* Charles W. Miller, a physician and state legislator from Waverly, Iowa, and strong critic of the AMA, was second vice-president. Its general counsel was a prominent Boston lawyer, John L. Bates, who had served as governor of the

> the protection of the people and not for commercial interests? What wouldn't he do to the adulterators, the lying advertisers, the manufacturers who use rotten and filthy material in their products and the men who swindle and cheat the public. What has been done so far wouldn't be worth mentioning in comparison to what Dr. Wiley and his bureau would do, if they were transferred to a department where he was not and could not be hampered by politics and commercial influence.[27]

The *Journal* showed no surprise the following month in reporting that a prominent advertising agency estimated the cost of the league's newspaper campaign at $50,000, and well understood why some business interests invested so heavily in the undertaking.[28]

The most noteworthy contribution that the Association made toward the establishment of a national health department in the presidential election year of 1912 was its agitation for the inclusion of a strong health-department plank in the major party platforms. The Committee on National Legislation told the Los Angeles session in June that never had the prospects for the integration of federal health agencies been brighter.[29] The Committee on National Legislation claimed considerable credit for the "health planks" in the Democratic and Republican platforms, but acknowledged that it was largely the work of one member, W. A. Evans. Although the Association was not pleased with the vague stand of the Republican party on the co-ordination of federal health services, the committee considered the Democratic health plank "by far the strongest and most satisfactory of all that have at any time been inserted in any platform." The *Journal* called it "a straight-forward endorsement of the principles of the present Owen Bill."[30]

While the Association was officially aligned with no party, most of its leaders felt that the Democratic victory of 1912 offered the brightest prospects for the integration of federal health services. There was considerable justification for this opinion. The Senate Committee on Public Health and National Quarantine allowed nearly a year to elapse before reporting on the second Owen bill, and then on April 13, 1912, submitted a much-amended measure to the upper house. There the delay of

state, 1903–1904. Paul A. Harsch to M. Bartlett, January 28, 1911, see letterhead. (League for Medical Freedom File, AMA, DI); Albert Nelson Marquis, ed., *Who's Who In America, 1914–1915* (Chicago: A. N. Marquis & Company, 1914), VIII, 142.

27 Editorial, *JAMA,* 58 (January 13, 1912), 121.

28 *JAMA,* 58 (February 3, 1912), 350.

29 HD, *Proceedings* (63 Annual Session, June, 1912), p. 44.

30 *JAMA,* 60 (June 28, 1913), 2082; *JAMA,* 59 (July 13, 1912), 126.

the committee was re-enacted, and not until February 3, 1913, was Senator Owen even able to get a vote on whether or not the bill would be considered. The failure of the bill to pass this hurdle was no great surprise to the AMA, which watched the measure die as the Sixty-second Congress expired.[31]

AMA and the Third Owen Bill

The last phase of the Association's early fight for a national health department began when the new Democratic administration took control. The AMA rejoiced when, on April 7, Owen introduced his third bill that reverted to the original plan of a department of health headed by a secretary. The *Journal* remarked that "The present bill is by far the best measure which has yet been presented on this subject."[32] A few days later representatives of the AMA met with delegates from 38 other organizations who assembled at the headquarters of the American Association for Labor Legislation to consider needed reforms in federal health activity.[33] More important, however, was a conference of leaders within the AMA, held at Washington, D. C., on May 5, to which a few prominent health department advocates were invited. Irving Fisher, together with Senators Owen and Joseph E. Ransdell, and Representative Martin D. Foster gathered with the leaders to plan the strategy for securing a national department of health.

Bitter experiences with long congressional delays led the conference to appeal directly to President Woodrow Wilson. It appointed a special committee to see the President the following day to solicit his support of the plan and of a few other health issues, including a presidential call for a national health conference and the establishment of a committee on public health in the House of Representatives. It also selected a committee to confer with Owen on amending his third bill.[34] Although Wilson looked favorably upon public health reforms, he was too en-

[31] The motion to consider the Owen bill resulted in a tie vote of 33 to 33 and the subject was dropped. See *JAMA,* 60 (May 3, 1913), 1384–85 for the legislative history of the different Owen bills.

[32] *JAMA,* 60 (April 26, 1913), 1308.

[33] *JAMA,* 60 (June 21, 1913), 2001.

[34] HD, *Proceedings* (64 Annual Session, June, 1913), p. 20. Besides members of the Council on Health and Public Instruction and the Special Committee on National Health Organization, other physicians invited to the conference were Surgeon General Rupert Blue of the United States Public Health Service, and officials of the AMA, including President Abraham Jacobi, President-elect John A. Witherspoon, Secretary Alexander R. Craig, and George H. Simmons.

grossed in other domestic issues, as well as important international problems, to offer the visiting committee any reason for immediate encouragement.[35]

Hardly had the leaders of the AMA recovered from the disappointment of the conference with the President, when news of the internal strife between the Committee on the National Department of Health and the trustees shocked the Sixty-fourth session of the House of Delegates meeting at Minneapolis in June. In characteristic fashion, the Association's aggressive battle against the enemies of a national health department turned into a civil war. The minority report of the committee suggests the intensity of feeling engendered against the trustees, whose co-operation, it contended, had been deficient. The report stated that the trustees refused to appropriate money for the political activities of the committee, and that they had attempted to make the committee no more than an adjunct of the Council on Health and Public Instruction. The report urged the appointment of a special lobbyist in Washington and charged that the trustees "have shown themselves entirely without the capacity for aggressive leadership necessary to win the fight."[36] In reply, the Reference Committee on Legislation and Political Action took the side of the trustees and asserted that all bills submitted by the committee were paid, and that the employment of a lobbyist in Washington was unwise. As the Committee on the National Department of Health asked that its work be either supported or discontinued, the reference committee "heartily concur[red]" in the latter alternative.[37]

Effect of World War I

All further efforts of the Association to secure a national health department before the outbreak of World War I were negligible, and during the war they were completely abandoned. The European conflict loomed only six weeks away when the Council on Health and Public Instruction told the Sixty-fifth session of the House of Delegates in June, 1914, that:

[35] No satisfactory report of the visiting committee's conference with the President has been preserved. Highlights of the meeting, however, are fairly well shown in later remarks in the *Journal* and in committee reports to the Sixty-fifth session of the House of Delegates. See, for example, *JAMA,* 63 (October 10, 1914), 1303; HD, *Proceedings* (65 Annual Session, June, 1914), p. 31.

[36] *JAMA,* 60 (June 28, 1913), 2082–83.

[37] *JAMA,* 60 (June 28, 1913), 2086.

It is hardly necessary to point out that the efforts of the administration for tariff and currency reform, as well as the amount of time devoted to the Mexican situation and the Panama Canal toll bill have made it practically impossible for this measure to be taken up as a part of the administration program.[38]

The approach of the war caught the AMA with its dream unrealized, and indefinitely postponed the prospect of the creation of a national health department. Not until the end of the decade did signs of revived interest in the idea appear within the organization.[39]

Scope of AMA's Interest

As World War I hastily brought the Progressive Era to a close, the American Medical Association had reason to look with pride on its contribution to the advance of legislation promoting social welfare. Although its agitation for a national health department brought no immediate success, its struggle for adequate food and drugs legislation had been in a large measure rewarding. Its insistence on strict enforcement of the legislation partially offset the work of forces seeking to destroy its effectiveness. Its bitter fight against the nostrum, discussed in the next chapter, also resulted in incalculable good. Neither had its untiring struggle for adequate vital statistics legislation in the states been in vain.[40]

Yet, a consideration of the great variety of social abuses confronting the United States in the new century leaves one as impressed with the comparative silence of the AMA on a significant number, as with its crusading fervor against a few. It showed no great interest in the growing slum and tenement problem and offered no leadership in the movement for the elimination of factory hazards, prohibition of child labor, or restriction on women's employment—all of which were vital health problems. It maintained an official neutrality in the prohibition struggle, and was drawn into the fight for narcotic control only after certain features of the Harrison Law of 1914 began directly to affect physicians.[41] The favorable experience of several foreign nations with such experi-

[38] HD, *Proceedings* (65 Annual Session, June, 1914), p. 31.

[39] *JAMA,* 72 (June 14, 1919), 1748.

[40] See pp. 22–23, 62–63, 65, 66n for an account of the Association's efforts to secure adequate vital statistics laws.

[41] For examples of the AMA's interest in the Harrison Law see *JAMA,* 63 (December 19, 1914), 2234; Editorials, *JAMA,* 64 (March 6, 1915), 834–35; *JAMA,* 72 (March 29, 1919), 942.

ments as compulsory sickness insurance, industrial accident insurance, old-age pensions, and minimum-hour laws made no great impression on the leadership of the AMA. Since the Association largely ignored many problems related to public health, it, naturally, rarely spoke out against abuses not connected with health and medicine.[42] It did not stray far from issues that were very intimately connected with the profession's interest and found its time largely consumed by crusading activities in these fields. Whether the Association would acquire a broader interest in problems of national welfare; remain a progressive organization along rather limited lines; or, later, join the forces fighting against the advance of social democracy were questions that only the future could decide.

[42] An exceptional case occurred in 1912 when the Los Angeles session of the House of Delegates adopted a resolution urging the state and federal governments to start extensive projects of reforestration. HD, *Proceedings* (63 Annual Session, June, 1912), p. 57.

Chapter 6

THE ANTI-NOSTRUM CRUSADE, 1906–1921

THE AMERICAN MEDICAL ASSOCIATION emerged from the successful food and drugs battle of 1906 determined to wage a bold and relentless campaign on medical quackery. Deficiencies in the new legislation convinced the AMA that it could not rely solely on the law or its enforcement to destroy the nostrum menace. Aware that earlier attacks on medical frauds had largely been the work of laymen, the Association moved forward to claim its rightful position of leadership in the struggle.

Fertile Nostrum Soil

Behind the façade of federal regulation, the Association found environmental forces that caused proprietary plants to flourish. Many areas far removed from centers of social and technological advance were particularly vulnerable to medical exploitation. Even after several decades of urban growth, the United States remained largely a rural nation that offered its agricultural population little more than a life of monotony and loneliness. Diseases and imaginary ailments besieged the wretched and decrepit creatures of the back country, whose desire for the healing virtues of some elixir did not surpass their thirst for its alcoholic content. The remoteness and isolation of many families also discouraged reliance on medical science when death so often arrived before a physician.[1]

[1] Thomas D. Clark, *Pills, Petticoats and Plows: The Southern Country Store* (Indianapolis: The Bobbs-Merrill Company, 1944), p. 224. The loneliness and anxiety of some country people of the twentieth century is described by one author who says, "It is not an uncommon thing, as rural postmasters will testify, for a man to ask for mail day after day, although no letter had ever come for him." David L. Cohn, *The Good Old Days* (New York: Simon and Schuster, c. 1940, by David L. Cohn), p. 561, used with permission of author's estate.

Among other factors making the nation a rich market for nostrum vendors was the uncritical thinking of a large portion of the population in which illiteracy stood at 10.7 per cent in 1900, with millions more barely above that level.[2] Likewise, the spirit of a generation that had defied the hardships of frontier conditions only reluctantly allowed the admission of physical frailties that passed beyond self-diagnosis and simple medication. Then too, the medical profession itself stood in no high repute, and the presence of a doctor at a patient's bedside gave no assurance that the remedy prescribed could not be found on the nostrum shelves of the nearest store. Also weighing heavily in favor of proprietary interests was the low economic level of the population that reduced medical expenditures to a minimum. Rural and urban families alike only slowly learned that the use of nostrums actually constituted the most costly type of medication, but quickly saw that it eliminated the expense of a doctor's visit.[3]

Preparation for the Crusade

Although the Association had done little toward attacking the proprietary industry before the passage of the Pure Food and Drugs Act, it had already established its most valuable machinery for the fight. The Council on Pharmacy and Chemistry that had earlier examined proprietaries sold only to physicians ("ethical") expanded its work of exposure to embrace the entire field of patent medicines.[4] The AMA compared the council's work to that of Dun or Bradstreet in commercial life. For the busy physician confronted with the increasing complexities of the pharmaceutical field, this body of experts provided "unbiased information" on the many pharmaceutical products appearing under "proprietary

[2] *United States Thirteenth Census,* 1910 (Abstract of the Census with Supplement for Illinois), p. 239. "The Bureau of the Census classifies as illiterate any person 10 years of age or more who is unable to write, regardless of ability to read." Illiteracy among Negroes was 44.5 per cent in 1900. For evidence that quackery held some sway over educated classes see Young, *Toadstool Millionaires,* p. 255.

[3] Much of the "medical democracy" that flourished before the Civil War outlasted the century and survived along with many forces that first produced it. For an account of self-medication in the earlier era see James Harvey Young, "American Medical Quackery in the Age of the Common Man," *The Mississippi Valley Historical Review,* 47 (March, 1961), 579–93.

[4] HD, *Proceedings* (65 Annual Session, June 1914), p. 5.

or brand names" and on all "newcomers to the pharmaceutical world."[5] For the public, the council became an agency of health protection in detecting and exposing many proprietary frauds.

The large volume of work that the Council on Pharmacy and Chemistry undertook brought about the establishment of the Association's Chemical Laboratory in the fall of 1906. During the preceding year the council had relied for aid upon several medical schools in checking on the composition of certain proprietaries, but the work had become too great to assign to outside agencies. Within a short time the laboratory became "a storehouse of chemical and pharmaceutical information" for doctors inquiring about the composition of ethical compounds. Gradually, like the work of the council itself, that of the laboratory expanded to include the investigation of many nostrums sold on the open market.[6]

Alerting the Public

Having established agencies for investigating the proprietary industry, the AMA turned to the task of publicizing nostrum exposures. Its own investigatory work had hardly begun when it secured permission to print and circulate in booklet form Adams's articles attacking quackery and nostrums. Within five years from the date of their original publication in *Collier's,* the AMA had printed 150,000 copies, which it sold at nominal prices to libraries and individuals throughout the nation. It later asserted that the extensive circulation of the evidence in *The Great American Fraud* had aided materially in destroying the worse abuses of fraudulent medical enterprises.[7]

To the Adams investigation, the AMA soon added its own, which it was just as eager to get before the public. Exposures that first appeared in the *Journal* were reprinted in pamphlet form for widespread circulation

[5] *The Propaganda for Reform in Proprietary Medicine* (Chicago: American Medical Association, 1922), II, 570. The Dun and Bradstreet firms had not merged at this time. For additional information on the organization and early work of the council see pp. 74–75 above.

[6] W. A. Puckner, "The Work of the American Medical Association's Chemical Laboratory," *Propaganda for Reform,* II, 322–23.

[7] *Nostrums and Quackery* (2nd ed.; Chicago: American Medical Association, 1912), I, 7. All subsequent references to Vol. I are to the 2nd edition. See also Editorial, *JAMA,* 54 (March 5, 1910), 796. As published by the AMA, *The Great American Fraud* contained 146 pages with 65 illustrations, and sold for less than cost. *JAMA,* 48 (May 11, 1907), 1617.

among the laity. In 1911 it brought a large number of exposures together in book form which appeared as *Nostrums and Quackery*. While the collected investigations of the AMA bore some similarity to Adams's work, the Association observed that *The Great American Fraud* gave a general treatment of many fakeries, whereas *Nostrums and Quackery* offered detailed treatment of a relatively few. Believing that medical charlatanry could thrive only behind a "veil of mystery," the Association's faith in the effectiveness of thorough exposures soon appeared justified.[8] The fine reception that the public gave the first edition of *Nostrums and Quackery* convinced the Association of the wisdom of its effort. In less than a year it had issued a second enlarged edition to meet the growing demand, and, in less than a decade, a second volume.[9]

Through the Propaganda Department which the Association had created to deal with the nostrum threat, the AMA accelerated its drive against proprietary abuses. In the first issue of the *Journal* for 1911, there appeared a new feature called "Propaganda for Reform," devoted to an exposure of fraudulent medical concerns. Although the *Journal* earlier contained a column entitled "Pharmacology," which principally exposed ethical proprietaries, the establishment of the new department demonstrated the growing aggressiveness of the Association. As the AMA aroused greater interest in the nostrum menace, the work of the department greatly increased. During 1912, it answered 2,450 letters from physicians and laymen, that increased to 4,200 in 1913, of which 1,213 came from the laity. In addition, the frequent inquiries of lay publications about the merits of many popular proprietaries indicated that some were giving more than nominal assent to the idea of clean advertising.[10]

As the work of investigating patent medicines and ethical proprietaries advanced, the Association decided to incorporate its findings about the

[8] *Nostrums and Quackery,* I, 11.

[9] *Ibid.,* p. 11. The 2nd edition, containing 708 pages, was 199 pages larger than the 1st. For the initial volume see *Nostrums and Quackery,* Vol. I (1st ed.; Chicago: Press of the American Medical Association). The 2nd volume contained 832 pages. Arthur J. Cramp, comp. and ed., *Nostrums and Quackery,* Vol. 2 (Chicago: Press of the American Medical Association, 1921).

[10] *JAMA,* 61 (January 7, 1911), 56–57; HD, *Proceedings* (65 Annual Session, June, 1914), p. 5. A few lay publications had awakened to the evils of nostrum advertising about this time, the most outstanding being *Printers' Ink.* This periodical published a model statute in November, 1911, for penalizing those engaged in false and fraudulent advertising. In the nineteenth century several agricultural papers seem to deserve most of the credit for even attempting feeble attacks upon nostrum advertising. See H. J. Kenner, *The Fight for Truth in Advertising* (New York: Round Table Press, Inc., 1936), pp. 26–27, 7–9.

latter in a book primarily designed for physicians. Although it had already learned that no clear lines of distinction separated ethical proprietaries from patent medicines, enough existed to warrant publication of *The Propaganda for Reform in Proprietary Medicines,* which soon appeared. This scientific work "strictly of professional interest" served as a fitting complement to the Association's exposure of medical frauds in *Nostrums and Quackery* and experienced a wide reception from the beginning. The popularity of the work accounted for the publication of nine editions, and for the appearance of a second volume which the Association published in 1922.[11]

Purging the Press

The Association waged no more effective attack on the nostrum industry than when it launched a movement to drive advertisers of fraudulent medical compounds from the press. Fully aware that the press held almost life and death power over the nostrum industry, the Association attacked publications that, by advertising nostrums, became accomplices in deception. In 1907, it adopted a resolution urging all medical journals to refuse advertising space to preparations of which the Council on Pharmacy and Chemistry had not approved. Five years later it denounced the entire business of patent medicine advertising, declaring that "there is no such thing as an unobjectionable 'patent-medicine' advertisement in a newspaper," and that "There can be no effective censorship of nostrum advertising."[12] It considered particularly deplorable the demands pressed by proprietary manufacturers upon editors that they publish nothing damaging to the sale of their products in the reading columns of their papers. The AMA realized, however, that its principal success at purging the secular press of patent-medicine advertisements lay in securing the enactment and enforcement of state and federal legislation that prohibited false or misleading advertisements of any type.[13] But it offered little more than general complaints against this widespread abuse.

[11] *The Propaganda for Reform in Proprietary Medicine* (9th ed.; Chicago: American Medical Association), I, 3. In the 7th, 8th, and 9th editions the AMA included a few exposures of popular nostrums. All subsequent references are to the 9th edition.

[12] *JAMA,* 50 (June 13, 1908), 2007; quotation, Editorial, *JAMA,* 58 (April 13, 1912), 1118–19.

[13] Editorial, *JAMA,* 58 (January 6, 1912), 36. Besides demanding that no matter critical of proprietaries could appear in the newspapers carrying their advertisements, some proprietary establishments forced newspapers to fight against government regulation of the nostrum business by the threat of stopping

With the medical press, however, the Association showed no inclination to temporize and mercilessly exposed offenders in the healing fraternity in spite of its earlier position among the transgressors. Sometimes it singled out an individual journal for attack, but frequently leveled its charges against a great number. The loose advertising standards of the *Charlotte Medical Journal* especially annoyed the AMA, but it also found the advertising policies of such organs as the *Illinois Medical Register,* the *Atlanta Journal of Medicine,* and the *International Journal of Surgery* particularly offensive. It described the advertising pages of the latter as "the gallery of nostrums."[14] In 1914, one issue of the *Journal's* Propaganda for Reform column criticized the advertising ethics of the "Big Six," but an editorial the next year cited 36 offenders.[15]

While attacking refractory periodicals, the Association did not forget to commend and encourage journals that chose to walk along the uncongested path of the just. The trustees attempted to comfort weak and vacillating publications with the disclosure that its own sacrificial conduct resulted in the loss of at least $25,000 during one year.[16] For losses others suffered the AMA expressed sympathy and appreciation. It commended the stand of the *South Texas Medical Record* for honest advertising and cited the *Medical World* of Philadelphia, the *Southern Medical Journal,* and the *Cleveland Medical Journal* as publications that had carried in their columns exposures of many nostrums.[17] The *Journal's* commendation of the advertising ethics of the secular press ranged from its praise of the *New York Tribune* and *Kansas City Independent* to public approval of the Oskaloosa (Iowa) *Times.* Even the *Royal Neighbor,* the publication of a fraternal order, received the Association's notice when it renounced its alliance with the nostrum vendors.[18]

---

their advertisements if hostile legislation was passed. Samuel Hopkins Adams, *The Great American Fraud* (4th ed.; P. F. Collier & Son, 1907), p. 143. In 1909 the editor of the *Journal* endorsed a New Zealand law that held the publisher along with the manufacturer liable for published misrepresentations of a proprietary. Editorial, *JAMA,* 52 (April 3, 1909), 1111. For the Association's criticism of the Pure Food and Drugs Act see pp. 84–85 above.

[14] *Propaganda for Reform,* I, 422–23; Pucker, in *Propaganda for Reform,* II, 15; *Propaganda for Reform,* II, 429, quotation p. 87.

[15] *JAMA,* 63 (October 31, 1914), 1594; *Propaganda for Reform,* I, 31. The "Big Six" were the *American Journal of Clinical Medicine* (Chicago); *American Journal of Surgery* (New York); *American Medicine* (Burlington, Vt.); *Interstate Medical Journal* (St. Louis); *Medical Council* (Philadelphia); and the *Therapeutic Gazette* (Detroit).

[16] *JAMA,* 48 (June 8, 1907), 1962.

[17] *Propaganda for Reform,* I, 440; Editorial, *JAMA,* 58 (January 6, 1912), 36.

[18] *JAMA,* 64 (January 2, 1915), 61; *JAMA,* 48 (February 2, 1907), 422; *JAMA,* 64 (April 24, 1915), 1430; *Propaganda for Reform,* I, 418–19.

More effective, however, than words of praise or criticism in purging medical journalism of the nostrum was the Association's establishment of the Co-operative Medical Advertising Bureau, December 1, 1912. This agency extended its services to the journals of state societies, in securing for them medical advertising that helped stabilize their income without degrading their standards. It encouraged improvements in their appearance and successfully promoted standardization in size. In addition, the bureau answered inquiries about acceptable advertising and provided co-operating journals with information about advertisers, credits, and business conditions. The fact that the bureau collected nearly $66,000 in 1920 to prorate among the co-operating state organs, after its own expenses were deducted, demonstrated no small degree of financial success. That 28 state journals had accepted the bureau's plan of clean advertising by 1920 indicated the popularity of its service as well.[19]

In handling the problem of nostrum advertisement in religious papers, the AMA did not consider that their spiritual function gave immunity from criticism. In fact, it readily pointed out the inconsistency of advocating prohibition on one page and advertising some highly alcoholic elixir on another. It had little sympathy for religious editors who raised the defense that nostrum advertising promoted a worthy cause. Early in 1907, it denounced the *Cumberland Presbyterian* (Nashville, Tennessee) for its low advertising standards and showed itself no respector of denominations by attacking the *Baptist Record* (Jackson, Mississippi) on the same grounds about three years later.[20] The Association realized, however, that the standards of medical advertisements had greatly im-

[19] HD, *Proceedings* (66 Annual Session, June, 1915), p. 3; *JAMA,* 76 (June 11, 1921), 1658. In 1917 the trustees announced that of all the journals owned by state societies only the Illinois journal refused to co-operate with the bureau; however, several state associations had no official organs. *JAMA,* 48 (June 9, 1917), 1714.

[20] *JAMA,* 48 (February 2, 1907), 435–36; *Nostrums and Quackery,* I, 267. The high alcoholic content of most proprietaries was sufficient ground in itself for the *Journal's* condemnation of them. That this was their chief appeal in a great many cases is quite certain. "Hostetter's Celebrated Stomach Bitters," which once contained 39 per cent alcohol (later reduced to 25 per cent), illustrates the point. "The *Baltimore Sun* of February 4, 1917, carried a news item from Danville, Va., to the effect that the police in that town had had to deal with a large number of 'drunks' each of whom admitted that he became intoxicated on 'a certain proprietary medicine which contained 25 per cent alcohol.' A telegram from the *Journal* to the Chief of Police of Danville asking for the name of the proprietary medicine in question, brought the laconic reply 'Hostetter's Bitters'," *JAMA,* 74 (May 29, 1920), 1535.

proved and reported in the fall of 1911 that "religious journals are practically free from the blight of 'patent medicine' advertisements."[21]

Attack on Supporters of Nostrum Business

Besides its attempts to purify the press, the AMA tried to silence the voices of individuals who openly sympathized with proprietary fakery and nostrum exploitation. Medical mavericks whose loose ethics, inferior training, or spirit of independence brought them in conflict with the Association's policies became the particular targets of attack. The *Journal's* exposure of these recalcitrants served as a deterrent against the defection of others. It referred to "W. T. Marrs, M.D., of Peoria Heights, Ill." as "our old testimonio-maniac friend," when he added the popular "Capudine" to the list of nostrums he publicly endorsed. In the same article the *Journal* mentioned a testimonial of "Dr. A. S. Reed of Naples, Maine" in which "the marvelous results achieved by the administration of Capudine are surpassed only by the still more marvelous spelling and composition of the testimonial." It even exposed a London doctor for his endorsement of proprietary frauds.[22]

Sometimes medically minded laymen incurred the wrath of the AMA for their support of nostrums and medical fakery. When Upton Sinclair replied to the *Journal's* attack on a California physician, Albert Abrams, with a defense of his unconventional methods, the Association attacked both. Asserting that Sinclair was no authority on medical matters, it charged that in earlier years he also became enthusiastic over "fast cures" and a "raw food fad" that he now rejected.[23] Occasionally a minister straggled across the *Journal's* firing range. It leveled strong criticism at Dr. Robert S. MacArthur, a prominent Baptist clergyman, for publicly commending the work of Andrew McConnell, founder of the "Society of Universal Science," whom it branded as a medical fake. When another promoter, C. H. Carson, whom the Association considered a charlatan, opened his "Temple of Health" in Kansas City, the *Journal* noted with disgust that a prominent local Congregational minister delivered an address.[24]

[21] *Nostrums and Quackery,* I, 328.

[22] *JAMA,* 51 (October 17, 1908), 1347–48; *Nostrums and Quackery,* I, 685

[23] *Propaganda for Reform,* II, 479–80.

[24] *Nostrums and Quackery,* I, 281, 329–30.

The Matter of Testimonials

Not only did the Association try to cut the major circuits through which knowledge about the nostrum reached the public, but it also attempted to inform the profession and laymen about the deceptions in most proprietary advertising. The AMA explained that few "unsolicited" nostrum testimonials were actually unsolicited, and that some sort of gift to a nostrum victim often produced an effusive recommendation of a product. The *Journal* pointed out that testimonial gathering had become a business of considerable importance and cited an advertisement in the *Chicago Tribune,* "MEDICAL TESTIMONIAL GATHERERS—Experienced; leads furnished; give references."[25] It also showed that the collection of letters written in response to nostrum advertisements constituted a widespread operation and gave the names and practices of some letter brokers. The *Journal* exposed the practices of the Woman's Mutual Benefit Company of Joliet, Illinois, which guaranteed confidential treatment of all letters addressed to Mrs. Harriet M. Richards, its advertising name, when the Guild Company, a letter brokerage, claimed to have 140,000 letters addressed to this firm available at five dollars a thousand. In the words of Samuel Hopkins Adams, it issued a warning to all who replied to the advertisements of many nostrum houses:

> You may know that all the things you have said about your health and your person—intimate details which you carefully conceal from your friends and neighbors—are the property of any person who cares to pay four or five dollars for the letters of yourself and others like you.[26]

The AMA also demonstrated the unreliability of testimonials. Some nostrum concerns resorted to the practice of exploiting the names of prominent physicians for the advancement of their products. In 1919, the *Journal* exposed the daring attempt of The Peneoleum Company to deceive the public by connecting the name of Alexander Lambert, president of the AMA, with its influenza nostrum. An investigation of the names affixed to testimonials sometimes revealed that they were actual forgeries. But, even if genuine, the Association contended that the mind untrained in medical science possessed little competence for appraising the value of a proprietary. Nostrum interests learned that the most

[25] *Ibid.,* pp. 681–82.

[26] *Ibid.,* pp. 646–47. Adams cites one letter brokerage in New York City that had a warehouse containing over 7 million letters. *Great American Fraud,* p. 143.

enthusiastic testimonials generally came shortly after the purchase of their products, when the buyer's hopes and imagination reached their height.[27] The *Journal* offered a psychological explanation for actual improvement in some instances. It cited a case of cancer reported by William Osler in which the patient, when assured of not having cancer by a trusted but mistaken consultant, added eighteen pounds of weight and lost all of the symptoms of the malady.[28]

Lure of Patent Medicine

The preparation of the nostrum with due regard for the expectations of the victim also increased the unreliability of testimonials. As nostrum consumers expected some quick effect, manufacturers graciously obliged. To the nostrum-buying public the words "change" and "action" were often synonymous with "improvement." Nothing served better than alcohol to effect the change and activate the system. Many a consumer, whose depressed spirits rose as he downed his favorite alcoholic elixir, gladly pointed others to his fountain of fulfillment. If his nostrum had the additional power of exciting the bowels, he affirmed its efficacy with all the more assurance.[29] While the popularity of compounds with these simple powers continued, the *Journal* repeatedly warned of their superficial effect and potential danger.

Another device of nostrum manufacturers that particularly impressed the layman was the technical verbiage used in describing their preparations. Of course, generous quantities of every-day language accompanied every nostrum, but proprietary concerns also satisfied the layman's expectation of finding some incomprehensible jargon. The *Journal* observed that nostrum makers described their products without revealing any facts that would "lift the veil of mystery" which remained their greatest asset.[30] Nostrum concerns even employed this device in promoting ethical proprietaries. The base of a simple clay poultice became "anhydrous and levigated argillaceous mineral" which, said the *Journal,* "sounds much more imposing than dry and finely powered clay." It also

[27] *Propaganda for Reform,* II, 442–43, 409. *Nostrums and Quackery,* I, 682.

[28] *Propaganda for Reform,* II, 440.

[29] Clark lists the four functions expected of tonics as "to ease pain immediately, give a cheerful warming glow to the whole body, taste strongly of herbs, and move the bowels." *Pills, Petticoats and Plows,* p. 231.

[30] *Propaganda for Reform,* II, 546.

cited one concern's description of a tablet with which it exploited the dental profession as "an anodyne, analgesic febrifuge sedative, exorcising [sic!] antineuralgic and antiheumatic action."[31]

For those who looked beyond nostrum chicanery for the foundation fallacies in proprietary theories, the *Journal* offered additional evidence. Repeatedly it cited one or more deficiencies in the system. As the technique of proprietary healing called for the administration of a "remedy" after an unskilled diagnosis, impersonal diagnosis, or none at all, it defied the most elementary scientific concepts. Since the proprietary industry constituted an "open shop," nothing precluded the entry of the untrained into the preparation and manufacture of medical compounds. The primary objective of the industry to exploit a medicine naturally increased its hesitancy to subject a preparation to scientific investigation. In addition, its oversimplification of pathological problems made treatment with proprietary compounds highly objectionable.

Allies of AMA

The Association's conflict with the proprietary business involved even more than refuting its theories, exposing its business methods, and attacking the nostrum-promoting press. In the true spirit of the muckrakers, it focused attention upon specific nostrums and their exploiters. Into the darkest recesses of the industry the Association probed, never hesitating to reveal the most sordid aspects of the business. No other organization in the nation after 1906 remotely rivaled the AMA in exposing the graft and ravages of the nostrum vendors.

Much of the Association's effectiveness in combating nostrums and quackery may be attributed to the success of its efforts in co-ordinating the work of its Council on Pharmacy and Chemistry with that of the Bureau of Chemistry of the Department of Agriculture. While the AMA's contact with the bureau dates beyond the establishment of the council in 1905, the struggle for the passage and enforcement of the Pure Food and Drugs Act closely integrated the work of the two agencies. In fact, as members of both, Wiley and Kebler rendered inestimable service to the AMA. As early as August, 1907, Kebler reported on 15 products that he had analyzed as a member of the council and expressed regret some three months later that the demands of

[31] *Ibid.* The bracketed word is in the source.

his government post reduced the amount of work he could do for the council. Moreover, the AMA frequently assisted the bureau in similar ways and carried its co-operation as far as recommending physicians to whom the bureau might send different medical remedies for approval.[32]

The close relation existing between the council and the bureau appears to have steadied and stimulated both. In 1908, Wiley raised objections to some of the compounds the *Journal* featured and two years later urged the editor to launch an attack on the fraudulent advertising of some whiskey producers. On another occasion he called upon the editor for greater moderation in his proposed attack upon the laxity of the courts in dealing with violations of the food and drugs legislation. Late in 1908, the editor, in turn, complained confidentially to Wiley of Kebler's tardiness in submitting reports on several products and asked the Chief to prod his associate along.[33] Close contact of the agencies, however, bred no contempt, and unity of purpose overcame whatever minor differences arose.

While relying heavily on the investigations of the Bureau of Chemistry, the AMA's council on Pharmacy and Chemistry co-operated with other agencies, organizations, and individuals that fought the nostrum. The work of the Postmaster's and Attorney General's Departments contributed to the strength of its crusade. Leading authorities in medical schools and universities assisted in some phases of research, and free exchange of information with the *British Medical Journal* and health organizations within the United States also proved helpful.[34]

Cases of Exposures

Strengthened by aid from many sources, the AMA carried on a continuous crusade against nostrums and quackery. Upon forms of medical charlatanry which it considered most harmful, it concentrated its heaviest attacks. For no aspect of the proprietary business did it have more contempt than for the "cancer cures," although "cures" for tuberculosis

[32] Kebler to W. A. Puckner, Aug. 6, 1907; Kebler to Simmons, Nov. 12, 1907; Kebler to Simmons, Feb. 20, 1906; Kebler to Simmons, Mar. 7, 1906, BCR.

[33] Wiley to Simmons, Oct. 15, 1908; Simmons to Wiley, Oct. 20, 1908; Wiley to Simmons, Nov. 3, 1910; Wiley to Simmons, Oct. 23, 1910; Simmons to Wiley, Dec. 19, 1908, BCR.

[34] *Nostrums and Quackery,* I, 8, 26; *Propaganda for Reform,* II, 394, 304, 171; *JAMA,* 50 (April 11, 1908), 1198.

were also bitterly fought.[35] Victims of tuberculosis, it observed, fell easy prey to ghouls of this nefarious trade. The pulmonary tubercular patient, more than any other, responded to psychic stimulus. The *Journal* referred to the experiments of a French physician, Albert Mathieu, who demonstrated the power of the mind over this disease. Patients, when convinced that a new serum injection they received would cure their disease, showed amazing improvement and lapsed into the former condition when the injection stopped. Actually the serum was only a salt solution.[36]

The Association's attack on a company in Columbus, Ohio, manufacturing and exploiting "Nature's Creation," illustrates the type of campaign it waged against medical quackery. The promoters owning this company were G. W. Campbell, formerly of Chicago, whom the AMA labeled as a medical quack, and a Mrs. J. M. Reynolds (later Cohen), whom Campbell branded later in a court dispute as a Chicago basement fortune teller.[37] Their wide publicity campaign brought heavy demands for their vaunted elixir. The public heard the news that it contained "at least one ingredient that the medical world knows nothing about . . . no chemist has ever been able to determine what it is." The bottle label bore the name "The Nature's Creation Co.'s Discovery" and the imprint of a beautiful waterfall. The price $5.00 also appeared, and below center, the statement, "A remedy for tuberculosis and weak lungs." Widely advertised testimonials impressed the public with the value of this mixture.

The exploitation of "Nature's Creation," however, impressed the AMA only with the gullibility of the public. It followed the company's activities and reported the findings. The Association's Chemical Laboratory found nothing in the compound to justify the company's claim, and the *Journal* charged that the product was only a "syphilis cure" that Campbell had once exploited in Chicago. The Association's check on many testimonials showed that all were either unreliable, untrue, or forgeries. The February 4, 1911, issue of the *Journal* carried the names and pictures of five persons whom "Nature's Creation" had "cured" not long before, who were then confined permanently in subterranean rest as victims of tuberculosis. It announced the findings of the Columbus Board of Health that 45 local residents "cured" of tuberculosis by "Nature's Creation" were not alive to testify two or three years later. It also reported the later admission of

[35] *Nostrums and Quackery,* I, 76.

[36] *Ibid.*

[37] *Ibid.,* pp. 131–32. This exposure includes pp. 131–46.

Campbell himself, that his nostrum, selling for $5.00 a bottle, never cost more than 24 cents to manufacture. While the Association felt the sting of Campbell's fierce retaliation against the editor of the *Journal,* it only intensified its campaign of exposure.[38]

The *Journal* attacked other consumptive-cure frauds with equal severity. It informed the profession that the publicity techniques of the sanctimonious "J. Lawrence Hill, A. M., D. D., M. D.," of Jackson, Michigan, followed the typical course of mail order quackery. First, the newspaper advertisement; second, "the series of follow-up letters, so prepared as to simulate communications"; third "the bait of a 'trial treatment' "; and finally, "the inevitable testimonials—the *sine qua non* of the quack." It showed that the $10.00 "cure," available after the fifth letter to an unresponsive patient for $3.20, possessed no value whatever in curing tuberculosis. It spoke of Hill as "one of those pious humbugs who work their church affiliation to the limit in the exploitation of fake 'cures,' " and cited a newspaper announcement of a message he delivered around Christmas, 1910, on "Christ the Wonderful One." The AMA found fraudulent Hill's claim that he had graduated from the University of Edinburgh, and proved untrue the testimony of a ministerial admirer that the promoter had been offered a position as assistant superintendent of the national Bureau of Chemistry.[39]

The Association's war on quackery also brought on its investigation of the crafty career of Orlando Edgar Miller whose trail of charlatanry extended into at least four decades. As early as 1900, he became interested in the idea of destroying the bacilli of tuberculosis by heating oxygen to 150 degrees, and maintained interest in the malady long enough to issue a publication entitled, "Consumption: Its Cause, Its Nature, Its Prevention, Its Cure." The *Journal* noted the long history of his interest both in religion and quackery, and the persistence of the former at Fort Leavenworth, as a Sunday school promoter, when a prison sentence for embezzlement temporarily interrupted his charlatanry

[38] In a sheet dated October 10, 1910, Campbell attacked Simmon's record as a practitioner in Lincoln, Neb. He reproduces what appears to be a local newspaper ad in which Simmons, who was then specializing in women's diseases, guaranteed cures "in all cases of Hemorrhoids, Piles, Fistula, Ulcer, Rupture, Itching Piles and all forms of Rectal disease no matter how long standing." Commenting on the seriousness of some of these ailments and criticising Simmon's for his promise to cure, Campbell added, "Even if only a *quack* Dr. Simmon's ought to be better informed." (Nature's Creation File, AMA, DI.)

[39] *Nostrums and Quackery,* I, 93–108; Joe Dowie to N. P. Colwell, Oct. 29, 1910 (Hill File, AMA, DI); Simmons to Wiley, Sept. 30, 1910, BCR.

in medicine.[40] Numerous other imposters exploiting consumptive victims faced the Association's withering blasts.

Even lower in the AMA's opinion stood the "cancer cure" pretender. Suffering and dying victims oftened turned to the ghouls of cancer quackery, who replaced their often meager savings with nothing but disillusionment and despair. The *Journal* described their two types of "cures" as those taken internally along with some antiseptic for external use, and the "paste" or "poultice" treatment in which a strong caustic was applied to the "ulcerating surface." The first treatment it considered worthless, and the second, "not only unreliable and painful but positively dangerous."[41] In the fight against this phase of exploitation, the AMA relied considerably on investigations by federal authorities and the Adams exposures. Governmental watch over the realm of cancer quackery reduced the functions of the AMA largely to that of publicizing its findings. In this capacity it alerted the medical profession and public to the nature and scope of the fraud.

The career of S. R. Chamlee in cancer-fakery well illustrates the chicanery of the trade. This bold promoter simultaneously operated concerns in St. Louis and Los Angeles, later keeping a step ahead of federal authorities at St. Louis by transferring his activities to Chicago. His extravagant advertising promised absolute cure for the letter-diagnosed user of the home-applied "Dr. Chamlee's Cancer Specific." The kind and gentle face on the letterheads bred confidence in the advertiser's honesty with his assurance: "Without Knife or Pain or Pay Until Cured." Newspaper advertisements carried his promise to give $1,000 for any failure in his treatment of tumor or cancer. In 1915 he urged doctors to buy his remedy, which had allegedly raised his income to $30,000 a year. The *Journal* watched his activities and publicized the worthlessness of his "Specific" that consisted of 99 per cent water and alcohol. It showed that he solicited money in advance of "cure" by a letter threatening to prepare one dissatisfied victim for a "complete set of teeth" if he appeared at headquarters for a financial refund.[42]

[40] *Nostrums and Quackery,* I, 115–30; some photostatic pages of Miller's pamphlet appear in Miller File, AMA, DI. In the same file a column from the *San Francisco Chronicle,* November 11, 1934, shows that Miller had just received a six-year federal prison sentence for using the mails to defraud. The AMA's fight against Miller was far from complete by the end of the second decade.

[41] *Nostrums and Quackery,* I, 25–26.

[42] *Nostrums and Quackery,* I, 37–45; *Chicago Examiner,* October 15, 1911, and Chamlee to A. S. Hawkins [1915] in Chamlee File, AMA, DI.

As the *Journal* demonstrated, Chamlee had no monopoly on the techniques of cancer quackery. It publicized the worthlessness of preparations that "Drs. Mixers" of Hastings, Michigan, sold as guaranteed cancer cures and the fact that the "Drs. Mixer" company included the father long deceased and the son, Charles W. Mixer, who was no doctor at all. It cited the efforts of the latter to mix religion, politics, and business. His advertisements urged the reader to perform a "Christian act" of sending addresses of all known cancer sufferers, while letters to some prospective Chicago victims in June, 1912, urged them to get in contact with him while he served as assistant sergeant-at-arms at the Republican National Convention. More concerned, however, about winning the confidence of the public than the friendship of the AMA, Mixer continued his work until death of cancer in 1934 closed nearly a half century of his medical charlatanry.[43]

Although quackery reached its worst in consumption and cancer fakery, its exploitation of many other ailments proved just as intensive if somewhat less destructive. Only the improbability of profits deterred expansion in any area, and this improbability lessened as clever promoters appealed to every human emotion and sensitivity. No field of exploitation better illustrated the appeal to pride than "obesity cures," so tantalizing to victims imprisoned within thick walls of fat. Nostrum advertisements, featuring monstrous figures with bulging breasts, mirrored to many overly-expanded females their plight and offered them hope. The path from homeliness to beauty, featured in feminine "before and after" advertisements, attracted weighty women and doubly appealed to heavily burdened men.

Extensive publicity explains the success of the Margorie Hamilton Company of Denver, Colorado, that offered a "Combination Quadruple System" effective in reducing fat without "horrible dieting" or "terrible gymnastic work." Reaching out for easy profits, "Margorie Hamilton" informed prospective victims that the success of her "Drugless Treatment" had enraged "jealous doctors" and had almost driven "off the face of the earth into the dark depth of oblivion would-be, make-believe, so-called fat reducing medical specialists. . . ." A statement listing the names of 14 doctors who allegedly approved of the treatment strengthened her testimony.[44]

[43] *Nostrums and Quackery,* I, 55–62; Releases in Mixer File, AMA, DI from (U.S. Department of Agriculture, Office of Information, Dec. 29, 1934) and from (Federal Trade Commission, Sept. 13, 1934).

[44] AMA, *Nostrums and Quackery,* I, 388–405 summarizes this case. Company form letter, April 1 (1912?); Sheet entitled "List of Physicians Giving Testi-

The AMA's investigation showed that this $15.00 cure called for dieting, purging, and exercises, and made use of only commonly known facts in effecting weight reduction. The Association felt that this remedy would be as effective as Sharp's "sure method of exterminating roaches," and for much the same reason:

> He would sell his secret with such apparatus as was necessary, to all who would remit $1. Those who "bit" received two small blocks of wood with the following instructions: "place the roach on the lower block, superimpose the upper block and apply pressure."

The Association's thorough exposure of Walter C. Cunningham and wife, Margorie Hamilton Cunningham, the promoters of this concern, brought about governmental investigation and their hurried departure for England.[45]

While exploiters of "obesity cures" thrived on the fat of the land, other promoters reversed the appeal to attract an emaciated market longing to possess modest quantities of well-distributed flesh. A Chicago firm operating as "Eloise Rae" promised to any concave-fronted, decrepit, or superannuated female "a full, firm, youthful bust" developed at home in 15 days.[46] An actress, Pearl La Sarge, lent her name to a firm that traced most family woes to the wife's poor complexion and offered a $10.00 remedy finally available to most patients for $1.00. "Dr. Howe & Co." of Chicago offered to "self-wrecked men" remedies for troubles that ranged from falling hair to failing memory.[47]

Neither the age nor general respectability of a proprietary deterred the AMA from attack. Through the years it had referred to the low value and high price of Lydia E. Pinkham's time-honored tonic. In 1915, the

---

monials for Margorie Hamilton Obesity Cure," (Margorie Hamilton File, AMA, DI).

[45] Quotation in *Nostrums and Quackery,* I, 401; see also 402–4; the *Denver Times,* June 7, 1912, p. 1. W. W. Grant, chairman of the Board of Trustees of the AMA, who lived in Denver, assisted the Association in the investigation of this case. Grant to Simmons, June 14, 1912 (Margorie Hamilton File).

[46] Cramp, *Nostrums and Quackery,* II, 64. In an unidentified newspaper clipping "Eloise Rae" advertised that "A Full Firm Bust is Worth More to a Woman Than Beauty" and added that although once "skinny, scrawny, flat and unattractive . . . I claim to be the highest priced artists' model in the United States, and what I did for myself I can do for you." (Eloise Rae File, AMA, DI).

[47] Cramp, *Nostrums and Quackery,* II, 63, 400. "Dr. Howe & Co." was one of the firms that the *Chicago Tribune* exposed in its campaign to destroy quackery in the city. It published a series of exposures from October 27 to November 29, 1913, and many of these were further published by the AMA. See *Nostrums and Quackery,* II, 359–62.

Journal exposed the business methods of the company in exploiting the name of its founder. Originally the friendly woman pictured on the package urged forlorn women to write her of personal problems and ailments. Although Mrs. Pinkham died in 1883, thirty years later the friendly face still appeared along with the same request. The company's reply that the daughter-in-law of the founder answered the letters left the AMA unimpressed.[48]

A Firm Fights Back

Most companies that the AMA attacked dared not seek damages through the courts, but the Chattanooga Medicine Company was a notable exception.[49] Its bulging coffers attested to the popularity of "Wine of Cardui" and left the company indisposed to tolerate opposition. Of high alcoholic potency, this preparation, designed for female ailments, satisfied the burning thirsts of women and men as well. Wretched personalities, inhibited by social and moral conventions, found relief in the effects of this compound that contained ingredients they could not otherwise respectably secure. The company's extravagant claims, supported by innumerable testimonials, heralded the arrival of a female utopia.[50]

When the AMA launched its attack on the sensitive sovereigns of this proprietary empire, reprisals were soon forthcoming. To the Association's charge "that the business had been built on deceit, and that Wine

[48] *JAMA,* 64 (May 15, 1915), 1674–75. As early as 1905 the company contended that it had made no effort to deceive the public into believing that Lydia E. Pinkham was still living and had publicly explained many times who was continuing her work. Living or deceased, however, Mrs. Pinkham retained devoted followers; one of whom, in the Midwest, found the compound powerful enough to produce her pregnancy when given to her husband. Company form letter, Dec. 1, 1905; letter to "Dr. Cramp," Oct. 28, 1927 (Lydia E. Pinkham File, AMA, DI).

[49] The *Journal* observed in 1916 that although a "dozen or more suits" had been filed against it and the AMA within the past ten years, only the one begun by the Chattanooga Medicine Company had come up for trial. *JAMA,* 66 (March 18, 1916), 900.

[50] One mute monument to the financial success of the company's sale of Wine of Cardui and other proprietaries is the Hotel Patten in Chattanooga. This hotel was named for Z. C. Patten, Sr., one of the originators of the business, who along with his son-in-law, J. T. Lupton, provided the money for building it. Jerome B. Pound, *Memoirs with Histories of Pound-Murphey-Willingham-Palmer-Pitts Families* (Chattanooga, Tenn., published by the author, 1949), p. 101. The *Journal,* from which this account is taken, began publishing the full proceedings of the trial beginning with *JAMA,* 66 (April 1, 1916), 1042–50.

of Cardui was a vicious fraud," the company responded with two libel suits: a personal suit for $200,000 that John A. Patten brought, and a partnership suit for $100,000 in which his brother, Z. C. Patten, Jr. was also a plaintiff.[51] Although the death of the former, April 26, 1916, stopped the progress of the personal suit, the other lasted through 13 weeks of stormy courtroom battle. While the jury gave a verdict for the Chattanooga Medicine Company, it assessed damages at only one cent. The *Journal* explained the Association's position as "Technically guilty; morally justified! To the Association a moral triumph; to the 'patent medicine' interests a Pyrrhic victory."[52] Unfortunately for the AMA, the suit that involved an expense of nearly $125,000 bore no comparison with the damages assessed and left it with an annual operating deficit for the first time in about 25 years. The Association deplored "The spectacle of a scientific organization, in its attempt to safeguard the public health, having to assume responsibilities that rightfully belong to the state and federal agencies. . . ."[53]

The extent of the Association's work in combating the nostrum menace embraced a field as large as the exploitation itself. As quackery also exploited victims of dope, nicotine, and alcohol, the Association came to their defense. It kept a watchful eye on promotional schemes in the field of electrotherapeutics, pointing out examples of fraud in treatments and mechanical devices. It warned the deaf and the blind of fakery in the promotion of sight restorers and hearing devices and befriended the victims of rupture, asthma, and hay fever by exposing a wide variety of fraudulent "cures." Frequently it called attention to the exorbitant price of proprietaries, well-illustrated by its exposure of "Murine," an eye wash, that sold for $1.00 an ounce but cost, it contended, about five cents a gallon to manufacture. Nor did the Association

[51] *JAMA,* 67 (July 1, 1916), 41; *JAMA,* 66 (February 19, 1916), 585. The AMA's attack, which provoked the Chattanooga Medicine Company to seek legal redress, appeared in *JAMA,* 62 (April 11, 1914), 1186–89, and *JAMA,* 63 (July 18, 1914), 258–62. *Harper's Weekly Magazine* also carried an exposure of the company's products at the same time, which involved it in a lawsuit.

[52] Clark, *Pills, Petticoats and Plows,* p. 251; quotation, *JAMA,* 67 (July 1, 1916), 41. Since the court allowed damages of one cent, the Chattanooga Medicine Company technically won the case and therefore could not have appealed it. For a further claim of the AMA's actual victory see Editorial, *JAMA,* 67 (July 15, 1916), 206. This decision, legally in favor of the medicine company, placed an impediment in the path of governmental agencies trying to enforce the food and drugs legislation. Kebler to Cramp, December 7, 1917, BCR.

[53] *JAMA,* 67 (July 1, 1916), 41; *JAMA,* 68 (June 9, 1917), 1718.

ignore diploma mills and irregular medical institutes, whose graduates often entered or supported the nostrum business.[54]

Problem of Ethical Proprietaries

While trying to protect the public from the widespread proprietary abuses, the AMA showed no less interest in guarding physicians against ethical proprietary frauds. The Council on Pharmacy and Chemistry framed a set of rules governing the admission of reports on proprietary, nonproprietary, and nonofficial products into the yearly publication, *New and Nonofficial Remedies.* This publication formed the basis for the two volumes, *Propaganda for Reform in Proprietary Medicines* and gave physicians a basis for judging the reliability of a compound. The establishment and publication of this standard served the additional purpose of bringing many concerns into conformity with higher ethics in manufacturing and advertising. The rules prohibited the admission of products of undisclosed composition or those for which the manufacturer supplied no tests for determining their identity or purity. Very few compounds advertised directly to the public found admission, and none that were accompanied by information suggesting self-medication. The council demanded the number of any patented or registered article and required that all poisonous compounds be so labeled. Other unacceptable articles included those with misleading names, those about which false or unwarranted claims were made, and products of no scientific usefulness.[55] While many firms sought the council's approval of their products, others supplied information, if at all, only on request.

Reference to a few specific cases will illustrate the council's problems in handling articles of special interest to physicians. Proprietary and pharmaceutical concerns often glaringly violated the rules for the admission of their products to *New and Nonofficial Remedies,* but frequently their subtle violations defied even the detection of physicians. The Association reduced the chances of deception even for the more unlearned physicians, however, by publicizing obvious and hidden violations.

The Council on Pharmacy and Chemistry found easily detectable

[54] *Nostrums and Quackery,* I, 195.

[55] "Official Rules of the Council on Pharmacy and Chemistry," (May 1, 1921), in *Propaganda for Reform,* II, 5–12. While revisions were made in the rules a number of times, fundamentally they remained the same during the first two decades of the century.

those products for which extravagant claims were made, but a business world so addicted to exaggeration could only gradually adjust itself to restraint. Yet, few were quite as extravagant as the manufacturer of "Somos," who listed a product as helpful in the cure of 158 diseases and ailments ranging from hallucinations to hydrophobia.[56] Some companies offered the council offensive products best described as "shotgun remedies," illustrated by "Tongaline" and "Peacock's Bromides," which it thoroughly exposed. Manufacturers of these compounds filled their products with many drugs with the idea that if one ingredient was ineffective, something in the complex mixture would prove beneficial. The *Journal* pointed out the potential danger of these compounds, charging that any such "mixture is just as preposterous in modern therapeutics as the blunderbuss would be on a modern battlefield." It described "Peacock's Bromides" as one of the "useless mixtures of well known drugs sold under grotesquely exaggerated claims," and placed "Tongaline" among the "preposterous therapeutic monstrosities."[57] Though well-acquainted with food fad exploitations, the council showed some surprise when "alfatone," which supposedly brought the rich properties of alfalfa to the human system, was advertised to the medical profession. It wryly commented that the future might hold in store "Tincture of Timothy Hay, Blue Grass tonic, [and] Cornhusk Wine!"[58]

The council's investigation of ethical proprietaries and articles, sold to both the profession and public, sometimes brought unfavorable publicity to prominent concerns as well as small establishments. The Chemical Laboratory considered almost worthless "Cin-U-Form Lozenges" that McKesson and Robbins advertised as valuable for the prevention of sore throat, colds, tonsillitis, pneumonia, and several other ills. The validity of claims for Eli Lilly and Company's "Catarrhal Vaccine Combined" and "Influenza Mixed Vaccine-Lilly" also weighed short in the balances.[59]

Friction between the Bayer Company and the Council on Pharmacy and Chemistry initiated one of the most important of the Association's exposures. In the advertisement of "Aspirin-Bayer," the objectionable practices of the company led to the elimination of its product from *New and Nonofficial Remedies*. In 1917, the Association also tried to

[56] *Propaganda for Reform,* I, 195.

[57] *Ibid.,* II, 398–99.

[58] *Ibid.,* pp. 29–30.

[59] *Ibid.,* pp. 237, 187.

prevent the renewal of the Bayer patent, monopolizing the manufacture and sale of acetylsalicylic acid of which patent it had never approved. It asserted that:

> . . . practically no other country in the world, not even the original home of the preparation, would grant a patent on either acetylsalicylic acid, the product, or on the process for making that product. The United States granted both! As a result, for seventeen years it has been impossible in this country for anybody except the Bayer Company to manufacture or sell acetylsalicylic acid, either under its chemical name or under any other name.[60]

The *Journal* demonstrated how the monopoly had greatly benefited the Bayer Company, but injured the public by comparing the prices an ounce charged druggists in the United States with several European countries.[61]

Austria-Hungary	4 cents	Holland	4 cents
British Isles	6 "	Norway	4 "
Denmark	4 "	Sweden	4 "
France	4 "	United States	43 "
Germany	4 "		

Through its long monopoly, the Bayer Company acquired other advantages that threatened to outlive the patent.[62] It secured a trademark for the name "aspirin," which the public came to consider the only name for acetylsalicylic acid. Even if the government granted no new patent, the Bayer Company held an advantage over all other potential manufacturers. The AMA contended that the company had no right to either the trademark or patent, but the company apparently retained the trademark several years after the patent expired in 1917. In the meantime, the *Journal* urged physicians to call for "acetylsalicylic acid" rather than "aspirin" in writing prescriptions.[63]

Naturally, the Association's exposure of medical quackery and exploitation produced both resourceful enemies and helpful allies. Reaction to its work varied from extreme hostility to wholehearted endorsement, which the *Journal* recognized, in 1912, by featuring a new department

[60] *Ibid.*, p. 481.

[61] The Drug Laboratory of the Bureau of Chemistry provided the AMA with some of the information it published about the Bayer patent. A. J. C. [Arthur J. Cramp] to Kebler, Sept. 25, 1909; Kebler to Simmons, Sept. 30, 1909, BCR.

[62] Since the Bayer Company was a branch of a German industry, the Alien Property Custodian took it over during World War I. It was sold to the Sterling Products Company of Wheeling, West Virginia. *Propaganda for Reform,* II, 485.

[63] *Ibid.*, pp. 480–82.

entitled "Knocks and Boosts" that carried "both bouquets and brick-bats."[64] Although the trustees confessed two years later that no other phase of the Association's work had ever encountered such opposition, the *Journal* had already designated the chief sources. Late in 1906, it identified the Association's principal enemies as the Proprietary Association of America, the "so-called 'ethical' proprietary medicine men," the nostrum-subsidized "privately-owned medical journals," and the firms publishing medical directories. The *Journal* described their attack as one of "Caricature, ridicule, invective, misrepresentation, half statements and distortions of the truth" aimed at nullifying the Association's work.[65] To the list of enemies it later added the petty medical organizations, largely composed of disgruntled, nostrum-supporting physicians, and a few low-grade medical schools that the Association had exposed.[66]

Although the names of the AMA's most outspoken enemies frequently varied, it believed that behind almost all attacks lay the financial might of the proprietary interests. The most annoying opposition came from such nondescript and misnamed organizations as the National League for Medical Freedom, the Medical Society of the United States (organized in 1916), and from irate editors of a few medical journals. The AMA, which had fought the national league over the health department bills early in the second decade, did not hesitate to attack the newer organization. It charged that the Medical Society of the United States had unsuccessfully attempted to interest general practitioners in "fee-splitting" and identified its president, A. H. Ohmann-Dumesnil, as the former editor of a nostrum-corrupted periodical and president of a "sundown" medical school. The *Journal* explained editor Edward C. Register's hostility by showing that as late as 1917, his own publication, the *Charlotte Medical Journal,* relied heavily on the support of nostrum enterprises.[67]

The opposition that the Association encountered in the struggle against medical exploitation was to some extent offset by the respectability of its allies. In the dissemination, as well as in the gathering of information

[64] *JAMA,* 58 (April 6, 1912), 1021. Since this material was only of transient interest it appeared in the advertising pages of the *Journal.*

[65] HD, *Proceedings* (65 Annual Session, June, 1914), p. 4; Editorial, *JAMA,* 47 (September 8, 1906), 778.

[66] *JAMA,* 56 (June 10, 1911), 1741; *JAMA,* 71 (October 5, 1918), 1158–59; Editorial, *JAMA,* 54 (March 5, 1910), 797–98.

[67] *JAMA,* 54 (June 4, 1910), 1876; *JAMA,* 71 (October 5, 1918), 1158–59; *JAMA,* 63 (September 19, 1914), 1038; *JAMA,* 71 (October 5, 1918), 1158; *JAMA,* 68 (February 24, 1917), 630–37. For the struggle with the National League for Medical Freedom over the health department bills see pp. 100–1 above.

that inflicted heavy damages on nostrum interests, the Association won the support of many reputable organizations, agencies, institutions, and individuals. Newspapers and lay journals frequently made use of materials which the Association prepared, and occasionally crusading organizations like the Woman's Christian Temperance Union gave extensive circulation to its literature. The AMA's work against the nostrum frequently found a place in the textbooks of public schools and colleges, and teachers of scientific subjects often made use of its findings. Public libraries became depositories of its exposures, and during World War I, the libraries of every military camp in the United States contained anti-nostrum literature.[68]

As the second decade came to an end, the AMA tried to evaluate the success of its battle against medical exploitation. The cautious statements of its leaders indicated no undue optimism. The Association realized that its exposures reached only a small portion of the population, and that proprietary interests matched each "dollar spent in behalf of rational medicine" with thousands for the advertisement of worthless and injurious preparations.[69] It remembered that the federal proprietary investigation, which it had urged President Wilson to initiate, had never occurred, and that only constant resistance prevented proprietary concerns from unloading worthless nostrums upon the army during the war. Serious problems also confronted the Association in the new era of "biologic therapy," when the opportunities for exploitation threatened even to exceed those of the older nostrum era. The AMA saw no reason to abandon its efforts of exposure against an industry so resistant to sweeping reforms.[70]

Nevertheless, the Association viewed with considerable satisfaction the accomplishments of a decade and a half of leadership in the proprietary fight. It had largely driven the nostrum from medical journals and had raised the standard of medical advertising to a position probably unsurpassed in Europe. A decided improvement appeared in the type of claims that proprietary concerns made for their products, and the growing num-

[68] *JAMA,* 68 (April 7, 1917), 1049; *JAMA,* 50 (April 11, 1908), 1196; *JAMA,* 76 (June 11, 1921), 1659; *JAMA,* 72 (June 14, 1919), 1741.

[69] W. A. Puckner, "The Council on Pharmacy and Chemistry, Present and Future," in *Propaganda for Reform,* II, 15. For evidence that the people most in need of enlightenment on the nostrum evil seldom read any exposures, see the letter of April 19, 1907, from J. E. Miller, a physician of Rogersville, Tennessee, to the editor of the *Journal. JAMA,* 48 (May 11, 1907), 1616–17.

[70] A. W. McAlester, Jr., HD, *Proceedings* (66 Annual Session, June, 1915), pp. 62, 64; *JAMA,* 72 (June 14, 1919), 1741; *JAMA,* 76 (June 11, 1921), 1659.

ber of states that had enacted a uniform law controlling advertising was also encouraging. The thousands of letters that it received from laymen showed rising interest in national health problems, as well as public recognition of the Association's service, and even abroad its struggle had not been ignored.[71] At the close of the decade the Association could look upon its unfinished work with no feeling of despair.

[71] *Ibid.*, p. 1659; Puckner in *Propaganda for Reform,* II, 323; Dwight H. Murray, *JAMA,* 76 (June 11, 1921), 1680; *JAMA,* 54 (June 11, 1910), 1965; HD, *Proceedings* (64 Annual Session, June, 1913), p. 6; Puckner, in *Propaganda for Reform,* II, 12. By June, 1921, 24 states had enacted a uniform law against untrue and misleading advertisements. Illustrating the interest that the AMA raised in nostrums and quackery was the fact that a large percentage of the 16,000 letters that the Propaganda for Reform Department received between 1913 and 1917, pertained to this problem.

Chapter 7 THE RISE OF THE COMPULSORY HEALTH INSURANCE ISSUE

THE SUCCESSFUL RECORDS of many movements agitating for far-reaching political and social changes in the early twentieth century have largely diverted attention from those that failed. Although many Progressive groups carried through their struggles against special privilege and tradition to total or partial victory, there were other movements, more controversial in character, that achieved no such success. Among groups whose agitations gathered significant support but resulted in disappointment were the early advocates of compulsory health insurance, whose work gained national notice during the second decade. While the American Medical Association showed little interest in several of the reform movements of the era, the health insurance agitation raised questions which it could not ignore.

Birth of the Issue

Many factors explain the rise of the compulsory health insurance issue at a time when the public had begun to deal with matters of political and economic reform. The nation's new role in world affairs brought a greater awareness of the internal development of other countries and the extent to which their social progress sometimes exceeded its own. The immigrant movement that reached tidal proportions soon after the new century began also accelerated the progress of economic democracy by bringing to the settlement of the nation's problems the benefit of European experience. Added to the outside forces influencing American thought was the continued march of industrialism, which enlarged the dimensions of many national problems. Rapid medical progress also indirectly strengthened the compulsory health insurance forces as the disparity between the advancement of medical science and the population's incapacity to afford its benefits became increasingly clear.[1]

Standing in sharp contrast to the medical and industrial progress of the new century was the legacy of insecurity that the new order bequeathed to the industrial worker. In the broad field of social insurance, no measures appeared more urgent than laws providing for old-age pensions, workmen's compensation, and for some form of health insurance. As proponents of social insurance pressed these issues on a largely apathetic public, they looked to the experience of several European nations that had already met in a large measure the newer challenges of industrialism. Germany's experiment with national social security legislation dated from the enactment of a compulsory health insurance law in 1883, to which Bismarck's government also added a workmen's compensation act the next year and a measure for old-age pensions in 1889. Not to be outdone in the struggle for economic reform, France began to adopt features of this system during the next decade, while the British Parliament enacted a workmen's compensation law in 1897 and an old-age pension in 1908, climaxing its program of economic legislation in that era with the establishment of a limited system of compulsory health insurance in 1911.[2]

While European insurance systems operated with a degree of success that soon assured their popularity and permanence, most Americans

[1] The first decade produced a number of noteworthy medical triumphs including victory over yellow fever in Cuba; the purifying and synthesizing of adrenalin, the first hormone isolated; first synthesizing of sulfanilamide; use of veronol, the first barbituate hypnotic; invention of the galvanometer for studying heart action; use of procaine as a local anesthestic; and the first knowledge of the importance of vitamins. In 1911, salvarsan was developed as a cure for syphilis and relapsing fever and throughout the second decade greater use was made of X-ray and radium. Joseph Hirsh and Beka Doherty, *The First Hundred Years of the Mount Sinai Hospital of New York, 1852–1952* (New York: Random House, Inc., 1952), pp. 96–101. For the social implications of improved medical technology see Iago Galdston, *The Meaning of Social Medicine* (Cambridge, Mass.: Harvard University Press, 1954), pp. 47–48.

[2] Walter Sulzbach, *German Experience with Social Insurance* (Studies in Individual and Collective Security, No. 2 [New York: National Industrial Conference Board, Inc., 1947]), pp. 10, 49, 58; Rubinow, *Social Insurance,* pp. 15–27, traces the social insurance movement in these and smaller European countries. For an account of the economic insecurity most Americans experienced in the early twentieth century see Burrow, "Political and Social Policies of the American Medical Association, 1901–1941," pp. 48–58.

showed little interest in a broad system of social insurance, though a large percentage fought futilely against the economic problems of sickness, disability, and old age. The federal government succeeded in largely ignoring their problems and, although 41 states had adopted workmen's compensation laws by 1920, only one (Arizona) passed an old-age pension law and this measure soon failed the judicial test.[3] The industrial labor force found little support among professional classes and, while the American Medical Association became quite interested in compulsory health insurance, it largely ignored other aspects of the social insurance movement. In fact, Alexander Lambert, a prominent spokesman of the AMA declared: "The laws were passed before the profession had waked up to its responsibilities that had come to it under the law or what its duties would be under the law."[4]

Association for Labor Legislation

Even the movement for compulsory health insurance had attained considerable importance before it attracted the interest of the AMA. While the Association was venting its earliest irritations over weaknesses in the Pure Food and Drugs Act, another body that convened in Madison, Wisconsin, in December, 1907, turned its attention to the health insurance idea. At the first annual conference of the newly established Association for Labor Legislation, Professor Henry Rogers Seager presented a broad program of social legislation, emphasizing the necessity of sickness insurance, but expressing preference for "subsidized and state directed sick insurance clubs" over compulsory plans. While this association gave further study to the sickness-insurance question, other organizations and foundations became interested in more comprehen-

[3] Robert Morse Woodbury, *Social Insurance: An Economic Analysis* (Cornell Studies in History and Political Science, Vol. 4 [New York: Henry Holt & Co., 1917]), p. 158; Abraham Epstein, *The Challenge of the Aged* (New York: Macy-Macius, The Vanguard Press, 1928), pp. 274–82; Sulzbach, *German Experience with Social Insurance,* p. 40; Abraham Epstein, *Insecurity, A Challenge to America* (2nd rev. ed.; New York: Random House, 1938), pp. 533–36. In 1908 the federal government enacted a measure providing compensation for some classes of government workers who sustained injuries in employment, but this law had only a narrow application. *JAMA,* 67 (October 28, 1916), 1307–8.

[4] "Medical Organization under Health Insurance," *American Labor Legislation Review* (March, 1917), p. 46, cited in A. M. Simons and Nathan Sinai, *The Way of Health Insurance* (The Committee on the Study of Dental Practice in the American Dental Association, Publication No. 6 [Chicago: The University of Chicago Press, 1932]), p. 188.

sive programs of social security. Financed by the Russell Sage Foundation, Lee K. Frankel and Miles M. Dawson went to Europe in 1908 and made a study of different social insurance systems which the foundation published in book form two years later as *Workingmen's Insurance in Europe.*[5]

The second decade opened with encouraging prospects for the proponents of social security legislation. Social issues that even most muckrakers ignored came to the forefront. Before the National Conference on Charities and Correction that met in June, 1911, the rising political figure, Louis D. Brandeis, stressed the urgency of the adoption of a broad plan of social insurance which the conference officially accepted the following year, when incorporated into a committee report. Members of the committee pressed these recommendations on the Progressive party at the Chicago convention in 1912, which resulted in their inclusion into the party platform. For the first time in American history the idea of compulsory health insurance received the official endorsement of a major party and retained its popularity for several years after the party collapsed.[6] Only a month after the Democratic triumph of 1912 shattered the Progressives' hope of victory, the Association for Labor Legislation, which at first seemed to favor a program of voluntary insurance, launched a drive to promote compulsory plans.

Convinced of the merit of compulsory health insurance and the possibility of its widespread adoption on the state level, the Association for Labor Legislation threw all of its energies into the fight. It appointed a committee on social insurance of nine members (later twelve), largely composed of well-known economists, statisticians, and physicians, which was responsible for advancing the compulsory sickness insurance movement.[7] While it attempted to arouse the interest of other organizations,

[5] Pierce Williams, assisted by Isabel C. Chamberlain, *The Purchase of Medical Care through Fixed Periodic Payment* (The National Bureau of Economic Research, Inc., Publication No. 20 [New York, 1932]), pp. 34–35; see foreword by John M. Glenn in Lee K. Frankel and Miles M. Dawson, *Workingmen's Insurance in Europe* (New York: Charities Publication Committee, 1911), pp. vii–viii.

[6] Williams and Chamberlain, *Purchase of Medical Care,* p. 35; Louise Wolters Ilse, *Group Insurance and Employee Retirement Plans* (New York: Prentice-Hall, Inc., 1953), 226–227. A program of medical care administered by the government had long been endorsed by Socialist groups.

[7] The only physician originally on the committee was Isaac M. Rubinow, who was also a statistician. The later enlargement of the committee brought into its membership two other physicians, Alexander Lambert and S. S. Goldwater. Williams and Chamberlain, *Purchase of Medical Care,* p. 36.

its principal function consisted of drafting a standard bill for compulsory health insurance along lines that the organization's study of the issue suggested.

The Model Bill

Nearly three years of careful work went into the preparation of the Standard Bill that appeared in tentative form in November, 1915, several months after the committee had publicized the general standards to which it believed a compulsory plan should conform. The Association for Labor Legislation considered the bill at its December meeting and, with a few changes, officially endorsed the measure in 1916.[8] The flexibility and precision of the model bill attested to the committee's familiarity with the subject and the thoroughness of its work.

While the Standard Bill did not propose to bring all economic classes under the operation of a compulsory plan, it offered coverage for the bulk of the population otherwise unable to bear the annual cost of illness. Every employed person earning $1,200 or less automatically fell under the compulsory plan, while home and casual workers and all other workers desiring to do so could subscribe to the scheme. No provision was made, however, for the unemployed or their dependents, who stood most in need of medical care and subsistence benefits. The expense of the system fell upon the employer, the employee, and the state. The employer bore two-fifths of the costs, matched by a similar amount from the employee (except in cases where the worker's wages fell below $9.00 a week), and a contribution of one-fifth from the state.[9] The bill provided for both cash and medical benefits. After an illness of four days, the insured became eligible for a cash payment equivalent to two-thirds of his weekly wages for any period of sickness that did not extend beyond 26 weeks in any one year. Any dependent whose condition required hospital treatment during the illness of his guardian also became eligible for a cash benefit of one-third of the weekly wages of the insured. The plan also provided for the necessary medical, surgical, and nursing care from the first day of sickness through any period of illness that did not exceed 26 weeks in any one year. It carried maternity

[8] *Ibid.*, pp. 39–40; Ilse, *Group Insurance and Retirement Plans,* pp. 226–27.

[9] Williams and Chamberlain, *Purchase of Medical Care,* p. 41. The state was also to bear the cost of operating the system. See p. 43. This bill appears in full in *JAMA,* 66 (June 17, 1916), 1979–81.

benefits and allowed a maximum of $50 a year for surgical appliances, medicines, eyeglasses, and other similar items, as well as the same amount for funeral expenses.[10]

In drafting the bill the committee tried to avoid the criticism often raised against compulsory health insurance plans. The measure provided for the insured's free choice of physicians from those listed on the panels or in the employ of the insurance carriers and recognized some grounds on which doctors might refuse medical service.[11] The committee omitted several important medical provisions in the tentative bill, in order that these might be drawn up in consultation with representatives of the medical profession.[12] By requiring that no panel doctor's list could include more than 500 insured families or 1,000 insured individuals, the committee hoped to maintain high standards of practice. It courted the favor of physicians by including a provision for the settlement of all medical disputes, arising under the system, by a medical advisory board that the professional organization of the state selected, while entrusting the proposed state social insurance commission with the power to handle all other disputes.

Agitation for Adoption

Having framed a concrete program for meeting the economic costs of illness, the Association for Labor Legislation proceeded to publicize the advantages of its plan. In 1916, the June issue of the *Labor Legislation Review* carried the association's "Brief for Health Insurance" that set forth basic concepts behind the compulsory health insurance movement. It charged that the sickness and death rates of wage earners were too high, and that their low incomes deprived them of treatment that advanced medical technology offered. It stressed the importance of an

[10] William and Chamberlain, *Purchase of Medical Care,* pp. 41–43; Ilse, *Group Insurance and Retirement Plans,* p. 226.

[11] Insurance carriers were allowed four methods of furnishing medical service. First, the panel system might be used in which every qualified doctor had a right to participate; second, physicians might be employed by the carriers, and from this number the patient had free choice; third, "District medical officers, engaged for the treatment of insured persons in prescribed areas"; and fourth, any combination of these methods. Williams and Chamberlain, *Purchase of Medical Care,* p. 42. While this system did not provide for a completely unrestricted choice of physicians, it probably provided for greater choice than that enjoyed by most families of limited means who had no health insurance.

[12] *JAMA,* 66 (June 17, 1916), 1950.

attack upon the problem of wage loss due to illness and of further advance in preventive medicine. Concluding that medical facilities existed for providing more adequate medical care, it offered its plan for compulsory health insurance as the most urgent step for meeting the nation's health problems.[13]

The agitation of the Association for Labor Legislation had not advanced far before several organizations and influential leaders either endorsed its proposal or joined the crusade for compulsory health insurance. Supporters of the movement represented a variety of professional and economic backgrounds. The economists, statisticians, and political scientists who figured prominently in the activities of the Association for Labor Legislation brought other organizations in touch with its work. In 1916, the association held the first session of its tenth annual meeting in conjunction with the American Economic Association, the American Sociological Society, and the American Statistical Association.[14] That it impressed several influential politicians is illustrated by the fact that Governors Hiram W. Johnson of California and Samuel W. McCall of Massachusetts became supporters of the compulsory health insurance idea. While Samuel Gompers opposed the principle, many industrial workers did not share his view and such prominent labor leaders as William Green, James Maurer, and John Mitchell favored a compulsory system.[15]

In 1916, a standing committee on social insurance, appointed by the National Convention of State Insurance Commissioners, reported in favor of a national program of compulsory health insurance, but the convention took no action on the report. Even the National Association of Manufacturers' committee on industrial betterment accepted the idea, although the association did not endorse the committee's report. A growing number of physicians approved of the movement for compulsory health insurance which drew considerable strength from public health officials, led by Benjamin S. Warren of the United States Public Health Service. In the initial stages of the crusade, the Medical Society of the State of New York openly endorsed the proposal.[16]

[13] Williams and Chamberlain, *Purchase of Medical Care,* pp. 37–39.

[14] *JAMA,* 67 (December 16, 1916), 1869.

[15] I. M. Rubinow to editor, *JAMA,* 68 (April 28, 1917), 1278–79; Williams and Chamberlain, *Purchase of Medical Care,* pp. 52–53.

[16] Williams and Chamberlain, *Purchase of Medical Care,* pp. 44–45; Rubinow to editor, *JAMA,* 68 (April 28, 1917), 1279; *JAMA,* 67 (September 9, 1916), 832; *JAMA,* 67 (December 30, 1916), 2032–33.

Interest of the AMA

The compulsory health insurance movement not only secured growing support from many sources, but attracted the interest of the AMA as well. Thoroughly identified with the forces of reform that had fought for public health legislation, the AMA made no effort to avoid the health insurance question. In fact the issue bore some kinship to other proposals for which the Association had fought. It had become an outspoken critic of the federal government's failure to give adequate protection against disease, the nostrum, and impure food, while also attacking the states' frequent delinquency in providing adequate health laws and regulating medical practice. It gave leadership to the movement for a federal department of health and the *Journal* favored the establishment of the Children's Bureau in 1912.[17] In order to correct the chaotic licensing situation that physicians encountered in moving from one state to another, the *Journal* approved of the establishment of a federal board of examiners whose accreditation would be recognized by all states. The *Journal* also endorsed the suggestion of state support for all worthy medical schools, maintaining that private endowments, while extensive, did not release the state from responsibility in this work. It showed no fear that government subsidization of training centers would lead to political domination of medicine.[18]

The compulsory health insurance issue, however, involved not only the question of the limit of governmental activity in the realm of preventive and therapeutic medicine but raised other problems as well. Years of experience with contract practice led the AMA to develop certain interpretations of ethical standards that applied also to the question of compulsory health insurance. Although it considered unobjectionable the practice, adopted by some industries and remote mining establishments, of contracting with physicians for the treatment of their patients, it strongly denounced most types of contract practice.[19]

[17] *JAMA,* 63 (April 27, 1912), 1288. The *Journal's* references to the Children's Bureau in the early years of the agency's existence are rare, even near the time of its creation. The AMA did feel that it allowed an overextension of lay influence in medical matters. See Michael M. Davis, *America Organizes Medicine* (New York: Harper & Brothers Publishers, 1941), p. 107.

[18] Editorial, *JAMA,* 38 (January 11, 1902), 108–9; Editorial, *JAMA,* 48 (March 9, 1907), pp. 879–80. The federal board was finally established and held its first examination in Washington, D.C., in October, 1915. William L. Rodman, *JAMA,* 64 (June 29, 1915), 2113–14.

[19] *JAMA,* 49 (December 14, 1907), 2028–29.

The AMA found particularly offensive the policies that lodges, fraternal orders, and benevolent societies sometimes adopted of levying small assessments against members, entitling them to the service of physicians which the intermediate agencies employed. The *Journal* denounced these plans as lay devices for medical exploitation, "buying a physician's services at wholesale and selling them at retail." It showed that the remuneration offered physicians under such plans was very small as compared with the pay that corporations allowed under reputable contracts and charged that the principle of remuneration that demanded an indefinite amount of medical service for a definite amount of pay only exploited the profession.[20] The *Journal* believed that the competitive bidding for contracts which this system promoted not only lowered the level of physicians' income, but restricted the patients' choice of physicians and dragged down the quality of medical service as well. Schemes providing equal salaries for participating physicians, regardless of the amount of work done, it also considered highly objectionable. When Zurich, Switzerland, adopted a municipal system of contract practice that combined most of these undesirable features, the *Journal* remarked that the "leveling down" process was a universal weakness of socialistic programs.[21]

When the agitation for compulsory health insurance showed no signs of abating, the AMA gave the issue more than passing thought. It had established no precedents of unalterable antagonism for compulsory health insurance and had formulated no doctrinaire position that precluded consideration of new approaches to the problem of meeting the costs of medical care. Its interest lay in guarding medical practice against the degrading features that any prepaid or tax-supported plan might include. It showed no disposition to stifle investigation or discourage discussion of plans as proposed in the United States or practiced abroad. The *Journal* published repeatedly the London correspondent's discouraging descriptions of the operation of the British system, but also carried articles that clearly supported a government-sponsored system of medical care. In the issue of July 18, 1914, James P. Warbasse, a New York physician, called attention to the growing number of governmental health functions and added:

[20] *JAMA,* 47 (December 8, 1906), 1923; *JAMA,* 57 (July 8, 1911), 145; *JAMA,* 49 (December 14, 1907), 2029.

[21] *JAMA,* 43 (October 8, 1904), 1067. See also the article of Malcom L. Harris, *JAMA,* 89 (November 26, 1927), 1871–72, in which he emphasizes many of the long-recognized defects of contract practice.

> The socialization of medicine is coming. The time now is here for the medical profession to acknowledge that it is tired of the eternal struggle for advantage over one's neighbor. The value of cooperation in science is proved. Medical practice withholds itself from the field of science as long as it continues a competitive business.[22]

About six months later, the *Journal* published an article favorable to social insurance written by Issac M. Rubinow, an outstanding authority on the subject and a leader in the movement for compulsory health insurance.[23]

Flirtation with the Issue

A few more months demonstrated that the Association's interest in compulsory insurance extended far beyond passing *Journal* references. The Judicial Council, headed by Alexander Lambert, gave the San Francisco session in June, 1915, a report on the European experience with social security, emphasizing particularly the British system. The report of the British experience stood in sharp contrast to the London correspondent's doleful descriptions.[24] The Judicial Council reported that, while instances existed of reduced incomes after the introduction of the system, the average annual income of physicians showed an increase ranging from $750 to $2,000. Not only did it emphasize the significant rise in income, but pointed out that for the first time millions of the British people had the advantage of medical care.[25] In November, 1915, the same month that the Association for Labor Legislation published its tentative bill for compulsory health insurance and called for any suggestions and criticisms, the *Journal* urged the profession to comply with this request. The Association for Labor Legislation planned to introduce the finished draft into the state legislatures the next year, and the *Journal* hoped "to avoid that lack of co-operation between the physicians and legislators which, for a time, marred some of the foreign legislation."[26]

[22] "The Socialization of Medicine," *JAMA,* 63 (July 18, 1914), 266.

[23] "Social Insurance and the Medical Profession," *JAMA,* 64 (January 30, 1915), 381–86.

[24] In 1915 the "London Letter" temporarily ceased to appear in the *Journal.* This was probably a disruption, however, that grew out of wartime conditions.

[25] *JAMA,* 65 (July 3, 1915), 85.

[26] *JAMA,* 65 (November 20, 1915), 1824.

The AMA's belated interest in compulsory health insurance gave it but little time to investigate either the merits of the issue or the distribution and deficiencies of medical service in the United States. It felt the need of additional information, however, many months before the organization of its Committee on Social Insurance early in 1916. Primarily responsible for the establishment of this committee were H. B. Favill, chairman of the Council on Health and Public Instruction, and Alexander Lambert, chairman of the Judicial Council, who, along with Frederic J. Cotton of Boston, became original members.[27] The committee's prestige rose when the Board of Trustees confirmed its organization in February, but no action was more significant than its selection of Isaac M. Rubinow as secretary at about the same time. The committee opened a bureau on East Twenty-third Street in New York City and undertook an ambitious long-range program that the Council on Health and Public Instruction described a few months later to the Detroit session, in a report that included the committee's own account of the growth of social insurance.[28]

The scope of the committee's plan indicated the earnestness and enthusiasm with which it approached its task. It hoped to educate the profession to the importance of social insurance and "particularly health insurance" and offered to serve as an information bureau for physicians desiring information about "facts or figures bearing on social insurance in any of its phases." It hoped to appear before legislative bodies "to protect the legitimate economic interests of the profession in the laws coming up for discussion concerning social insurance."[29] Besides serving these immediate purposes, the committee planned to undertake other functions that would require a longer time to perform. Among these were the compilation of a bibliography on social insurance, the inauguration of correspondence with European health insurance organizations, and the conducting of statistical studies of the medical facilities of the United States, including also the status and earnings of the American medical profession.[30]

[27] *JAMA,* 66 (June 17, 1916), 1950. The committee lost a faithful member when H. B. Favill died before the June session of the House of Delegates convened. *JAMA,* 66 (June 17, 1916), 1942.

[28] *JAMA,* 66 (June 17, 1916), 1951. In 1916, interest in compulsory health insurance also appeared on the state society level, and was discussed, for example, at the meeting of the Texas association. Nixon, *History of Texas Medical Association,* p. 296.

[29] *JAMA,* 66 (June 17, 1916), 1951.

[30] *Ibid.,* pp. 1951–52.

Along with the presentation of this comprehensive program, the committee left the AMA in no doubt of its position on the health insurance issue. Its praise of the British plan clearly revealed its sympathy for a compulsory health insurance system. While disclaiming any intention of "arguing for or against health insurance," it reminded the profession that the British experiment had focused attention on the fact that many formerly uninsured workers, who struggled against the economic burden of sickness, lived "an existence in civilized communities little better than savages." Furthermore it added: "However one may criticise the details, the insurance act has unquestionably improved the condition of the working classes which have come under the law." Its preference for compulsory over voluntary health insurance clearly appeared in additional comments on the European situation:

> . . . it is evident . . . that voluntary insurance as seen in Germany and Great Britain previous to the adoption of compulsory insurance secures protection against sickness only to the thrifty and well paid industrial worker. It does not reach those who need it most.[31]

The committee felt that only a system of state compulsory insurance reached the poorest classes.

A third of a century later, the Bureau (later Department) of Medical Economic Research of the AMA, in its contention that the Association never opposed voluntary insurance, concluded from this committee's report that it "did not discuss the desirability of any insurance system."[32] While the committee made no recommendation for the adoption of health insurance systems in the United States, the bureau's statement is somewhat misleading. The committee not only described the operation of the European compulsory health insurance systems, but expressed approval of compulsory schemes which it considered far superior either to voluntary insurance or to none at all. From specific European experiences with compulsory health insurance, it drew broader

[31] *Ibid.*, pp. 1953, 1985, 1952.

[32] Frank G. Dickinson, "A Brief History of the Attitude of the American Medical Association toward Voluntary Health Insurance" (American Medical Association, Bureau of Medical Economic Research, Bulletin 70 [Chicago, 1949]), p. 7. In later footnotes, citations to material prepared by the AMA's Department of Medical Economic Research and its predecessors, the Bureau of Medical Economics and Bureau of Medical Economic Research, the first reference to the American Medical Association is omitted. The full report of the Committee on Social Insurance appears in HD, *Proceedings* (67 Annual Session, June, 1916), pp. 17–52, as well as in the *Journal*.

conclusions that it indicated would apply to the United States as well. Its delay in making any formal recommendations resulted from its uncompleted study of the issue, and probably from the realization that a large portion of the profession was not ready for any revolutionary proposals.[33]

Even before the Council on Health and Public Instruction submitted the social insurance committee's report to the House of Delegates in June, 1916, the compulsory health insurance controversy had already reached the legislative chambers. The *Journal* quickly reported the introduction of compulsory insurance bills into the New York and Massachusetts legislatures in January, adding that the Association for Labor Legislation drafted the bills with the aid of the AMA's social insurance committee. Then followed a favorable comment on the principles of social insurance:

> Much of the best informed opinion of the country is in favor of these proposals. . . . The introduction of these bills marks the inauguration of a great movement which ought to result in an improvement in the health of the industrial population and improve the conditions for medical service among the wage earners.[34]

Compulsory insurance agitation quickly spread to other legislative bodies and even reached Congress in 1916. Although hearings were conducted on a resolution that called for a federal plan providing unemployment, invalidity, and sickness benefits, Congress took no further action.[35]

The increasing gravity of the international crisis did not at once retard the progress of the compulsory health insurance movement or check the interest of the AMA. Just before Germany's renewal of unrestricted submarine warfare, which quickly wrecked the chance of better relations with the United States, the *Journal* of January 27, 1917, showed unusual interest in the insurance question. While reminding the profession that the United States stood practically alone among the large industrial

[33] It is not surprising that the committee's report showed sympathy for compulsory health insurance. I. M. Rubinow was an original member of the social-insurance committee of the American Association of Labor Legislation, and Alexander Lambert was later a member. Lambert's favorable views on compulsory health insurance are expressed in "Health Insurance and the Medical Profession," *JAMA,* 68 (January 27, 1917), 257–58. Michael M. Davis maintains that the early favorable attitude of the AMA's Committee on Social Insurance toward compulsory health insurance was due in a large measure to Lambert's "views, prestige, and diplomatic skill." *Medical Care for Tomorrow* (New York: Harper & Brothers Publishers, 1955), pp. 275–76.

[34] *JAMA,* 66 (February 5, 1916), 433.

[35] Williams and Chamberlain, *Purchase of Medical Care,* p. 45.

nations that had not adopted compulsory health insurance, it looked upon the spread of workmen's compensation laws as the "entering wedge" for this type of legislation.[36] The same issue carried an article by Alexander Lambert who charged that "self-respecting people of small means who pay their bills" could not afford needed medical care in the United States and suggested compulsory health insurance as the answer. Six weeks later the *Journal* carried Irving Fisher's address before the Medical Society of the State of New York, which referred to the backwardness of the United States in providing for compulsory health insurance and urged the profession's support of the compulsory health insurance bill then before the state legislature.[37]

When the Council on Health and Public Instruction presented the social insurance committee's report to the New York session of the House of Delegates in June, that body found the committee just as favorable as the year before to the idea of compulsory health insurance. The report stressed the point that whatever political reasons accounted for the enactment of these laws in Europe, the principle beneath compulsory health insurance was no less valid, and cited proof of the widespread admission that voluntary schemes had failed, but that compulsory plans had proved successful. While still making no recommendation for the profession's support of compulsory health insurance, it did offer a resolution embodying certain principles that it felt any system should include. This resolution called for:

> . . . freedom of choice of physician by the insured; payment of the physician in proportion to the amount of work done; the separation of the functions of medical official supervision from the function of daily care of the sick, and adequate representation of the medical profession on the appropriate administrative bodies.[38]

Although the House of Delegates endorsed these principles, the committee's report indicated that it sensed a rising spirit of unreasoning opposition to the idea of compulsory health insurance and warned that:

> Blind opposition, indignant repudiation, bitter denunciation of these laws is worse than useless; it leads nowhere and it leaves the profession in a position of helplessness if the rising tide of social development sweeps over them.[39]

[36] *JAMA,* 68 (January 27, 1917), 292.

[37] *JAMA,* 68 (January 27, 1917), 257–58; *JAMA,* 68 (March 10, 1917), 801–02.

[38] *JAMA,* 68 (June 9, 1917), 1745–47, 1755.

[39] *JAMA,* 68 (June 16, 1917), 183; quotation, *JAMA,* 68 (June 9, 1917), 1755.

Growth of Opposition

A large portion of the profession apparently did not heed the warning of the committee, whose faint suspicion of growing opposition soon proved justified. Whether acting on reason or prejudice, an increasing number of physicians definitely identified themselves with the group opposing compulsory insurance, a group that included insurance companies, much of the labor movement, and most employers.[40] Yet, perhaps the proponents of compulsory health insurance encountered their greatest obstacle in the public's dwindling interest in the issue when the nation's entry into World War I hastily turned popular attention from problems of domestic reform and disrupted the work of the Committee on Social Insurance as well.

The *Journal,* which for years had favorably publicized the compulsory health insurance question, turned noticeably toward the other side in the early months of 1917. The issue of February 10 carried a letter from Frederick L. Hoffman, statistician of the Prudential Life Insurance Company, to the editor of the *Journal* who concluded from a study of comparative vital statistics that the level of health of the American people rivaled that of countries with compulsory health insurance and considered such a scheme "wholly unnecessary" in the United States.[41] As articles favorable to the issue became quite rare, unfavorable comments increased until June, 1917, when the pressure of wartime medical problems probably accounted for the exclusion of the question from the *Journal.*[42]

The most noteworthy attack on the system came from Eden V. Delphey, a New York physician, chairman of the Health Insurance Committee of the Federation of American Economic Leagues, who wrote denouncing compulsory health insurance in general and the Standard

[40] Williams and Chamberlain, *Purchase of Medical Care,* p. 51; Rubinow to editor, *JAMA,* 68 (April 28, 1917), 1278–79.

[41] *JAMA,* 68 (February 10, 1917), 480.

[42] The *Journal* did carry a letter already referred to that was favorable to health insurance from Rubinow to the editor. *JAMA,* 68 (April 28, 1917), 1278–79. The AMA was not alone among professional organizations which displayed a favorable attitude toward compulsory health insurance and then turned against it. The American Pharmaceutical Association followed precisely the same course between 1917 and 1918. "Report of the Special Committee on Compulsory Health Insurance of the Chicago Branch of the American Pharmaceutical Association," *Journal of the American Pharmaceutical Association,* 6 (March, 1917), 314–16; 7 (April, 1918), 381–85; and 7 (October, 1918), 899–900.

Bill in particular. His 18 objections to compulsory health insurance, based on 26 years of "active private practice among the wage earners," covered most criticisms of the system. Some of his objections grew out of his belief that "more is paid for 'movies' and 'rum' than is paid for medical attendance and treatment"; "the loss per year due to sickness is much less than that due to compulsory and involuntary holidays"; the worker wants free choice of a physician rather than one "forced on him by the insurance carrier," and desires to avoid all other technical complications of the system.[43] While Delphey's arguments were not new, they largely embodied the substance of the Association's attack on compulsory health insurance for the next three decades.

Nearly two years elapsed before the revived issue again brought discord within the Association. A *Journal* editorial entitled "The Failure of German Compulsory Health Insurance" appeared in the issue of February 1, 1919. This was soon followed by another article against compulsory health insurance which indicated that the *Journal* had experienced no change of heart since cooling off to the idea.[44] The reorganization of the Committee on Social Insurance, whose work had been disrupted during the war, also gave promise of a more conservative policy. Isaac M. Rubinow no longer continued as secretary for the committee and, while Alexander Lambert remained as chairman, the presence of Malcom L. Harris of Chicago, who soon became an outspoken opponent of compulsory health insurance, eased fears of the committee's sympathy for the idea.[45]

Although signs appeared that the Association's interest in the question had declined, the Atlantic City session in June offered convincing proof of the persistence of the compulsory health insurance issue. The Committee on Social Insurance again prepared an exhaustive report on the subject that appeared less sympathetic than those submitted before and followed the pattern of earlier reports in offering no recommendations. The strength of the sentiment against compulsory health insurance, however, appeared in no way to influence the attitude of the Council on Health and Public Instruction. It felt that the profession had as yet ac-

[43] *JAMA,* 68 (May 19, 1917), 1500–1.

[44] *JAMA,* 72 (February 1, 1919), 347; *JAMA,* 72 (April 26, 1919), 1246–47.

[45] *JAMA,* 72 (June 14, 1919), 1750. Other new appointees on this committee were S. S. Goldwater of New York and Frederick Van Sickle of Olyphant, Pennsylvania. In the absence of information on the exact time when Rubinow's work was discontinued, it may be assumed to have been about the time of the reorganization. For additional information see Fishbein, *History of AMA,* p. 318.

cepted no worthy criteria for rationally evaluating the merits of the issue and observed that:

> The attitude of the majority of physicians up to date has been one of unqualified and often unreasoning opposition, without any effort to study the question or to consider the arguments put forward in favor of the proposed plan. Unreasoning opposition or sweeping and often erroneous general arguments against the measure will not prevent its adoption nor will it enhance the influence of physicians.[46]

Its report also pointed out four possible procedures of dealing with the economic burden of illness. The first lay in raising family incomes so that each could meet its own sickness problem; the second embodied a program of preventive medicine that reduced the incidence of illness; the third consisted of dividing the costs between industry, the wage earner, and the state; and the fourth was that of *laissez faire,* leaving existing conditions undisturbed. The council considered the first three procedures, in order, "the economic remedy," "the state public health remedy," "social insurance," and added the fourth as "no remedy at all."[47] That friendliness toward the compulsory health insurance principle had not become heresy appeared further from the fact that Alexander Lambert, formerly chairman of the social insurance committee and head of the Judicial Council, served at that time as president of the Association. That the compulsory health insurance issue still retained considerable popularity was indicated when the Reference Committee on Legislation and Political Action refused to submit, for the consideration of the House of Delegates, a resolution of the Medical Society of the State of New York condemning the proposal.[48]

Although both friend and foe of compulsory health insurance had some reason for claiming victory at the Atlantic City session, the outcome of the movement within the Association became quite clear even before the House of Delegates met again. Lambert's new position probably safely removed him from any connection with the health insurance agitation, while the termination of Rubinow's services curtailed the agitation itself. Occasional articles critical of compulsory health insurance continued to appear in the *Journal,* and not many months passed before several state journals attacked the Council on Health and Public Instruction for failing to oppose the issue.[49] Enemies of the movement received

[46] *JAMA,* 72 (June 14, 1919), 1750.
[47] *Ibid.*
[48] Fishbein, *History of AMA,* pp. 744–47; *JAMA,* 72 (June 21, 1919), 1836.
[49] *JAMA,* 74 (May 1, 1920), 1241–42.

additional aid when one of their number, Malcom L. Harris, a new appointee on the social insurance committee, began an attack on compulsory health insurance in the *Journal* on March 27, 1920.

In substance, Harris's articles attacked the principles behind compulsory health insurance, charged that the plan degraded medical practice without solving the economic problems of illness, and proposed his own solution. He denied that the theory of workmen's compensation, which assumed that the expense of accidents occurring in production were chargeable to the cost of production, had any application to compulsory health insurance.[50] He maintained that the establishment of such a system inevitably brought some type of contract practice in which the state "proceeds to contract for [physicians'] services just as it would for so much coal or groceries or any other commodity, failing to appreciate the fact that medical services cannot be measured by the ton or bushel."[51] Compulsory health insurance also ignored important aspects of the health problem such as "working conditions which cause fatigue; morbidity and mortality statistics according to occupation; effects of irregular employment on health; inadequate diet, bad housing conditions and overcrowding, and unfavorable community environment." His own proposed solution did not appear either as clear or definite as his criticism of compulsory health insurance.

> Shall the state by a system of compulsory medical treatment simply attempt to cure the ills of the unfortunate, or shall it, by proper preventive measures and by aiding in the adjustment of sociological and industrial conditions, enable the people to rise to or above the normal income point, so that they may, by their own resources, fulfill their responsibilities and obligations in life?[52]

Collapse of a Movement

Less than three weeks after the publication of Harris's second article, the fateful Seventy-first session of the AMA began in New Orleans. As the first postwar general election year turned popular attention to the serious question of the United States' role in world affairs, the House of Delegates also confronted a problem of exceptional gravity. The fact that this session received no report from the Committee on Social

[50] "Compulsory Health Insurance," *JAMA,* 74 (March 27, 1920), 907.

[51] *JAMA,* 74 (April 10, 1920), 1041.

[52] *JAMA,* 74 (March 27, 1920), 907, 908.

Insurance, whose demise dated from this meeting, indicated that the issue might die unnoticed. The Council on Health and Public Instruction did not press the matter, and told the delegates that the failure of the compulsory health insurance issue in New York left "no state in which this question is at present up for discussion in any concrete form. . . ."[53] As the movement practically collapsed before the defection of friends and the contempt of foes, forces stirred beneath the surface of the meeting that hoped to dramatize the death of the issue and prevent its revival.

The Reference Committee on Legislation and Political Action at the preceding session blocked a resolution anathematizing compulsory health insurance, but the new one traveled a different route. The Reference Committee on Hygiene and Public Health approved with almost no change the resolution against compulsory health insurance that Edward L. Hunt of New York submitted and referred it to the House of Delegates.[54] With no other alterations, on April 27, this body approved the measure that was submitted to it in the following form:

> *Resolved,* That the American Medical Association declares its opposition to the institution of any plan embodying the system of compulsory contributory insurance against illness, or any other plan of compulsory insurance which provides for medical service to be rendered contributors or their dependents, provided, controlled, or regulated by any state or the Federal government.[55]

The AMA at last had officially spoken, but hardly in time to hasten the death of the general movement for compulsory sickness insurance. Although health insurance advocates introduced the Standard Bill into the legislatures of 15 states between 1916 and 1920 and secured for their measure the favorable report of investigatory commission in four of the nine states that appointed commissions, the movement had about run its full course by 1920.[56] The zeal that its leaders displayed proved

[53] *JAMA,* 74 (May 1, 1920), 1242.

[54] *JAMA,* 74 (May 1, 1920), 1256, 1319.

[55] *JAMA,* 74 (May 1, 1920), 1319. The numerical vote of the House of Delegates is not given. The following year, however, Frederick R. Green, secretary of the Council on Health and Public Instruction, referred to it as "a practically unanimous vote." "The Social Responsibilities of Modern Medicine," *JAMA,* 76 (May 28, 1921), 1481. For interesting comments on the significance of committees in the AMA's history see Garceau, *Political Life of AMA,* pp. 81–82.

[56] Elizabeth W. Wilson, *Compulsory Health Insurance* (Studies in Individual and Collective Security, No. 3 [New York: National Industrial Conference

no match for the implacable opposition that developed. The movement came a little too late to be pushed far along by the Progressive Movement and appeared too early to avoid the distracting influences of the war. The wage worker, taxpayer, and employee shied away from the idea of expanding governmental activities that substantially increased operational costs and allied readily with employers, the insurance business, the medical profession, some labor unions, and other groups against the movement.[57]

Board, Inc., 1947]), pp. 2, 15. The nine states that appointed commissions to study the subject were Calif., Conn., Ill., Mass., N.J., N.Y., Ohio, Penn., and Wis. Wilson further states that the four states in which the committees made favorable reports were Calif., N.J., N.Y., and Ohio. John A. Lapp says that the commissions in six states reported in favor of compulsory health insurance by January, 1920, namely, Calif, Col., Mass., N.J., N.Y., and Ohio. "The Findings of Official Health Insurance Commissions," *American Labor Legislation Review* (March, 1920), p. 27, cited in Simons and Sinai, *The Way of Health Insurance,* p. 193. Epstein, *Insecurity: A Challenge to America,* p. 448, says that the commissions in five states favored compulsory health insurance and lists these as Calif., Mass. (first commission reports), N.J., Ohio, and Pa. Additional information is supplied by Green, *JAMA,* 76 (May 28, 1921), 1478.

[57] I. M. Rubinow, *The Quest for Security* (New York: Henry Holt and Company, 1934), pp. 210–14.

Chapter 8

POLITICAL PROBLEMS IN THE REPUBLICAN ERA, 1921–1933

THE AMERICAN MEDICAL ASSOCIATION derived little comfort from the Republican party's campaign promises in 1920, knowing that the appeal for "normalcy" instead of nostrums had no reference to medical nomenclature. As the search for something impressive passed the victorious candidate by, the *Journal* found in the house of Harding some reason for a glimmer of hope. Soon after the November election it informed the profession that Warren Gamaliel Harding's father, George T., had long practiced medicine in Marion, Ohio, and that his brother, George T. Jr., followed the same profession in Columbus. Keenly aware that politicians found matters of national health among the easiest to neglect, the Association hoped that favorable hereditary influences would dominate over natural political indifference.[1]

Postwar Problems

Whatever might be the new administration's policy on major medical issues, the Association's attitude toward the federal government underwent a noticeable change. The beginning of the new century presented the picture of a weak and threatened organization of 8,400 members seeking governmental assistance in its struggle against many foes. Two decades later, however, when fellowships in the Association reached over 47,000 and membership exceeded 83,000, and when state and federal legislation

[1] *JAMA,* 75 (November 13, 1920), 1348. Harding's appointment of a homeopath, Charles E. Sawyer of Marion, Ohio, as his personal physician with the rank of brigadier general, probably did not enhance the President's position with the AMA. John D. Hicks, *Republican Ascendancy, 1921–1933* (New York: Harper & Brothers Publishers, 1960), p. 79, refers to this appointment.

had greatly weakened medical quackery and cultism, the Association found the greatest threat to professional security in the national government itself.[2] As opposition in the medical world recoiled before its growing strength, the AMA moved in confident defiance of threats that came from political sources.

The Association's fear of expanding governmental influence over medical practice partially arose from the spirit and problems that World War I bequeathed. The AMA shared the general disillusionment of a nation that had found the fruits of victory bitter and that glanced with growing suspicion on compulsory health insurance and other social experiments of recent European origins. Besides the potential threat of the health insurance issue, the unfolding of the government's plan of veterans' benefits aroused the anxiety of the AMA. Not only did it watch the development of a federal program of medical care for the sick and wounded among the 1,390,000 who served on the battlefront, but also the enlargement of the program to include others from a discharged army of 4,500,000 who needed medical service.[3] While the AMA found in the veterans' medical program serious inroads on private medical practice, it also faced another threat. Proposals for federal subsidization of state health programs concerned with infant- and maternal-welfare problems raised the fears of the AMA early in the postwar decade.

Specter of Compulsory Health Insurance

Among the major tasks that confronted the Association when the twenties began, none appeared more urgent than preventing a revival of interest in compulsory health insurance. Having officially denounced

[2] *JAMA,* 74 (May 1, 1920), 1233. For an explanation of the difference between "members" and "fellows" see p. 49 above.

[3] Charles Seymour, *Woodrow Wilson and the World War* (Vol. 48 of The Chronicles of America Series, Allen Johnson, ed. [New Haven: Yale University Press, 1921]), p. 227; Harold U. Faulkner, *From Versailles to the New Deal* (Vol. 51 of The Chronicles of America Series, Allan Nevins, ed. [New Haven: Yale University Press, 1950]), p. 21. The total estimate of the number of American soldiers engaged in military service during World War I, including those who were only in training camps, has been set by the Veterans Administration at 5,338,475. *The World War Veterans and the Federal Treasury* (New York: National Industrial Conference Board, Inc., 1932), p. 59. The nation's effort to divorce itself from Europe's postwar problems is described in Frederic L. Paxson, *American Democracy and the World War* (Berkeley: University of California Press, 1948), III, 20–39.

the proposal in 1920, the Association sought justification for its action at home and abroad. Impressed by the London correspondent's criticism of the British system as published in the *Journal,* the AMA solicited a more authoritative account by an official of the British Medical Association. It called upon the secretary, Alfred Cox, for his impressions of the system, which the *Journal* published in three installments beginning May 7, 1921.[4] To a profession long acquainted with the reports of the "London Letter," this authoritative account of the operation of the British program brought needed light.

While Cox noted the profession's early hostility to the system, he showed that most opposition had turned into enthusiastic support. He charged that the widely circulated criticisms of the system came from the yellow press, and from some eminent physicians whose business among the wealthier classes removed them from close contact with the system. While showing that rural physicians and those in industrial areas had received the greatest financial benefit from the scheme, he concluded that "financially the Insurance Act has been a blessing to the medical profession. . . ." and seriously doubted "that the program has reduced the income of a single doctor in the country."[5] Far from being a mechanical system unresponsive to the wishes of the British Medical Association, he noted that the plan had incorporated most of the profession's demands. The chief criticism that he offered of the British system was the increased liability of the medical profession to become a *"pawn in a political game."*[6]

Cox believed that although the British system had brought many advantages to the medical profession, it had bestowed its principal benefits upon the public. For the lowest income groups, he contended, it had provided medical care unavailable before, except through charity, and had considerably increased medical services for a great portion of the population. He denied the charge that the extension of service had resulted in its deterioration and even maintained that the quality had improved. Besides stating that the administration of the act had been financially successful, he attempted to show that most of the defects of the program were not inherent weaknesses and that many objections raised against the system had not the slightest validity.[7]

[4] Editorial, *JAMA,* 76 (May 7, 1921), 1313.

[5] "Seven Years of National Health Insurance in England," *JAMA,* 76 (May 21, 1921), 1397–98.

[6] *Ibid.,* p. 1401; *JAMA,* 76 (May 7, 1921), 1310.

[7] *JAMA,* 76 (May 14, 1921), 1350; *JAMA,* 76 (May 21, 1921), 1399–1400; *JAMA,* 76 (May 7, 1921), 1310.

While Cox's observations seemed damaging to the AMA's position, the *Journal* moved quickly to blunt its impact upon the profession. An editorial appearing in the same issue with his first installment offered no denial of the successful operation of the British plan, but maintained that the British system initially confronted conditions that had almost no counterpart in the United States. It referred to the degrading effect of contract practice by friendly societies and lodges on British medical service as problems that only a small portion of the American medical profession had confronted.[8] The editor found nothing in the article that required a serious re-evaluation of the Association's policies.

The *Journal* quickly followed publication of the Cox report with a vigorous attack upon the sickness insurance program proposed by the American Association of Labor Legislation. Frederick R. Green, secretary of the Council on Health and Public Instruction, presented the case for the AMA. Maintaining that the plan was neither health insurance nor insurance, he contended that it had as its chief purpose the "maintenance of the productive efficiency" of industrial workers rather than their health, and that employers, while required to share its risks, were excluded from its benefits.[9] He also contended that justification for compulsory health insurance rested upon the validity of four assumptions, none of which rested on sufficient evidence. These he listed as the insistence that a disproportionate amount of illness among the employed classes necessitated a special type of aid; that the average employee could not bear the financial burden of sickness; that existing methods for controlling disease and promoting health were inadequate; and that compulsory health insurance under government supervision provided the best solution. Nor did he forget the Association's contention that the United States had little to learn from the British experience, although he supported the argument somewhat differently. Green saw stationary economic classes in England, maybe permanently in need of medical care beyond their means, but in the United States, he asserted, "The employee of today is the employer of tomorrow and the member of the leisure class of the day after."[10]

The controversy over compulsory health insurance in May, 1921, contributed much to the tension that characterized the deliberations of the House of Delegates that convened in June. Frank Billings, a trustee of the AMA and twice its president, was called to account for his earlier

[8] Editorial, *JAMA,* 76 (May 7, 1921), 1313–14.

[9] *JAMA,* 76 (May 28, 1921), 1479–80.

[10] Ibid., pp. 1480–81.

advocacy of compulsory health insurance. While his skillfully worded reply constituted no actual denial of the charge, the Association seemed satisfied when he announced that his public statements for several years showed his disapproval of the system.[11] The excitement of the session further appeared in resolutions offered by state societies that sought to commit the Association against all types of "State Medicine," "Diagnostic Clinics," "Health Centers," "Group Practice," and "Compulsory Health Insurance," that were "wholly or partly controlled, operated or subsidized by the State or National Government." While these resolutions did not come up for vote, the House of Delegates did approve of a substitute offered by the Reference Committee on Legislation and Public Relations that proposed close limitations on the right of the state to treat disease.[12]

The Boston session of 1921 provided convincing proof that danger lurked in the path of any important physician who publicly showed sympathy for any such plan of compulsory health insurance. Still stunned by the shock of the Cox report, the *Journal* continued to publish the critical articles of the London correspondent and assure the profession that the British experiment offered no example for the United States. Six months after publishing the favorable installments on the British system, the *Journal* contended that:

> . . . the unavoidable conclusion from the entire mass of evidence is that health insurance, even in England, after being in force for nearly ten years, is still an experiment, and a costly and by no means a universally satisfactory experiment at that. It has not bettered public health conditions.[13]

The Association's hostility to compulsory health insurance gradually became even more pronounced. The speaker of the House of Delegates,

[11] *JAMA,* 94 (May 24, 1930), 1677; *JAMA,* 99 (October 1, 1932), 1187–88; Fishbein, *History of AMA,* pp. 1189–90; HD, *Proceedings* (72 Annual Session, June, 1921), p. 40. Billings was the only man besides Nathan S. Davis who served twice as president.

[12] HD, *Proceedings* (72 Annual Session, June 1921), pp. 34, 38. The adopted resolution declared that the AMA "opposes the state treatment of disease, except (a) in the institutional care of the delinquent, diseased and defective; (b) the treatment of those diseases whose treatment is essential to prevention; (c) the recognition and securing the correction of common defects of school-children." *Ibid.,* p. 43. State societies submitting resolutions not voted on were those in Ill., Mich., and N.H. For resolutions offered by individuals defining or condemning state medicine, see HD, *Proceedings* (72 Annual Session, June, 1921), pp. 34, 38–39.

[13] Editorial, *JAMA,* 77 (November 19, 1921), 1657.

F. C. Warnshius, demonstrated the rising temper of the organization as he assured the Seventy-third session in May, 1922, that:

> Compulsory health insurance never will and never can become an American institution. As our campaign of public education broadens, this fantastic, un-American machination and the fancies of its proponents will fail to arrest legislative attention and consideration or draw unto it public demand and support.[14]

Resolutions that never reached the floor at earlier sessions seemed no more extreme than one which this session adopted. The House of Delegates not only offered a definition of "state medicine," but placed almost any further extension of governmental influence over medical care in this category. The resolution stated that:

> The American Medical Association hereby declares its opposition to all forms of "state medicine," because of the ultimate harm that would come thereby to the public weal through such forms of state practice. "State Medicine" is hereby defined for the purpose of this resolution to be any form of medical treatment, provided, conducted, controlled, or subsidized by the federal or any state government, or municipality, excepting such service as is provided by the Army, Navy, and Public Health Service, and that which is necessary for the control of communicable diseases, the treatment of the indigent sick, and such other services as may be approved by and administered under the direction of or by a local county medical society, and are not disapproved by the state medical society of which it is a component part.[15]

The Sheppard-Towner Issue

The Association directed its resolution attacking "state medicine" not only against the compulsory health insurance issue but also against another that developed. It appeared as a protest against the passage the year before of the Sheppard-Towner Act, which provided federal subsidies for states that would conduct infancy and maternity welfare programs. While the administration hoped that this measure would appeal to the newly enfranchised women voters, it had a repelling influence on the AMA.

The Association, having officially spoken against compulsory health insurance in 1920, showed no disposition to allow the extension of

[14] HD, *Proceedings* (73 Annual Session, May, 1922), p. 2.
[15] *Ibid.*, p. 44.

governmental control over medical service by another route. The compulsory insurance idea itself hardly appeared more repugnant to the *Journal* than the provisions of the proposed Sheppard-Towner bill.[16] The *Journal* considered particularly dangerous the increased power that the measure gave the federal government over the public health problems of the states, and the necessity of their compliance with requirements of the national government in securing federal grants. It showed that even the funds that the states contributed under the program fell under federal supervision and control. The co-operative method of financing, calling for contributions from both state and federal governments, appeared unsound to the *Journal,* which also maintained that the limited funds provided could produce no important results. Its contention that no emergency existed that justified the measure bordered closely on the idea that there were no results to produce. Nor did it agree that the Children's Bureau should administer the act rather than the United States Public Health Service.[17]

In fighting the bills that became the Sheppard-Towner Act, the Association's agitation consisted in part of supplying congressmen with material against the proposed legislation. Despite the fact that this measure became law November 23, 1921, the AMA got some consolation from defeat. The *Journal* maintained that the measure as finally enacted represented an improvement over the original Senate bill and described it as an appropriations act that made federal funds available to the states on an optional basis. While appearing in no way reconciled to the measure, it felt that many of its worst features had been deleted.[18]

Veterans' Issues

Unlike many issues related to the extension of governmental control over matters of medical care and public health, the friction between the AMA and the federal government over veterans' medical benefits did not begin very soon after the war. Not until the middle twenties did this

[16] A measure considerably like the Sheppard-Towner bill was introduced in Congress in 1918, but the AMA showed no particular interest until after the introduction of the latter. For the background of the measure and its provisions see Harry S. Mustard, *The Government in Public Health* (New York: The Commonwealth Fund, 1945), pp. 72–75.

[17] Editorial, *JAMA,* 76 (February 5, 1921), 383; *JAMA,* 76 (May 28, 1921), 1504.

[18] *JAMA,* 87 (February 11, 1922), 435.

question, which soon outweighed many others in significance, become a major problem for the AMA. The principal conflict between the Association and the federal government arose after the passage of the World War Veterans' Act of 1924. Relying on the patriotic sentiments of the nation and supported by a mighty army of voters, powerful forces pushed through legislation upsetting the principles that had governed the administration of veterans' medical benefits.[19] This measure, altering the standards for the disposal of medical aid to veterans, just as sharply clashed with the Association's attitude toward the veterans' medical program.

The AMA was thoroughly convinced that the passage of the measure represented a betrayal of public interest. The act allowed veterans of all military occupations and expeditions since 1897 with nonservice-connected disabilities the use of all beds in veterans' hospitals that veterans with service-connected disabilities did not occupy. While offering no criticism of the principle of federal hospitalization for veterans with service-connected disabilities, the Association strongly condemned federal provision of medical service to veterans whose disability had no such connection. It considered that the measure discriminated against private practitioners and denied the patient the free choice of physicians by providing medical care only by physicians in government service. Although patients were not compelled to choose medical service that the government provided, the AMA considered that the appeal of medical service at government expense would serve effectively in turning veterans from private practitioners. Since the act allowed medical benefits for many able to pay, the Association charged that this tended "to pauperize an independent, self-supporting part of the citizenship" and to overburden the population in general with excessive taxation.[20] Besides

[19] The AMA offered very little criticism of the administration of veterans' benefits in the first few years after the war. The annual session of 1922 tabled a resolution that criticised the extent of lay control over medical matters in the Veterans' Bureau. Resolution, B. B. Shurly, HD, *Proceedings* (73 Annual Session, May, 1922), p. 46. H. H. Shoulders, a prominent leader in the AMA's struggle over veterans' issues, maintains that veterans' organizations never pressed for nonservice-connected hospitalization benefits, but that the agitation came from bureaucrats who had much to gain from the expansion of the system. HD, *Proceedings* (95 Annual Session, July, 1945), p. 4.

[20] H. H. Shoulders, "An Insurance Plan of Benefits vs. a Hospital Plan of Benefits for Ex-Soldiers of the United States," *AMA Bulletin,* 26 (October, 1931), 146–47; United States Veterans' Bureau, *Medical Bulletin,* 2 (June, 1926), 616; Resolution, Ben R. McClellan, HD, *Proceedings* (76 Annual Session, May 1925), pp. 36, 47.

setting forth the Association's grievances against this measure, the Atlantic City session in 1925 announced its intention of seeking an amendment to the act that would eliminate these features.[21]

The *Journal* gave the profession no opportunity to forget the alleged menace of this measure and repeatedly called attention to its dangers, until the pressure of other legislation obnoxious to the *Journal* temporarily diverted its attention. Early in 1926 it announced that:

> Through paragraph 10 of section 202 of the World War Veterans' Act of 1924, the federal government planted the germ of state medicine in our body politic and entered directly into competition with the private practitioners and private hospitals of the country.[22]

The *Journal* not only attacked the act as providing for state medicine, but also pointed out the existence of plans to expand the services allowed under this measure. It observed that bills then before Congress proposed the extension of federal hospitalization benefits to veterans of all wars, as well as their free access to the outpatient clinics of government hospitals.

When the Dallas session convened in June, the trustees expressed alarm over the growth of federal competition with private medical practice. They informed the delegates that during the first fiscal year in which the new act operated, 13,243 veterans with nonservice-connected disabilities (17 per cent of the total) received treatment in hospitals directed by the Veterans' Bureau, at a cost to the government of about $5,000,000.[23] The next month the *Journal* declared:

> State medicine in this obnoxious form is with us, and is tending to grow under the patronage of the federal government. . . . How long such unfair competition will continue is uncertain. But unless the present movement is checked, the outcome is sure; a greater and greater encroachment on the rights of the individual patient and physician.[24]

The *Journal* also warned that this new policy could just as easily be broadened to include federal medical care for government employees.

Revived Sheppard-Towner Issue

While the AMA never conceded any justification for the expanded program that the act of 1924 authorized, its agitation against the meas-

[21] HD, *Proceedings* (76 Annual Session, May, 1925), p. 60.
[22] *JAMA*, 86 (January 23, 1926), 278.
[23] HD, *Proceedings* (77 Annual Session, April, 1926), p. 15.
[24] *JAMA*, 86 (June 12, 1926), 1840.

ure seemed hardly as pronounced after the appearance of an older issue. By self-limitation the Sheppard-Towner Act, passed in 1921, expired on June 30, 1927, unless Congress extended its life.[25] The harassed Association, long provoked by the threat and reality of federal competition with private medical practice, renewed its attack upon the measure. Since, like the veterans' act, it called for federal subsidization of medical service and the granting of benefits to certain groups along no clearly defined lines, the AMA found that its criticisms of one act applied also to the other.

With the appearance in Congress of bills designed to extend for two years the life of the Sheppard-Towner Act, the Association began its agitation early in 1926 to prevent their passage. Repeating some of the organization's objections to the Sheppard-Towner law, the *Journal* requested all physicians to write or wire the President and their United States senators and representatives protesting its extension.[26] As excitement over the matter again stirred the Association, the AMA offered its ablest explanation for opposing the measure. In a restrained and cogent article, William C. Woodward, executive secretary of the Bureau of Legal Medicine and Legislation, set forth the principles behind the measure, the history of its operation, and an appraisal of its success.[27] That the issue continued to disturb the Association became even clearer late in the year, when a December issue of the *Journal* published a telegram protesting the measure which the Association had sent to "the President, the Vice President and certain interested senators." While Congress considered the extension of the act, the Association sent pamphlets condemning the measure to members of the House and Senate.[28]

When, early in 1927, Congress extended for two years the operation of the Sheppard-Towner Act, the Association, though disappointed, showed little discouragement. It determined to prevent additional extensions and continued its agitation against the measure. Additional articles criticizing the act appeared in the *Journal,* and Woodward launched another attack in the *Bulletin.*[29] The Association kept alert to the introduc-

[25] *JAMA,* 86 (February 6, 1926), 421.

[26] *Ibid.*

[27] "The Sheppard-Towner Act: Its Proposed Extension and Proposed Repeal," *AMA Bulletin,* 21 (May, 1926), 126–33.

[28] *JAMA,* 87 (December 18, 1926), 2098; HD, *Proceedings* (78 Annual Session, May, 1927), p. 16.

[29] See Editorial, *JAMA,* 91 (November 3, 1928), 1721–22; *JAMA,* 92 (May 4, 1929), 1525; "The Threatened Extension of the Sheppard-Towner Act," *AMA Bulletin,* 24 (February, 1929), 74–75. Woodward's attack on the effects of

tion of all bills that proposed to perpetuate federal aid for infant and maternal welfare and brought its influence directly to bear on Washington.

As the AMA expected, proponents of the Sheppard-Towner legislation intensified their efforts to extend the benefits of the act as the date for its expiration approached. The bills that it found most dangerous were twin measures that Senator Wesley L. Jones of Washington and Representative John G. Cooper of Ohio introduced on April 18, 1929. Since the Association felt that these bills extended the Sheppard-Towner legislation "in every essential particular" except for no time limitation, it found them "open to every objection ever raised against the Sheppard-Towner Act."[30] While the extended law did expire, the agitation for its revival did not. The *Journal* noted that the early advocates of federal aid for maternal and infant welfare contended that the original act was only temporary, and primarily designed to stimulate state activity in this work. Over eight years after the measure became law, the *Journal* observed that "If the act stimulated the states in this manner it accomplished its purpose and there is no reason for resurrecting it. If it did not, the act was a failure and there is even less reason for doing so."[31]

By the time of the Detroit session in June, 1930, the AMA showed signs of growing irritation over the vitality of the Sheppard-Towner issue. Considering the term "state medicine" no longer adequate to describe federal programs authorized by the measure, it searched for a more odious epithet. The House of Delegates showed no hesitation in condemning the system "as unsound in policy, wasteful and extravagant, unproductive of results and tending to promote communism. . . ."[32] Not only did the governing body brand the program as a move toward communism, but also notified the President and Congress of its action, and urged all component medical societies to support its position.

The Association found another opportunity to strike at the principles of Sheppard-Towner legislation when over 3,000 representatives of

---

Sheppard-Towner Act did not go unchallenged. T. Swann Harding cites the obvious mistake of comparing infant and maternal mortality rates in states that adopted the program with those that did not. He shows that, generally, states with the lowest death rates adopted the programs and that the others had a much broader area in which to show improvement. See Harding, *Degradation of Science* (New York: Farrar & Rinehard Incorporated, 1931), p. 248.

[30] *JAMA,* 92 (May 4, 1929), 1525–26; Editorial, *JAMA,* 94 (April 19, 1930), 1241.

[31] Editorial, *JAMA,* 94 (April 19, 1930), 1340.

[32] HD, *Proceedings* (81 Annual Session, June, 1930), pp. 35, 41.

many professions and interests assembled in November for President Herbert Hoover's White House Conference on Child Health and Protection. The matters discussed included the federal policy of subsidizing state health activities and unifying federal health agencies, topics of great interest to the AMA. Though representatives of the Association attended the conference, they expressed displeasure with the outcome. When Committee A of Section II of the conference submitted its report, recommending further federal appropriations for federal aid to state health work and for its administration at the federal level exclusively by the United States Public Health Service, the spokesmen for the AMA raised objections. While favoring the unification of federal health agencies, they vigorously opposed a renewal of the principles of the Sheppard-Towner Act. Consequently, the published report of the committee carried the dissent of Olin West, secretary of the Association, and Warnshuis, still speaker of the House of Delegates, to the recommendation of further federal aid for state health activities.[33]

Hardly had the AMA time to recover from some of the disappointing results of the White House conference, when it heard the news that the United States Senate on January 10, 1931, passed the Jones-Cooper bill embodying the general provisions of the Sheppard-Towner Act. The new decade had started badly for the AMA, and offered promise of little more on the political front than a struggle over the revival of the principles of the Sheppard-Towner legislation and the maintenance and extension of veterans' benefits. Although the House of Representatives did not pass the new measure, the activity of the AMA seems to have been little more than to urge all physicians to encourage their representatives to vote against it.[34] The next year the Association tried to kill a similar state subsidy bill even before it came up for Senate vote. On February 4, 1932, six prominent physicians, at least two of whom were influential leaders of the AMA, appeared before the Senate Committee on Commerce to speak against a measure practically the same as that which the Senate had passed the year before. They tried to convince the committee that the operation of the Sheppard-Towner Act had not appreciably reduced infancy and maternity death rates, and that the new

[33] *JAMA,* 95 (December 6, 1930), 1765; *Report: Public Health Organization* (White House Conference on Child Health and Protection [New York: The Century Co., 1932]), pp. 332–38. Unlike West, who voted negatively on the report, Warnshuis accepted it but protested against the idea of further subsidies for state health activities.

[34] *JAMA,* 96 (January 24, 1931), 274.

bill was actually more objectionable than its predecessors. Although the committee approved the measure with some modifications, seven of its members drafted a dissenting report clearly showing the favorable impressions the physicians had made.[35] The failure of Congress again to enact this legislation neither allayed the fears of the Association nor completely discouraged proponents of the bill.

The success of the AMA's efforts to prevent the enactment of maternity and infant welfare legislation during the Hoover era largely resulted from factors more important than its own influence. The deepening shadows of the depression and the ineptitude of a confused administration brought to the front issues even more urgent than federal health subsidies. As unemployment figures soared and bread lines lengthened, a divided and struggling administration rocked almost helplessly in the currents of a major crisis. Offering more sympathy than assistance for those afflicted either by hunger or disease, it bequeathed its mounting problems to the new administration.

Persistence of the Veterans' Issues

While worried throughout the Hoover era by the continued agitation for a revival of the principles of the Sheppard-Towner law, the Association watched the increasing liberalization of veterans' legislation with great alarm. The measures that Congress repeatedly enacted, providing for the enlargement of the government's hospital facilities and the agitation for bonuses to hospitalized veterans, troubled the Detroit session of 1930. The AMA had predicted that the granting of hospitalization privileges to veterans with nonservice-connected disabilities would lead to other infringements on private medical practice and it now faced the reality of their existence. The government no longer offered veterans with nonservice-connected disabilities the use only of beds not needed by veterans who incurred disabilities in service, but had begun to build additional facilities for both. The trustees reported to the House of Delegates that the situation was "grave," and secured their approval of a resolution condemning such a policy as "communistic," in language

[35] HD, *Proceedings* (83 Annual Session, May, 1932), p. 44; Editorial, *JAMA,* 99 (September 3, 1932), 836. During the period from 1929 until 1935, when the Social Security Act revived the program of maternal and infant welfare, the Children's Bureau conducted only educational work and studies. Mustard, *Government in Public Health,* p. 77.

similar to that adopted by the same session in denouncing the principles of the Sheppard-Towner legislation.[36]

AMA's Hospitalization Proposal

Despite the Association's strong objection to many features of the veterans' program, it began to learn that a purely negative policy could not succeed. That its own strategy for correcting the alleged dangers in the program had undergone considerable change became quite evident by the time of the Philadelphia session a year later. The House of Delegates adopted a resolution that Harrison H. Shoulders of Nashville, Tennessee, proposed, calling for a discontinuance of the existing policy of governmental hospitalization for veterans with nonservice-connected disabilities, and substituting in its place a proposal for a disability insurance program financed and administered by the federal government. The plan proposed the payment of a weekly cash benefit during the period of total disability, in addition to a liberal hospitalization payment for periods when veterans with nonservice-connected disabilities were hospitalized. The scheme also provided for veterans with service-connected disabilities, and, while in no way interfering with the benefits they received for disabilities incurred in service, placed any additional disabilities under the operation of the insurance system.[37]

A few months after the House of Delegates adopted this proposal, Shoulders offered convincing proof in the *Bulletin* of its advantages over the hospitalization plan in force. He showed that the government's program called for an expenditure of about $200,000,000 for the maintenance of veterans' hospitals in operation and others to be constructed, which did not include the initial construction costs for either type, the cost of equipment, or the expense of transporting veterans to and from such hospitals. Careful calculations convinced him that for an annual expenditure of $92,400,000 the government could adequately provide disability payments and hospital benefits under the Association's plan. Since 70 per cent of the veterans treated in government hospitals in 1930 had nonservice-connected disabilities, a great part of the expenditure would go for their treatment.

[36] HD, *Proceedings* (81 Annual Session, June, 1930), pp. 14, 35, 39.

[37] HD, *Proceedings* (82 Annual Session, June, 1931), pp. 32, 34. An elaboration of the scheme appears in Shoulders, *AMA Bulletin,* 26 (October, 1931), 146–54.

Shoulders believed that this plan had many advantages over the older program. It eliminated the expense of further hospital construction and the excessive travel expenses that the government paid for many veterans who went to distant government hospitals, by providing for their treatment in local private hospitals as well as in government institutions. It offered the veteran a cash income payment to defray the cost of physicians' services or for supporting dependents or both. It allowed more of the money that Congress appropriated to go directly for veterans' assistance, avoiding the enormous costs of new government hospitals and the likelihood of their operation long after their usefulness had ceased. In addition, the plan allowed the unrestricted choice of physicians and the personal payment for their services through the cash benefit provision.[38]

Not only did the Association show some willingness to adjust its policy to a changed situation, but it established contacts with the American Legion in order to win its approval. Olin West and Shoulders, along with four other representatives of the AMA, met with leaders of the American Legion on November 19, 1931, in a conference that seemed to draw the two organizations a little closer together. On December 30, the AMA scheduled another meeting at its own headquarters that brought together the Board of Trustees, West, Woodward, Morris Fishbein, and a few other leaders of the AMA, besides prominent officials of the American Legion. The Association seemed to have impressed the representatives of the veterans' organization with the feasibility of stopping additional hospital construction and with the idea of treating veterans in private hospitals, but a later meeting in February, 1932, brought out some very real differences. In a conference at Washington, D.C., that included also representatives of the Veterans Administration and the American Hospital Association, the legion made a stand against the Association's disability insurance plan. While serious conflicts appeared, the conference appointed a committee to help reconcile the differences and serve a liaison function between these organizations. The recommendations of this committee failed to endorse all of the proposals of the AMA, but accepted its view that some use should be made of private hospitals.[39]

When the House of Delegates met in New Orleans in May, the Association further clarified its program for disability insurance. It reaffirmed

[38] *AMA Bulletin,* 26 (October, 1931), 147–51.

[39] HD, *Proceedings* (83 Annual Session, May, 1932), pp. 42–43.

its endorsement of the disability insurance proposal of the preceding session, but elaborated more fully on what it thought this proposal should include. It adopted a resolution submitted by Shoulders which proposed coverage under the insurance plan to veterans of all wars, military occupations, or expeditions whose active service lasted at least 90 days. The resolution called for a cash weekly benefit of $12.50, covering the entire period of total disability, and an allowance of $4.00 a day for periods of hospitalization. Carefully prepared to avoid conflict with the administration of service-connected benefits, it also guarded against many possible abuses of such an insurance system.[40]

During the closing months of the Hoover administration, the AMA continued its effort to correct certain features of the veterans' program, and to secure the adoption of its own plan. Its agitation appeared to have borne some fruit when a congressional committee, before which its representatives had appeared, reported a bill in April, 1932, that greatly restricted government hospitalization and medical service to veterans with nonservice-connected disabilities. The Association had reason for disappointment when the measure became a law with these restrictive features omitted. The action of the House on May 31, in creating a committee to investigate governmental competition with private business, however, encouraged the Association and gave its representatives an opportunity to air their grievances before this group. In a prepared statement Woodward and Edward H. Cary traced the alleged unwarranted encroachments on private practice even back to a minor infringement in a veterans' act of 1922, and showed that between 1925 and 1931, the percentage of veterans with nonservice-connected disabilities treated in government hospitals jumped from 17 per cent of all veterans treated to 77 per cent. They offered strong evidence from the plans for additional hospital construction that even this percentage would increase.[41]

While standing firmly against certain features of the government's program for veterans, the Association nevertheless maintained contact with the legion, and three AMA leaders attended its Portland session in September. This session resulted in the formation of a committee that included two physicians, which was established to give advice to the legion's National Rehabilitation Committee. A few weeks later the same

[40] HD, *Proceedings* (83 Annual Session, May, 1932), pp. 32, 44–45.

[41] HD, *Proceedings* (84 Annual Session, June, 1933), p. 15. Joint Congressional Committee on Veterans' Affairs, Seventy-second Congress, second session, *Hearings* (Washington: Government Printing Office, 1933), I, 238–39.

three leaders attended a conference in Washington, called by the Veterans Administration.[42] Despite the Association's strenuous effort to check the encroachments on private medical practice, it had little reason to be encouraged when the Hoover administration closed.

Lesser Issues

The AMA's fight against some features of the veterans' legislation, as well as its opposition to the maternity and infancy welfare program and a revival of the compulsory health insurance movement, did not completely exhaust its political activities. Although largely occupied by these problems, it showed some interest in other political and social questions. It did not abandon its idea of the unification of federal health activities in an executive department or lesser agency, but did little toward its realization.[43] Its interest in the experiment with national prohibition largely centered in its attempt to secure a relaxation of restrictions in the Volstead Act, regulating the medical use of alcohol. Its concern over the evolution controversy of the middle twenties was based primarily on its belief that legislative restrictions on the teaching of evolution might seriously retard the advancement of medical science.[44]

The Role of Leadership

Although the period from 1920 to 1933 found the AMA politically active, it did not try to restore much of the nation-wide legislative machinery that had disintegrated by the end of the war. It fought the political battles of these years without the use of some of the channels through which its pressure had once been effectively exerted on local societies. It did attempt, however, to maintain contact with the principal officials of state medical associations, including their legislative committees. Early in the third decade, the secretary of the Council on Health and Public Instruction reported several meetings in states where legislatures were soon to convene for the mapping of political strategy

[42] HD, *Proceedings* (84 Annual Session, June, 1933), p. 32.

[43] *JAMA,* 80 (January 27, 1923), 262; HD, *Proceedings* (78 Annual Session, May, 1927), p. 58.

[44] HD, *Proceedings* (78 Annual Session, May, 1927), p. 16; (82 Annual Session, June, 1931), p. 41; and (76 Annual Session, May, 1925), p. 59.

with the legislative committees of state associations.[45] Through its Bureau of Legal Medicine and Legislation, created by the St. Louis session of 1922, the Association sought to gather information from state societies about medical bills that various state legislatures had under consideration, but found many associations un-co-operative. Later it relied on a legislative reporting service for knowledge of bills introduced in state legislatures, and passed its information on to the principal officials of state associations.[46] But upon these state organizations fell the responsibility of building and maintaining their own constituent societies and organizing the machinery for exerting political pressure, without much assistance from the AMA.

The Association, however, had effective means of uniting most of the profession behind its leadership, and increasing its influence in political affairs. The *Journal* and the *Bulletin* carried its views to the medical profession, while *Hygiea,* first published in 1923, had a growing popular appeal.[47] By the middle of 1924, the Association had found the radio a convenient medium of publicity on a limited scale. The newly-established Woman's Auxiliary of the American Medical Association, which enlisted women physicians and doctors' wives, also drew public attention to the Association's work.[48]

Individual personalities, however, cannot be ignored in accounting for the organization's growth. When the devoted editor and general manager of the Association, George H. Simmons, retired from active duties, September 22, 1924, the AMA's new editor, Morris Fishbein, energetically advanced the Association's interests along with Olin West, who became its general manager the same year.[49] As a faithful spokesman of the AMA, Fishbein's services extended far beyond his editorial duties. The trustees' report of 1928 that referred to 58 addresses he had delivered the preceding year, four of which were before state medical

[45] HD, *Proceedings* (73 Annual Session, May, 1922), pp. 19–20.

[46] HD, *Proceedings* (74 Annual Session, June, 1923), pp. 19–20; (77 Annual Session, April, 1926), p. 13; *AMA Bulletin,* 20 (February, 1925), 33; HD, *Proceedings* (81 Annual Session, June, 1930, p. 14.

[47] *JAMA,* 100 (April 1, 1933), 1036–37. For the circulation of the Spanish issue of the *Journal* in 1923 see HD, *Proceedings* (74 Annual Session, June, 1923), p. 12.

[48] HD, *Proceedings* (75 Annual Session, June, 1924), pp. 16, 45; see *AMA Bulletin,* 25 (November, 1930), 205, and 25 (December, 1930), 237 for the origin of the Woman's Auxiliary and the nature of its work.

[49] HD, *Proceedings* (76 Annual session, May, 1925), p. 9.

associations, partially illustrates the extent of his activities.[50] Against developments that appeared to threaten its security during the Republican era, the Association brought determined leadership, growing medical backing, and considerable popular support.

[50] *Ibid.,* (79 Annual Session, June, 1928), p. 7. The position Fishbein held gave him great influence over the Association's policies. As early as 1909, President Hubert L. Burrell told the Sixtieth session that the one who held the office of secretary, editor, and general manager (then held by one person) was "largely responsible for the policies of the Association." *JAMA,* 52 (June 19, 1909), 2031.

Chapter 9

CHANGING PATTERNS IN THE ADMINISTRATION AND PURCHASE OF MEDICAL CARE

As THE AMERICAN MEDICAL ASSOCIATION struggled against political encroachments on private medical care in the early postwar era, traditional forms of medical service were also being shaken by more elusive developments. The rapid progress of technology and medical science after the war, together with the problems created by peacetime adjustment, greatly upset patterns of medical care that had remained largely unchanged for centuries. While the Association welcomed the impressive advance of scientific medicine, it looked apprehensively upon other trends affecting the organization and administration of medical service.

Rise of Group Practice

Among developments that gave the AMA cause for some anxiety was the rapid growth of group practice. While the organization of medical groups often served the best interest of at least a portion of the profession and public, their popularity seemed to imperil the future of individual practitioners. The co-operative medical experience that World War I gave many physicians, as well as the growing fame of such institutions as Mayo Clinic, greatly increased the appeal of organized medical service. Physicians, returning to private practice in areas where the supply of medical facilities lagged far behind scientific advancement and public need, found the idea of group practice even more attractive. In many localities only a physicians' merger movement held promise of providing the type of facilities that few acting alone could afford.[1] Another factor accounting for the growing popularity of joint service schemes was the impetus they received from federal subsidies for state health programs that led to the establishment of group practice centers.

Early in 1921, the *Journal* referred to the combination movement in medical service as a "most important innovation," and while giving reasons for its development, showed considerable concern for the effect it would have upon traditional medical practice. It asked:

> . . . what of the outcome of this new development? What of the physicians outside the group? Some evidently are seeing the advantages and are forming other groups—perhaps in some instances forced to do so in self-defense! Will not this mean group against group? May it not be one more step toward the complete elimination of the medical practitioner—of the family adviser—of him who heretofore has reflected to the public the altruistic motives of the medical profession? Does it mean that the family physician is being replaced by a corporation?[2]

The trend toward group practice after the war showed some signs of slowing down in the early twenties, but its revival in 1928 convinced the Association that it was more than a passing problem. Although no cases attracted as much publicity as the Mayo Clinic, and such combinations as the Battle Creek (Michigan) Sanitorium and the Ross-Loos Medical Group of Los Angeles, less publicized medical centers sprang up in all sections of the land.[3]

[1] Bureau of Medical Economics, "Group Practice" (Chicago: American Medical Association), pp. 40–41. Group practice frequently offered other advantages, such as the removal of administrative and financial duties from group physicians and reduction in cost of treatment when the service of several doctors was required. C. Rufus Rorem, *Private Group Clinics* (The Committee on the Costs of Medical Care, Publication No. 8 [Washington, D. C.: The Committee on the Costs of Medical Care]), pp. 110–11.

[2] *JAMA,* 76 (February 12, 1921), 452–53.

[3] Bureau of Medical Economics, "Group Practice," p. 41; Esther Lucile Brown, *Physicians and Medical Care* (New York: Russell Sage Foundation, 1937), pp. 155–56. One authority, writing in 1927, stated that there were then nearly 6,000 clinics in the United States, more than half of which had been established in the preceding twelve years. His use of the word "clinic," however, is broader than the privately operated establishments referred to in this chapter. Michael M. Davis, in collaboration with other staff members of the Committee on Dispensary Development of the United States Hospital Fund of New York, *Clinics, Hospitals and Health Centers* (Harper's Public Health Series, Allan J. McLaughlin, ed. [New York: Harper Brothers Publishers, 1927]), p. 37.

Reconciling itself to the probable permanence of group practice, the American Medical Association hoped for little more than to prevent the movement from endangering the profession's cherished standards. Its interest lay in eliminating influences that encouraged economic rivalry among physicians, degraded medical service, and unfairly jeopardized the position of the individual practitioner. In 1922 it amended the Principles of Medical Ethics to govern the growth of group adventures. The revised sections denounced the activities of "any individual, or any institution, private or public, or corporation, or association, or group of individuals under whatever name" that used "advertisements to the general public" or circulars for the solicitation of patients. Also branded as unethical were any efforts to advertise "a small group of physicians to the detriment of the whole profession. . . ."[4]

While the Association took responsibility for revising and interpreting the Principles of Medical Ethics, to local societies largely fell the problem of enforcement. The preponderance of individual practitioners in professional ranks, however, gave some assurance that the worse competitive features of group practice would not develop. As constituent societies watched developments on the local level, the AMA remained alert to national trends. In 1922 it made a survey of private medical clinics in the United States and promised to keep its records up-to-date.[5]

Growth of Contract Practice

Not only was the Association somewhat disturbed by the growth of group-medical units, but showed greater concern over the renewed threat of contract practice. In fact, the development of contract schemes appeared as a fitting complement to the growth of group affiliations. A few daring physicians urged the establishment of both before the decade had passed. R. C. Burrow of Kentucky recommended group and contract practice as the best method of providing the nation's middle class with adequate medical care, maintaining that if these forms

[4] HD, *Proceedings* (73 Annual Session, May, 1922), p. 42.

[5] HD, *Proceedings* (74 Annual Session, June, 1923), p. 24. Disputes arising among physicians and local societies are nearly always settled there. A board of impartial physicians is chosen, or preferably, use is made of the Board of Censors of the component medical society of the AMA. Bureau of Medical Economics, "Economics and the Ethics of Medicine" (Chicago: American Medical Association, 1926), pp. 41–42.

were unethical then the ethics should be disregarded.[6] The Association was much less inclined to accept either innovation, however, and assumed the role of protecting medical practice against their real or imagined dangers.

While contract schemes dated as far back as the colonial era, by the 1920's they had lost most of their original simplicity. For the AMA they no longer possessed only those harmless features that made them unobjectionable as methods of providing medical service to employees of remote railroad, lumbering, and mining enterprises of the West or to members of a few philanthropic organizations.[7] The newly-adopted workmen's compensation laws had carried contract schemes far beyond their original purposes without eliminating all dangerous tendencies. The simple negotiations between industries and physicians in western areas became less frequent as local hospitals, often under lay control, secured these contracts and then initiated ruinous competition among physicians by bargaining for medical services with the lowest bidder. By combining contract practice with hospitalization benefits, a number of unethical medical contract plans found ready acceptance in some regions. As the exploitation of the profession through contract schemes proved highly rewarding, especially in the lumbering regions of Washington and Oregon, resourceful promoters persuaded other industries in a number of states to adopt such systems.[8] In 1931, the Judicial Council of the AMA noted with alarm that many schemes no longer limited their

[6] Burrow stressed the advantages of group and contract practices for meeting the medical needs of the medium income family which, he insisted, "is certainly up against it if one of the family develops a case of Typhoid Fever or Pneumonia, or even an ordinary obstetric case." He maintained that the poor could receive free ward care in hospitals but that the moderate income class was hard pressed. He contended that a group practice unit could profitably remove tonsils in his area for $35.00 but that the cost to the public under prevailing methods was $85.00. The establishment of contract plans, he believed, would further lighten the burden of medical care. "Group Practice," *Kentucky Medical Journal,* 27 (June, 1929), 257–58. For the AMA's earlier experience with contract practice see pp. 139–40 above.

[7] R. G. Leland, "Contract Practice" (Chicago: Bureau of Medical Economics), pp. 1–2. George Washington employed the contract system in administering medical care to the employees of his estate and prearranged contracts for medical service were occasionally found on Southern plantations up to, and in some instances, after the Civil War. Frederick D. Mott and Milton I. Roemer, *Rural Health and Medical Care* (New York: McGraw-Hill Book Company, Inc., 1948), pp. 437–38.

[8] Leland, "Contract Practice," pp. 3–4. I. S. Falk, C. Rufus Rorem, and Martha D. Ring, *The Costs of Medical Care* (The Committee on the Costs of

benefits to industrial workers, but offered protection to all groups without regard to occupation. Even earlier a number of local medical societies in the West had begun to organize their own contract plans to combat the sinister influence of lay-administered programs.[9]

Alert to the dangers that threatened in contract practice, in 1926 the Judicial Council defined this form of medical service and prepared to make a thorough investigation of contract systems. The council identified this form of practice as:

> . . . the carrying out of an agreement between a physician or group of physicians as principals or agents and a corporation, organization or individual, to furnish partial or full medical service to a group or class of individuals for a definite sum for a fixed rate per capita.[10]

While studying the development of contract schemes, the council in 1927 listed features that made any plan unacceptable, without repeating the Association's familiar criticisms that such schemes offered a definite amount of pay for an indefinite amount of work, and resulted in retailing medical service secured at wholesale prices.

The council considered unethical any system that compensated physicians at a rate below that usually charged by the profession in the locality, or that offered remuneration so low that competent service became impossible. If such schemes encouraged physicians to underbid for contracts or led to the solicitation of patients, they constituted unethical forms of practice. The Judicial Council also considered as intolerable any plan which failed to provide for "a reasonable degree of free choice of physicians." Three years later, in an effort to destroy lay control over physicians' earnings, the Association urged the profession to avoid all contact with hospitals that had adopted any system of collecting fees for medical service.[11]

Medical Care, Publication No. 27 [Chicago: University of Chicago Press, 1933]), pp. 453–55, explains how the medical profession was exploited by such systems. Additional information is supplied in "New Forms of Medical Practice" (Bureau of Medical Economics, American Medical Association), pp. 11–19.

[9] Leland, "Contract Practice," pp. 18–19; Louis S. Reed, *Blue Cross and Medical Service Plans* (Washington, D.C.: Federal Security Agency, U.S. Public Health Service, October, 1947), pp. 136–37. For examples of some contract schemes see R. G. Leland, "Some Phases of Contract Practice" (Bureau of Medical Economics, American Medical Association), pp. 7–26.

[10] HD, *Proceedings* (77 Annual Session, April, 1926), pp. 27, 48.

[11] HD, *Proceedings* (78 Annual Session, May, 1927), pp. 25–26 and (81 Annual Session, June, 1930), p. 36.

After the AMA had established rather definite standards for appraising an ever increasing number of contract schemes, it found the *Journal* a powerful medium for publicizing their merits and weaknesses. In the early thirties this organ warned the unwary physician of alleged dangers lurking in most contract plans and followed carefully their spread in many areas.[12] During 1932, the Association established other criteria for determining their acceptability. Besides conforming to the principles already formulated, R. G. Leland, director of the newly established Bureau of Medical Economics, emphasized that no such plan should exploit the profession or ignore preclinical or preventive medicine. He also insisted that in any system of contract practice the medical profession must assume "full responsibility for the determination of professional qualifications and ethics and adequacy of medical care," and allow changes in medical practice only after thorough investigation.[13]

The Association did not confine its fight against unethical forms of contract practice to the simple formulation of principles, but found other means of holding the profession in line. Its Judicial Council received reports of irregular developments in medical practice and frequently advised state associations on a course of action. When the Dallas County (Texas) Medical Society suspended two of its members in 1932 for practicing under what it considered were unethical contracts, the state association as well as the Judicial Council of the AMA upheld its action. Organized pressure further developed when the trustees in February, 1933, asked that all component bodies declare their views publicly on "general social, legislative and economic relationships of medical practice only through approved channels of the American Medical Association."[14]

The Group Hospitalization Movement

In addition to the Association's struggle against the alleged evil influence of group and contract practice, it looked upon the growth of group hospitalization schemes as a dangerous development. These schemes served as the layman's counterpart of the medical profession's group practice plans and often tied in with contract practice systems.

[12] In the fall of 1932, practically every issue of the *Journal* carried an exposure of some contract scheme or an attack upon the alleged evils of contract practice.

[13] Leland, "Some Phases of Contract Practice," pp. 27–28.

[14] HD, *Proceedings* (81 Annual Session, June, 1930), p. 23; Falk, Rorem, and Ring, *Costs of Medical Care,* p. 466; quotation, *JAMA,* 100 (March 4, 1933), 668.

Of the three periods that marked the progress of the movement to the end of World War II, the first dating from 1890 to 1928, witnessed the origin and development of industrial and single hospital plans.[15] Like the system of contract practice, group hospitalization schemes proved very useful as a method of providing hospital service for employees of mining, railroad, and lumbering companies operating in isolated areas. In this period, mutual benefit associations and mutual insurance companies offered limited hospitalization benefits to employees of a widening group of industries, but usually at excessive rates. Later, individual hospitals found in local hospitalization plans the promise of economic security.[16]

Few group hospitalization plans that single hospitals offered appeared earlier than that which the Hospital Service Association of Rockford, Illinois, established after its organization in 1912. Restricting its coverage to local residents over 15 years of age, without chronic illnesses or bodily defects requiring hospitalization, it offered a plan of limited hospital service at moderate cost. The Grinnell (Iowa) Community Hospital, organized in 1921, promoted a similar prepayment plan, followed by one that the Brattleboro (Vermont) Benefit Association instituted soon after its organization six years later. No early scheme, however, achieved greater success or popularity than the Baylor Hospital Plan in Texas that Justin F. Kimball established in 1929, which became the actual forerunner of the more comprehensive plans that developed a few years later.[17]

The successful operation of single hospital group payment schemes, as well as the need for a much broader population coverage, led to the establishments of several non-profit hospital plans in the period from 1929 to 1936, followed by the initial operation of the Blue Cross plans. Several multiple hospital schemes, operating at points as widely separated as Newark, New Jersey, and Sacramento, California, proved advantageous to the public and to hospitals alike.[18] The rise of these

[15] J. T. Richardson, *The Origin and Development of Group Hospitalization in the United States, 1890–1940* (University of Missouri, Studies, Vol. 20, No. 3 [Columbia, University of Missouri Press, 1945]), p. 14.

[16] *Ibid.*, pp. 14–15; C. Rufus Rorem, *Non-Profit Hospital Plans* (January, 1940), p. 4; see the report of the Committee on Miscellaneous and Unclassified Plans in *Report* (Commission on Medical Care Plans [Chicago: American Medical Association, 1958]), Part II, pp. 4–5.

[17] Reed, *Blue Cross and Medical Service Plans,* pp. 9–10; Richardson, *Origin and Development of Group Hospitalization,* pp. 15–17.

[18] Richardson, *Origin and Development of Group Hospitalization,* pp. 17–18.

new forms of group hospitalization not only added prestige to the movement, but also offset much of the reproach cast upon it by some disreputable schemes that had also emerged.

Objections to Group Hospitalization

Faced with a development that threatened to revolutionize the financial arrangements for hospital care, the Association could not remain indifferent. Despite its belated interest in the movement, its attitude toward hospitalization insurance had crystallized before the beginning of the New Deal era. While the highest oracle, the House of Delegates, issued neither curse nor blessing, other forces within the Association determined its direction.

Among these was the Judicial Council, whose report to the legislative body in 1926 called attention to the growth of prepayment plans, some of which provided only for medical care, while others included surgical and hospitalization benefits. Convinced that no scheme could provide these services for the low dues that some assessed, it looked upon such schemes as unethical. It also reminded the profession of the revision of the ethics in 1922 that prohibited the solicitation of patients by "individual physicians, by groups, by institutions, or by organizations of physicians."[19]

Although the late twenties witnessed the spread of group hospitalization schemes, the Association for several years after 1926 seemed almost oblivious to their development. This subject received almost no consideration at the annual sessions and only rare mention in the *Journal.* The principal reminder of alleged evils in health insurance schemes came from the London correspondent. His attacks upon the British compulsory medical system appeared more numerous and severe especially after British workers, whose doctors' bills were already covered under the national insurance act, entered schemes offering hospitalization benefits, and as agitation increased in England for the expansion of national health legislation.[20] The Association's retiring

[19] HD, *Proceedings* (77 Annual Session, April, 1926), p. 28.

[20] The British health insurance legislation of 1911 did not provide for hospitalization benefits and the movement for this type of coverage through contributory hospital schemes was greatly encouraged by the depression. Bureau of Medical Economics, "New Forms of Medical Practice," p. 41. For examples of the London correspondent's attacks see *JAMA,* 94 (May 17, 1930), 1642; *JAMA,* 94 (May 31, 1930), 1772–73; *JAMA,* 95 (August 16, 1930), 543.

president, Malcom L. Harris, warned the Detroit session in 1930 of developments that threatened to create a "socialized" profession and urged local societies to avert the danger by organizing medical centers that offered services to the lowest income groups at whatever price they could pay. The House of Delegates showed little interest in this recommendation, however, and, while offering no solution for the economic problems of medical care, heard the new president, William Gerry Morgan, refer to the voluntary schemes of sickness insurance as having "paternalistic aspects."[21]

Four months later, a *Journal* editorial branded all forms of health insurance as failures among the schemes designed to provide the public with adequate medical care at a price it could afford, saying:

> It is strange that physicians, who themselves distrust panaceas for diseases of the human body, should continually venture panaceas for the indispositions of the body politic. It is strange that public men who distrust one track systems in their commercial ventures should be willing to support similar systems for the solution of the problem of the cost of medical care.[22]

In the following year the Judicial Council again called attention to the problem. Charging that most schemes providing for medical care and hospitalization benefits were financially insecure, it reported that:

> In the cases presented to it the Judicial Council has advised against the adoption of such plans by community hospitals because it is believed that they are not economically sound in that they may be unfavorably affected by conditions entirely beyond control under which contracts cannot be fulfilled.[23]

At the New Orleans session of 1932, President Edward Starr Judd reaffirmed the Association's confidence in the sufficiency of medical service. While suggesting a more careful study of new plans of medical practice, he thought that current service was generally "satisfactory and adequate."[24]

Not until the last quarter of 1932 did the question of prepayment plans for hospital and medical service receive much attention from the AMA. Its sudden interest took the form of a critical survey of plans in operation, which the *Journal* began to publish in the issue of October 8.

[21] *JAMA,* 94 (June 28, 1930), 2037.
[22] Editorial, *JAMA,* 95 (October 25, 1930), 1267.
[23] HD, *Proceedings* (82 Annual Session, June, 1931), p. 24.
[24] HD, *Proceedings* (83 Annual Session, May, 1932), p. 2.

For a period of several months its case-method treatment of group plans drew attention largely to the more disreputable types and, by emphasizing their defects and minimizing their virtues, placed the whole development in an unfavorable light.[25] The process of educating the public to the disadvantages it found in group health insurance might have been a gradual one but for an incident that occurred in late November.

The Committee on the Costs of Medical Care

At this time the independent Committee on the Costs of Medical Care, organized May 17, 1927, and financed by eight philanthropic foundations, closed it monumental five-year study of the health needs and resources of the nation and published its final reports.[26] Composed of 23 members with medical degrees, drawn from both public health work and private practice, as well as five prominent economists, 11 representatives from the general public and a few others, the varied composition of this committee of 45 members justified confidence in the impartiality of its work.[27] It had already published some of its 26 fact-finding studies and issued other reports that challenged faith in the adequacy of hospital facilities and medical care. Its alarming disclosures confirmed the findings of other authorities whose publications failed to arouse much national interest.[28]

[25] The *Journal's* survey of prepayment plans appeared under the heading "New Forms of Medical Practice." *JAMA,* 99 (October 8, 1932), 1267–68. The first cases considered were largely nondescript schemes that frequently combined medical and hospitalization benefits. Not until the issue of January 14, 1933, did it begin to discuss purely hospitalization schemes considering first the Baylor plan. *JAMA,* 100 (January 14, 1933), 121–23.

[26] *Medical Care for the American People: the Final Report* (The Committee on the Costs of Medical Care, Publication No. 28 [Chicago: The University of Chicago Press, 1932]), pp. vi–viii. The committee first referred to itself as the Committee on the Cost of Medical Care but later used the plural, "Costs."

[27] *The Five-Year Program* (The Committee on the Cost of Medical Care, Publication No. 1 [Washington, D. C.]), p. 6. Ray Lyman Wilbur, who held a medical degree and was Secretary of Interior during the Hoover administration, was appointed chairman of the committee, and Harry H. Moore became the director of the study. Besides Wilbur, who was elected president of the AMA in 1923, two other members of the committee later served as president, namely, Malcom L. Harris (1929) and Nathan B. Van Etten (1940). Olin West was the secretary of the AMA at the time of his appointment to the committee. Fishbein, *History of AMA*, pp. 1190, 334, 384.

[28] Michael Davis in *Paying Your Sickness Bills* (Chicago: University of Chicago Press, 1931), presented a dark picture of the inadequacy of medical care

With an astonishing mass of data that almost defies summarization, the committee's studies showed the inadequacies and inequalities of medical and hospital service, and the inability of a large percentage of the population to purchase it. Whereas one of its studies set the required number of physicians for adequate medical service at 134.71 for each 100,000 population, it found that the distribution among states in 1927 ranged from 71 in South Carolina to 200 in California. Accepting a ratio of 462 general hospital beds to 100,000 as the need, it found a disparity in 1930 varying from 142 in Mississippi to 654 in Colorado, with a total of nine states below 200.[29] Another study noted that 30.3 per cent of the families in the United States had incomes of $1,400 and under in 1928, and that in the twenties one-fourth of the persons treated in hospitals (exclusive of those treating mental and tubercular patients) could provide no payment for medical care.[30]

Viewed in the light of the convincing evidence of its exhaustive survey, the committee's majority report appeared quite moderate, although calling for substantial changes in the administration of medical care. It recommended the disposal of medical services "largely by organized groups of physicians, dentists, nurses, pharmacists, and other associated personnel" whose work should be centered around a hospital.[31] It advocated the enlargement of all basic health services and recommended "that the study, evaluation, and co-ordination of medical service be considered

---

and the inability of many people to pay for it, while the next year, A. M. Simons and Nathan Sinai, *The Way of Health Insurance,* urged compulsory health insurance as the only adequate solution for American health problems.

[29] Lee and Jones, *Fundamentals of Medical Care,* pp. 114–16; 119–21. The AMA's attention had already been called to very serious problems arising from the poor distribution of medical service. The National Grange, in session at Cleveland, Ohio, sent a telegram to the House of Delegates on November 24, 1927, urging it to "avert a general breakdown in rural medical service, which, unless present tendencies are arrested and corrected, appears to be inevitable." *AMA Bulletin,* 23 (April, 1928), 100.

[30] Louis S. Reed, *The Ability to Pay for Medical Care* (The Committee on the Costs of Medical Care, Publication No. 25 [Chicago: University of Chicago Press, 1933]), pp. 11, 1. The author cites the source of the figures on family income and shows how they were determined.

[31] *Medical Care for the American People,* p. xvi. Besides the majority report, there were several minority reports. The first minority report, signed by nine physicians including Malcom L. Harris, Olin West, and Nathan B. Van Etten, leaders of the AMA, disapproved of the idea of voluntary health insurance. Kirby S. Howlett and Robert Wilson, two other signers, approved of most of the first minority report but favored compulsory health insurance. Two dentists issued a separate report and Walton H. Hamilton and Edgar Sydenstricker each prepared separate statements. Their reports and statements are given in *ibid.,* pp. 150–201.

important functions for every state and local community. . . ." Stressing the need for better trained physicians, its most startling recommendation urged the adoption of group payment "through the use of insurance, through the use of taxation, or through the use of both these methods" for meeting the costs of medical care. While expressing approval of the idea of group payment plans, the committee cautiously recommended the continuation of the individual fee method for those who preferred it, and a clear distinction in all group plans between the costs of medical service and the cash benefits that the schemes provided.[32]

The Journal Attacks the Committee

Publication of the majority report quickly alarmed the *Journal* whose editor, Morris Fishbein, had long been irritated by the committee's work.[33] Even before reviewing much of the evidence upon which the committee based its report, and without waiting for any action of the House of Delegates, he launched a bitter attack upon the committee. Noting the "personal bias" for health insurance schemes of Harry H. Moore, the director of the studies, he wrote that the majority recommendation for group insurance came as no surprise. Observing that reports which the committee had already published indicated its final conclusions, he added:

> So definite was the trend of the committee's studies in this direction that one must review the expenditure of almost a million dollars by the committee and its final report with mingled amusement and regret. A colored boy spent a dollar taking twenty rides on the merry-go-round. When he got off, his mammy said: "Boy, you spent yo' money but where you been?"[34]

The editor then called the recommendation for the administration of

[32] *Ibid.,* p. xvi.

[33] See Editorial, *JAMA,* 95 (October 25, 1930), 1267. Other signs had already appeared of a sentiment within the AMA unfavorable to the Committee on the Costs of Medical Care. At the Philadelphia session of 1931, an unsuccessful attempt was made to get the Association to object officially to the name of this committee and to try to have it changed. Some thought that the very name of the committee attached too much significance to physicians' fees rather than other costs of illness. See Albert Soiland, HD, *Proceedings* (82 Annual Session, June, 1931), pp. 31, 34. One physician, L. B. McBrayer, criticised the name of the committee as early as 1929 in *AMA Bulletin,* 24 (December, 1929), 244.

[34] Editorial, *JAMA,* 99 (December 3, 1932), 1950.

medical service by organized medical groups as service rendered by "medical soviets."[35]

Nor did Fishbein's instant outburst quickly subside. Commenting upon the announced plans for carrying out, with practical demonstrations, the recommendations of the committee's majority report, the editor remarked in the next issue of the *Journal* that:

> As might be expected, the economists, particularly those with socialistic leanings, who have found in the Committee on the Costs of Medical Care an outlet for views which they could not express in business, as well as employment for more statisticians and economists, are already active in developing a new group.[36]

Avoiding any serious refutation of the committee's case, he then proceeded to attack those who planned to experiment with the committee's recommendations.

Criticisms of Specific Plans

Aiding the editor's efforts to discredit the committee and its proposals, another section of the *Journal* continued to review cases of group insurance. Turning finally to those that provided only for hospitalization benefits, it drew up 15 weaknesses in such schemes in the issue of January 21, 1933, while listing only four advantages. Contending that the growth of group hospitalization plans resulted from the desperate efforts of many hospitals to find "any port in a storm," several of its objections stressed the alleged disastrous effects of commercialism, competition, and lay influence over hospital service under such schemes, which, it felt, would soon defile medical standards. It charged that such plans divided the medical profession as well as hospitals, and loosened the control of local societies over medical service. It also contended that hospitals became "preferred creditors" for many patients who did not understand that their hospitalization benefits did not include physicians' services, and that such plans offered protection only to wage earners, and to them only when employed. Standing out among other

[35] *Ibid.* Even the medical book review section of this issue took an excursion into politics. Along with reviews of medical books there appeared, on page 1974, a very favorable one on James Montgomery Beck, *Our Wonderland of Bureaucracy: A Study of the Growth of Bureaucracy in the Federal Government, and Its Destructive Effect upon the Constitution.*

[36] Editorial, *JAMA,* 99 (December 10, 1932), 2034.

objections was the Association's contention that such plans generally led to compulsory health insurance. It did not find the system, which it conceded could be actuarially sound and also economically stabilizing to both patients and hospitals, able to overcome what it considered its serious weaknesses.[37]

While the Association did a great deal to discredit the Committee on the Costs of Medical Care, the committee actually had a positive influence on the AMA. President Malcom L. Harris called attention to the merit of its earlier work in 1930 and told the Detroit session that some of the Association's most serious challenges lay in dealing with the economic problems of medical care. He urged the House of Delegates to establish a bureau of medical economics, which would investigate the economic aspects of medical problems and make its studies available to the profession. Although not immediately established, the new bureau commenced its work between the annual sessions of 1931 and 1932.[38]

From the time the Association began to notice the growth of group hospitalization schemes, until the end of the Hoover era, it obstructed their development. While the AMA had no *official* policy, the leaders in its most influential positions improvised an unauthorized one of their own. The *Journal's* criticism of the theory and operation of group hospitalization schemes had so broadened by the later part of January, 1933, that probably no plan could have escaped its condemnation. While the Association had much more to say about the voluntary insurance question, its attitude, as later discussed, matured during the New Deal era.

[37] "New Forms of Medical Practice: Hospital Insurance Schemes," *JAMA*, 100 (January 21, 1933), 192–94. For another treatment of alleged defects in voluntary plans, which repeats most of these listed here, see the paper presented by R. G. Leland to the Annual Congress on Medical Education and Licensure, February 14, 1933, "Prepayment Plans of Hospital Care," *JAMA*, 100 (March 25, 1933), 871.

[38] HD, *Proceedings* (81 Annual Session, June, 1930), pp. 2–3; Fishbein, *History of AMA*, p. 389.

Chapter 10 RESPONSE TO THE NEW DEAL, 1933–1937

WHEN THE NEW ADMINISTRATION took control in Washington in March, 1933, the American Medical Association had not overcome the shock brought on by the revival of health insurance agitation. While the *Journal* opposed the voluntary health insurance movement and attacked the Committee on the Costs of Medical Care, the Association had done little to develop a constructive approach to the health problems that faced the nation. Relying largely on conventional forms of practice and payment for meeting the nation's medical needs, its policies had remained virtually unshaken by the ravages of the Great Depression.[1]

Crisis in Medical Care

Although the Roosevelt administration sought the co-operation of the AMA in launching some of its basic programs, it required no professional assistance to discover the magnitude of the national crisis in medical care. In fact, the growing ranks of unemployed that probably exceeded 14,000,000 early in 1933 offered adequate proof that the medical crisis was only one of many.[2] In the absence of professional

[1] A few county medical societies began to experiment with plans for providing the needy with medical care during the early years of the depression, but in 1935 the Bureau of Medical Economics noted that county societies offering such programs, or planning to, did not exceed 100. HD, *Proceedings* (86 Annual Session, June, 1935) p. 12.

[2] The Bureau of Labor Statistics of the United States Department of Labor set the unemployment figure in 1933 at about 12,634,000 in an estimated potential working force of 50,403,000. The Labor Research Association's estimate of unemployment was 16,138,000. Broadus Mitchell, *Depression Decade: from New Era through New Deal, 1929–1941* (Vol. 9 of *The Economic History of the United States,* Henry David and others, eds., [New York: Rinehart & Company,

leadership in advancing broad and effective programs of medical care, great social pressures swelling behind the dams of governmental inertia had moved the nation in directions that presented formidable dangers to the profession.

The depression not only created grave national problems, but brought into clearer view a great number that had long existed. It set before a troubled public the striking contrast between the nation's technological advance and its social progress. Little of the wealth that the twentieth century created ever reached the masses, and the age of machine production left with the working classes as many burdens as it lifted. Low wages and long hours still accompanied industrial advances, while the threat of sickness, unemployment, and the likelihood of insecurity in old age loomed ever before a struggling army of wage earners.

The nation matched its failure to deal with the problems of industrialization with equal unconcern for protecting its health resources. Statistical proof of declining national death rates from most major diseases, coupled with an unsteady but rising expenditure for public health, appealed more to the nation's pride than to its desire for greater improvement.[3] Accumulating evidence from many sources, however, supported the disturbing conclusions of the Committee on the Costs of Medical Care. Although the measurement of public health facilities on a city or county basis has only limited validity, it roughly presents the general picture. While the nation had 1,208 cities of 8,000 population or over in 1930, it had only 1,511 child health centers for its 3,072 counties, and one-sixth of these were located in one state.[4] Only

---

Inc., 1947]), pp. 92, 451, 453. For other estimates ranging from 13,577,000 to over 16,000,000 see Paul Webbink, "Unemployment in the United States, 1930–1940," American Economic Association, *Papers and Proceedings,* 30 (February, 1941), 250–51, in David A. Shannon, ed., *The Great Depression* (Englewood Cliffs, N. J.: Prentice-Hall, Inc., 1960), p. 6. The AMA recognized that "about seventeen million persons were in need of assistance beyond their own resources to provide the necessities of life." Bureau of Medical Economics, "Care of the Indigent Sick" (Chicago: American Medical Association), p. 46.

[3] *Historical Statistics of the United States, 1789–1945* (U. S. Bureau of Census [Washington, D. C.: Government Printing Office, 1949]), pp. 48, 52. There was a considerable increase in the ratio of deaths for each 100,000 persons resulting from diseases of the heart and from cancer and other types of malignant tumors. The expenditures of the United States Public Health Service increased from $2,858,628 in 1915 to $12,080,211 in 1933, and reached $16,130,841 in 1932. In 1920, 1921, and 1922, it exceeded any of these figures.

[4] *United States Fifteenth Census, 1930, Population,* Vol. 2, p. 9; *The World Almanac* (1931), p. 485; *Child Health Centers: A Survey* (White House Conference on Child Health and Protection [New York: The Century Co., 1932]), pp. 6–7, 3.

519 counties had full-time county health organizations in 1933, and in these the average annual per capita expenditure amounted to only 28 cents, a sum that showed a slight drop from the figures reached in the late twenties. So limited was the interest of some states in problems of social welfare that not until 1933 did the birth and death registration area of the United States Bureau of Census embrace the entire population.[5]

Added to the nation's apathy toward problems of public health were wide sectional disparities in the quantity and quality of medical facilities. Although 14 of the Southern states from West Virginia to Texas had nearly as large a population as 11 others north of the Potomac (besides the District of Columbia), their capital investment in hospitals in 1928 amounted to hardly more than a third, and the total number of hospital beds a little less than one-half that of the latter group.[6] The disparity in the distribution of medical facilities among sections, however, did not appear nearly as great as that among races. Two terms of the Roosevelt administration had passed when Florida, which led the Southern states in the number of general, nonfederally-owned hospital accommodations for Negroes, reported only 1.5 such beds for each thousand population, with 3.2 for its white population against the recommended minimum of 4.62 general hospital beds, whether federally, state, or privately owned. But even this low standard exceeded Mississippi's ratio which stood at 0.5 and 3.2 for its Negro and white population respectively. Added to this disparity was the great dearth of Negro physicians, that threatened to become worse when a 30 per cent decline in enrollment in Negro medical schools set in between 1926 and 1937.[7]

Not only did the Great Depression and the inadequacy of health and medical facilities make the population more receptive to novel ideas for

[5] Harry S. Mustard, *Government in Public Health,* p. 133; *Historical Statistics of the United States, 1789–1945,* p. 45.

[6] C. Rufus Rorem, *The Public's Investment in Hospitals* (Chicago: The University of Chicago Press, 1930), p. 43. The states included in the Southern group are Ala., Ark., Fla., Ga., Ky., La., Miss., N.C., Okla., S.C., Tenn., Tex., Va., and W. Va. Those in the area north of the Potomac included Conn., Del., Me., Md., Mass., N.H., N.J., N.Y., Penn., R.I., and Vt., as well as the District of Columbia.

[7] Mott and Roemer, *Rural Health and Medical Care,* p. 239; Bernhard J. Stern, *American Medical Practice in the Perspectives of a Century* (New York: The Commonwealth Fund, 1946), p. 134. Although the ratios cited for hospital beds in Florida and Mississippi include accommodations only in general, nonfederally-owned hospitals, whereas the ratio of 4.62 beds for each thousand population includes also accommodations in federally-owned, general hospitals, the federally-owned general hospital beds in these states were probably too few to change significantly the ratios given.

meeting national health problems, but the public's stake in the ownership of health facilities increased its concern. In 1934, 66 per cent of the nation's hospital beds were in governmental institutions, and 14 per cent of a total health bill of $3,500,000,000 was paid through taxation. Aware of its hospital investment, which reached $3,000,000,000 by 1930, the public sought a responsibility for deciding the economic problems of medical care somewhat in proportion to its financial investment. In addition, the 1,500,000 Americans employed in various health and medical services on the eve of the depression began to challenge the position that 210,000 physicians and dentists occupied in largely representing the nation's entire health forces on matters of health and medicine.[8]

Response to Emergency Legislation

Amid pressures that threatened traditional approaches to problems of medical care, the American Medical Association stood guard for the protection of the profession's welfare. The passage in May, 1933, of the Emergency Relief Act, which created the Federal Emergency Relief Administration, provided an occasion to test the AMA's response to the emergency features of the New Deal program. This act allowing the use of federal funds for medical relief in cases where the destitution of the sick and injured and the exhaustion of local resources deprived them of medical care, vitally touched the Association's interests. Bidding for the medical profession's support of this emergency program, Harry L. Hopkins, the relief administrator, discreetly sought the AMA's cooperation in formulating rules regulating the disposal of federal medical relief funds. After collaborating with officials of the AMA, he issued FERA "Rules and Regulations No. 7," which showed indications of the Association's influence.[9]

This program, conforming to standards for administering indigent medical care that the local medical societies had already endorsed in Webster County, Iowa, and elsewhere, received the AMA's support. Adequate safeguards protected the "traditional family and family phy-

[8] N. W. Faxon, "Half-Empty Hospitals," *Survey Graphic,* 23 (December, 1934), 604; William Trufant Foster, "Medicine's Right to Control . . . ," *ibid.,* p. 588; Michael M. Davis, foreword in Rorem, *Public Investment in Hospitals,* p. x; Simons and Sinai, *The Way of Health Insurance,* p. 174.

[9] HD, *Proceedings* (85 Annual Session, June, 1934), p. 15.

sician relationship" and preserved the profession's freedom. The medical profession became an integral part of the organization, providing the service and sharing the responsibility of determining the fee schedule necessary for the receipt of emergency funds. The ruling, largely based on economy, that no hospital fees would be paid from the $500,000,000 appropriated in the Emergency Relief Act strengthened the traditional pattern of house visitation and prevented professional subservience to lay administered hospitals.[10] The AMA approved the government's policy of not requiring membership in a local society of physicians participating in the program and raised no objection to the small medical fees that the government allowed. Although the advance of the program brought growing criticism from the Association's leadership, the plan lost little of its popularity among physicians in general, and by the fall of 1935 embraced 4,359 practitioners, dentists, and druggists in the Los Angeles area alone. While becoming increasingly fearful of the government's role in the provision of medical care, the AMA found its interests well protected and soon regretted the regulation that allowed no expenditure of federal funds for hospitalization when adequate home treatment became impossible.[11]

Other instances of the Association's willingness to co-operate with the New Deal emergency relief program soon appeared. The Civil Works Administration, which commenced operations in November, 1933, incorporated the idea of work relief and bestowed some of the privileges of permanent federal employees on those engaged in its projects. Since employees of the CWA became eligible, under the United States Employees' Compensation Act of 1916, for medical care and hospitalization

[10] *Ibid.*, p. 15; Bureau of Medical Economics, "Care of Indigent Sick," pp. 40, 47–49; Pierce Williams, "Alternatives to Compulsory Public Health Insurance," The American Academy of Political and Social Science, *Annals,* 170 (November, 1933), 132–33.

[11] Editorial, *JAMA,* 102 (January 13, 1934), 133; *The Literary Digest* (August 10, 1935), 15; HD, *Proceedings* (85 Annual Session, June, 1934), p. 15; Bureau of Medical Economics, "Care of Indigent Sick," pp. 112–14. One writer, noticing the growth of unfavorable comment of the FERA from the Association's leadership, suspects that the initial popularity of the program among local physicians accounts for the AMA's support before the program had been well tested. David Gordon Bridgman, "The American Medical Association and the Great Depression," (unpublished Ph.D. dissertation, Harvard University Library, 1956), pp. 166–68. The inadequacy of the program is described by another who says that it was "virtually swamped in the twenty-six states attempting it." Dixon Wecter, *The Age of the Great Depression, 1929–1941* (Vol. 13 of *A History of American Life,* Arthur M. Schlesinger and Dixon Ryan Fox, eds. [New York, The Macmillan Company, 1948]), p. 274, used with permission.

at government expense for injuries and diseases acquired in or directly attributable to their employment, the matter concerned the AMA. The approximately 4,000 physicians already registered for providing medical service under the act could not administer to about 4,000,000 scattered employees of the CWA, and the Association wanted the government to recognize any of its members as approved for such practice. Although the government rejected this idea, it nevertheless relied upon the AMA for advice in drawing up regulations and worked closely with state and county medical societies in recruiting qualified physicians to handle medical cases arising from CWA employment.[12]

The National Recovery Act of June 16, 1933, provided for a complex system of business codes and for the Public Works Administration, but its passage created no immediate problem for the Association. Unlike the works program established by the CWA, that of the PWA and of the Works Progress Administration of 1935 (later Works Projects Administration) offered none of the benefits of regular federal employees to their workers.[13] The Association's immunity from the pressure of NRA regulation seemed to have disappeared in July, however, when the administration promulgated the supplementary President's Re-employment Agreement. Months before industrial trickery and evasion had largely wrecked the NRA program, the government called on all employers to accept blanket operational codes. Some 2,333,000 employers of 16,000,000 workers soon displayed the Blue Eagle, which became in many instances no more than a decoy.[14]

The rapid growth of the falcon family, however, made a strong impression on some parts of the medical profession. Many physicians throughout the nation signed codes prescribing the hours and wages of their employees. Others, with more reluctance, asked the Association for advice. Mounting professional interest spurred the Association into action, as the Executive Committee of the Board of Trustees turned its attention to the matter on August 4, 1933. A letter of August 7 to the National Recovery Administration called for the government's interpretation of the relation of the NRA to the medical profession, but the

[12] HD, *Proceedings* (85 Annual Session, June, 1934), p. 15.

[13] The fact that the CWA "operated straight from Washington . . . avoiding local red tape" probably explains why its workers came under the Employees' Compensation Act of 1916, whereas the PWA and WPA were state and federal co-operative adventures. See Wecter, *Age of Great Depression,* p. 74, for an account of the CWA.

[14] Mitchell, *Depression Decade,* pp. 239–47.

reply, over two weeks later, left most of the Association's questions unanswered.[15]

Occupying a fringe area in the application of NRA legislation, the bewildered Association passed the problem on to the local societies. While determined to violate neither the "spirit" nor "letter" of the code agreement plan, it found difficulty in reconciling parts of the program with medical ethics. Professional display of the Blue Eagle brought the threat of unfair competition and public discrimination against nonsigners of blanket codes. While the trustees of the AMA declined to enter into the President's Re-employment Agreement, they did not advise local societies against such action. Instead, they urged all societies disturbed by this matter to consult the National Recovery Administration about changes in their code that would eliminate unfair competition and induce all doctors in a locality to sign it.[16]

In addition to the administration's careful concern for medical interests in launching its emergency program, the AMA had other reasons for looking with favor on some of the President's policies. It seemed particularly pleased when the new administration, among its first acts, defied enormous pressure and greatly reduced the appropriation for veterans' benefits. The passage of an act that deprived all veterans of World War I with nonservice-connected disabilities of pensions, except those who had served at least 90 days and were totally disabled, harmonized well with the AMA's ideas. When Congress soon passed a measure over the President's veto that allowed free medical service and transportation for impecunious veterans with nonservice-connected disabilities, the Association regretted that Roosevelt's views had been rejected.[17]

Committee on Economic Security

A period of growing tension between the AMA and the administration, however, followed more than a year of rather cordial relations.

[15] HD, *Proceedings* (85 Annual Session, June, 1934), pp. 13–14.

[16] *Ibid.*, p. 14. The AMA offered no explanation of what changes might be secured in the codes under which many physicians practiced to make them acceptable to all doctors. It seems merely to have shifted a difficult problem to local societies without offering any really helpful advice.

[17] Katherine Mayo, *Soldiers What Next!* (Boston: Houghton Mifflin Company, 1934), pp. 199–201; HD, *Proceedings* (85 Annual Session, June, 1934), p. 16. See p. 32 for very favorable comments on the administration's veterans' policy.

In June, 1934, the President created the Committee on Economic Security, which was to report by December on a sound program of social legislation for consideration by the first session of the Seventy-fourth Congress. This committee, headed by the Secretary of Labor, included also the Attorney General, the Secretary of Treasury, the Secretary of Agriculture, and the Federal Emergency Relief Administrator, and was provided with a technical staff under the direction of the prominent labor economist, Edwin E. Witte. In addition, the President's plan called for an advisory council on economic security that included a special medical advisory committee (known as the Medical Advisory Board) composed of prominent American physicians.[18]

Although the administration appointed 11 members to this committee, without the assistance of the AMA, the Association did not object to its creation. The Secretary of Labor, Frances Perkins, discreetly informed the organization of the administration's plans and quickly received assurance of its willingness to co-operate with the Committee on Economic Security. The AMA offered the committee access to information on health and medical problems that the Bureau of Medical Economics had compiled, and made the bureau's staff available to the committee for consultation and advice.[19]

While harmony prevailed between the Association and the Committee on Economic Security during the earliest stages of the latter's work, friction between the two finally developed. A meeting of the Medical Advisory Board in Washington, D.C., November 14–15, 1934, attended also by R. G. Leland and A. M. Simons of the AMA's Bureau of Medical Economics, and Edgar Sydenstricker and I. S. Falk of the technical staff of the Committee on Economic Security, brought out differences in the thinking of the AMA and the advisory board on one

[18] Francis Perkins, "The Way of Security," *Survey Graphic,* 23 (December, 1934), 620; *JAMA,* 103 (November 10, 1934), 1454.

[19] *JAMA,* 103 (November 10, 1934), 1454. Those appointed to this committee were Walter L. Bierring (Iowa), Rexwald Brown (Calif.), James D. Bruce (Mich.), George W. Crile (Ohio), Harvey Cushing (Conn.), Robert B. Greenough (Mass.), J. Shelton Horsley (Va.), James A. Miller (N.Y.), Thomas Parran, Jr. (N.Y.), George M. Piersol (Pa.), and Stewart R. Roberts (Ga.). This list included several prominent physicians. Bierring was president of the AMA; Miller, of the American College of Physicians, and Greenough of the American College of Surgeons. A daughter of the prominent physician, Harvey Cushing, was married to James Roosevelt, son of the President, on June 3, 1930. Editorial, *JAMA,* 103 (November 24, 1934), 1627; *JAMA,* 103 (November 10, 1934), 1455. Elizabeth H. Thomson, *Harvey Cushing: Surgeon, Author, Artist* (New York: Henry Schuman, 1950), p. 274.

hand and the representatives of the administration on the other. While the group contemplated means of expanding government health services and providing medical care at government expense for dependents and classes with certain diseases, it encountered greater difficulty in discussing the health insurance issue. The Medical Advisory Board asked for an extension of time to consider this question and the technical staff agreed to co-operate with Leland and Simons in further health insurance studies.[20]

The passage of a few weeks, however, seemed to confirm the Association's fear that the administration had inclined itself toward a legislative program out of line with the organization's interest. It found the report that the Committee on Economic Security, submitted to the President in December, particularly disturbing. While disavowing intention of recommending any health insurance plan, the committee stressed the value of state health insurance systems that provided medical care for all, and a partial income replacement for losses wage earners sustained in periods of illness. While the committee referred to payroll deductions as the method for meeting the major costs of the program, it mentioned the probable need of federal subsidies and supervision for the safe and solvent operation of compulsory schemes.[21] Some of the 11 principles upheld in this report, as a basis for adequate medical care, reminded the AMA of earlier political battles and revived issues which it had fought against for many years.

As the President's recommendations to the first session of the Seventy-fourth Congress would probably include many proposals of the committee, the Association awaited the delivery of his message on January 4, 1935, with considerable anxiety. The *Journal,* a week later, however, found encouragement in the fact that the address made no direct mention of health insurance, although it dealt at length with social insurance issues and the matter of subsidies for welfare programs, and added:

> More than anything else the medical profession fears hasty action and the setting up of some scheme which, once established, will ride, like the old man of the sea, on the back of medical progress and impede its advancement.[22]

While many physicians opposed the President's comprehensive program, his omission of recommendations for compulsory health insurance met

[20] *JAMA,* 103 (November 24, 1934), 1627.
[21] HD, *Proceedings* (Special Session, February, 1935), pp. 3–4.
[22] Editorial, *JAMA,* 104 (January 12, 1935), 122.

with general approval. Two days after the address, Harvey Cushing of the Medical Advisory Board, commended the President for omitting direct reference to compulsory health insurance.[23]

Attitude Toward Social Security Legislation

The AMA watched political developments in the national capital with increasing interest and showed no surprise that bills proposing a broad social security system soon appeared in the Seventy-fourth Congress. On January 17, when the President submitted another congressional message Senator Robert F. Wagner of New York introduced the "Wagner Bill" (S. 1130) that had as its counterparts in the House, H. R. 4120 and H. R. 4142, introduced respectively by Representatives Robert L. Doughton of North Carolina and David J. Lewis of Maryland. In addition, the President submitted along with his message the report of the Committee on Economic Security, which increased the Association's fear that this report might add to the popularity of proposals for compulsory health insurance.[24]

The *Journal* quickly recognized the revival of old issues in these new measures and saw in them the ghost of the old Sheppard-Towner Act. It denounced the principle of federal subsidies to the states for the maintenance of health and welfare programs and the extension of federal control over such state activities. It deplored the fact that the Wagner bill provided for no centralization of the scattered health functions of the federal government, and showed that it actually more widely dispersed responsibility for the government's public health work.[25] Despite some objections to all these measures, however, the AMA officially endorsed many of their provisions, and Walter Bierring, president of the Association, told the House Committee on Ways and Means on January 31, that Title VII of H. R. 4120 (for expanding health facilities), should be supported. Nevertheless his view appeared in striking contrast to a communication from the Illinois State Medical Society submitted by Representative Everett M. Dirksen of Illinois, which charged that the bill threatened the very foundations of private medical practice.[26]

[23] Thomson, *Harvey Cushing,* p. 301.

[24] HD, *Proceedings* (86 Annual Session, June, 1935), p. 15; HD, *Proceedings* (Special Session, February, 1935), p. 9.

[25] Editorial, *JAMA,* 104 (January 26, 1935), 319–20.

[26] House Committee on Ways and Means, Seventy-fourth Congress, first session, *Hearings on H. R. 4120* (Washington: Government Printing Office, 1935), pp. 650, 1140.

Convinced that the Seventy-fourth Congress would probably enact far-reaching social legislation, the trustees felt that the Association should officially declare its views on several current national issues. To accomplish this, they resorted to the unusual expedient of convoking the House of Delegates in special session.[27] The group, assembling in Chicago, February 15, 1935, heard J. H. J. Upham, chairman of the Board of Trustees, summarize the political problems that confronted the organization. He insisted that the Association must once again declare its position on the extension of federal or state subsidized medical service outside the branches of the military services, beyond the classes that normally received public-supported medical service, and beyond the experiments in government-subsidized medical service that had met the approval of local medical societies. He maintained that the House of Delegates should announce its position on the 11 principles of medical care that the Committee on Economic Security had endorsed. He urged the body to express its view on the question of federal subsidies for state medical services and the provision of the Wagner bill that placed medical affairs under a lay board in the Department of Labor. He also suggested that the Association take some action on the Epstein bill, a compulsory health insurance measure that had aroused the interest of some state legislatures, and concluded with the vague proposal that the Association perfect plans for the further improvement and better distribution of medical services.[28]

The response of the House of Delegates to Upham's suggestions could hardly have been more gratifying. A special committee that the session appointed to "crystallize the expressions of the delegates and bring recommendations to the House for final action" hurriedly carried out its assignment and presented a report that the body adopted.[29] This report ignored the basic philosophy underlying proposals for social security programs, but actually offered no objection to much that was fundamental within the bills. While agreeing that emergency conditions sometimes justified federal aid for the care of indigents, it implied opposition to the extension of such aid under ordinary conditions. It deplored the fact that the Wagner bill provided for the creation of a

[27] The special session in 1935 was only the second in the AMA's history. The first occurred during World War I. HD, *Proceedings* (Special Session, September, 1938), p. 6.

[28] HD, *Proceedings* (Special Session, February, 1935), p. 4.

[29] *Ibid.*, p. 5. The members of this committee were Harry H. Wilson (Calif.), N. B. Van Etten (N.Y.), E. H. Cary (Tex.), W. F. Braasch (Minn.), Warren F. Draper (Va.), F. S. Crockett (Ind.), and E. F. Cody (Mass.).

social insurance board with many functions of a medical nature without specifying the qualifications of members of this board. It also criticized those provisions of the bill that placed the lay controlled Children's Bureau in charge of federal medical expenditures for child and maternal health.[30]

The committee did not concentrate its attack solely on the Wagner bill. It referred to the "inconsistencies and incompatibilities" of the studies of the Committee on Economic Security and called the Epstein bill a "vicious, deceptive, dangerous and demoralizing measure." It charged that this bill encouraged multiple taxation, extravagant administration, and inordinate costs, opening the way to "social and financial bankruptcy."[31] Although the report offered no refutation of arguments advanced for a comprehensive system of social security, it served the purpose of hurriedly setting forth the Association's attitude on important proposed legislation.

The special February session not only gave authoritative sanction to the opinion that AMA leaders had expressed about the Wagner and Epstein bills, but threw additional light upon the growth of unfriendly relations between the Association and the national administration. The trustees charged that the administration refused to reveal the names of physicians it had selected to serve on the Medical Advisory Board of the Committee on Economic Security until just before the board's first meeting. They inferred that the presence of such compulsory health insurance advocates as Isidore Falk, Michael M. Davis, and Nathan Sinai on the technical staff pretty well offset the later addition of R. G. Leland and A. M. Simons of the AMA's Bureau of Medical Economics. The trustees also referred to the administration's appointment of a former member of the Committee on the Costs of Medical Care, Edgar Sydenstricker, as director of the technical staff's medical service division, whose liberal views on social security caused him to reject even the final majority report of that committee.[32]

[30] HD, *Proceedings* (Special Session, February, 1935), p. 4. The House of Delegates worked out no clear position on most social insurance issues. While maintaining that aid to the indigent should come normally from state rather than federal sources, the social security legislation included much more. It called for an old-age assistance and an old-age insurance program and a system of state-administered unemployment compensation. The AMA raised no objections to the principles behind these programs aimed at reducing indigency. Unfortunately, the House of Delegates left the matter unclarified and the centennial history speaks of the AMA's opposition to the Wagner Act. Fishbein, *History of AMA,* pp. 416–17.

[31] HD, *Proceedings* (Special Session, February, 1935), p. 5.

[32] *Ibid.,* pp. 2–3.

Growing popular approval of a broad program of social security confronted the AMA, when the House of Delegates opened its Eighty-sixth annual session at Atlantic City in June. The legislative body, however, showed no intention of modifying its official attitude toward what was now called the Wagner-Doughton-Lewis bill. Declining to wrestle with most basic social security issues, the trustees' report, which the House accepted, repeated the Association's standard objections to the measure, advancing in addition only a few novel, tangential criticisms. Among these was the contention that the bill empowered the proposed social insurance board with the responsibility of making recommendations on such questions as social insurance, which convinced the delegates that this measure could lead directly to a federal compulsory health insurance system. The report also pointed out that the measure provided for the alleviation of the hazards of illness as well as of old age, unemployment, and dependency, but observed that the bill had been redrafted to provide for a social security instead of a social insurance board.[33]

Supplementing the trustees' comments on the alleged weaknesses of the bill, the Committee on Legislative Activities reported on prospects for the enactment of a comprehensive social security law. From its strategic observation posts, it concluded that the administration would press no sickness insurance proposal in the first, or probably the second, session of the Seventy-fourth Congress. It did report however that the administration would probably later present such a measure as a "trial horse" to observe popular reaction.[34]

Two months after the delegates adjourned, presidential approval of the amended Wagner-Doughton-Lewis bill on August 14 closed the first stage of the revived social insurance struggle. The AMA, however, dared not stack arms as long as the administration seemed disposed to risk a renewal of hostilities by testing the strength of the "trial horse." Yet, the beginning of the armed truce gave the Association a chance to reflect on the salients it had successfully defended and those it had lost. The AMA rejoiced that health insurance found no place in the measure and noted that even the word "illness" had been deleted from the title of the original Wagner-Doughton-Lewis bill. It believed that the establishment of a social security board rather than a social insurance board farther removed the nation from the threat of a federal compulsory

[33] HD, *Proceedings* (86 Annual Session, June, 1935), p. 16.

[34] *Ibid.*, p. 51. Members of the Committee on Legislative Activities closely watched political developments and frequently consulted with congressional leaders about various measures.

health insurance system.[35] On the other hand, the Association felt that the government had framed much of its permanent program on policies that should be reserved for emergencies only. Although the AMA largely ignored the plan of state and federal co-operation in the old-age and unemployment compensation systems that the act established, it was shocked at the provisions of federal aid for maternal, widow, and child welfare. The authorized annual appropriation of $24,750,000 for aid to dependent children, and $3,800,000 for maternal and child health,[36] as well as other large appropriations, made the old Sheppard-Towner Act appear almost innocuous.

The AMA saw some effective checks to the successful operation of the program. It warned that much of the act might be scrapped by the Supreme Court. Another difficulty that appeared especially formidable was the inadequate supply of trained and experienced medical assistants for administering the law. Yet, despite these problems, the AMA pledged the support of the medical profession in attempting to carry the law into effect.[37]

Attack on British System Challenged

Although disturbed by certain features of the social security legislation, the AMA had other reasons for fearing the gradual extension of government control over private medical practice. Growing interest in the operation of the British health insurance program threatened to undermine the Association's propaganda against it and weaken resistance to the compulsory health insurance movement in the United States. For many years the AMA attempted to convince the medical profession and the public of the failure of the British plan, supporting its contention with the frequent publication of derogatory letters from the London correspondent. Although authoritative British sources occasionally denied the truthfulness of these charges,[38] no thorough exposure of the Association's tactics occurred until 1934. In December, 1933, the American College of Dentists and the Michigan State Medical Society

[35] Editorial, *JAMA,* 105 (August 24, 1935), 601; J. William Holloway, Jr., "The Seventy-fourth Congress, First Session, and the Medical Profession," *AMA Bulletin,* 31 (January, 1936), 19.

[36] Wecter, *Age of Great Depression,* p. 181.

[37] Editorial, *JAMA,* 105 (August 24, 1935), 601.

[38] In 1926, after a careful investigation of the British health insurance system, a Royal Commission concluded: "We can say at once that we are satisfied that the Scheme of National Health Insurance has fully justified itself and has, on the whole, been successful in operation. . . . We are convinced that National Health Insurance has now become a permanent feature of the social system of this

financed Nathan Sinai and H. A. Luce in a study of the British system. Their extensive survey not only provided overwhelming testimony from prominent British physicians and others about the success of the compulsory system, but also revealed the source of the AMA's misinformation. The report disclosed that the Association's London correspondent was "neither in regular practice nor . . . a member of the British Medical Association."[39]

Gradually the lay press carried to the public favorable information about the British plan that had long been denied physicians in most of their professional organs. Sometimes direct refutations of the AMA's attacks on the British system by officials of the British Medical Association reached the public through the daily press. Periodicals started more frequent discussions of compulsory health insurance and reported on experiments abroad. The *Survey Graphic* devoted most of an issue in 1934 to the health insurance question and opened its pages to Michael M. Davis, who risked offending national pride in reporting on "How Europeans Pay Sickness Bills."[40]

---

country, and should be continued on its present compulsory and contributory basis." Representatives of the British Medical Association appeared before this commission expressing equally high approval. Among other things, they said, "Large numbers, indeed whole classes, of persons are now receiving a real medical attention which they formerly did not receive at all." G. F. McCleary, "Health Insurance in Europe," The Milbank Memorial Fund, *Quarterly,* Edgar Sydenstricker, ed., 12 (January, 1934), 13–14. See also Simons and Sinai, *The Way of Health Insurance,* p. 152, and Hugh Cabot, *The Doctor's Bill* (New York, Morningside Heights: Columbia University Press, 1935), pp. 174–75. Not all physicians were misled by the AMA's attack upon the British system. At the Annual Conference of Constituent State Medical Associations in Chicago, November, 1930, J. Rosslyn Earp of Colorado said: "If you will read the discussion at the last meeting of the British Medical Association, not through the columns of the London correspondent of Dr. Fishbein's little sheet, but through the official report in the British Medical Journal, I think that you will quickly realize that national health insurance is not so unpopular as it is generally imagined to be in this country." *AMA Bulletin,* 26 (February, 1931), 43. See remarks also of Henry O. Reik of New Jersey and W. C. Rappleye of Connecticut, pp. 46–47.

[39] HD, *Proceedings* (85 Annual Session, June, 1934), p. 40. Despite this exposure, the AMA seems to have exerted little effort for several years to acquire authoritative information about the British system. In 1938, the trustees' report finally noted that "arrangements . . . have been made whereby officials of the British Medical Association contribute regularly important statements on the medical economic conditions in Great Britain and as to the manner in which the British Medical Association is attempting to solve its problems." HD, *Proceedings* (89 Annual Session, June, 1938), p. 8. But see also p. 346 below for account of the London correspondent who continued to report.

[40] James Rorty, *American Medicine Mobilizes* (New York: W. W. Norton & Company, Publishers, 1939), p. 203; *Survey Graphic,* 23 (December, 1934), 617–19, 627–28.

Compulsory Health Insurance Agitation

While growing interest in European health insurance systems and the existence of regrettable features in the Social Security Act provided the Association with sufficient cause for alarm, it had other reasons for fearing the widespread adoption of compulsory health insurance. The trustees told the Atlantic City session in June, 1935, of the introduction of the Epstein bill and a similar measure into four state legislatures, and referred to the health insurance battle in California. Three months earlier, following a stormy session, the medical association of this Western state submitted a bill to the legislature providing for both voluntary and compulsory health insurance.[41] This incident not only increased the health insurance threat, but tended to discredit the AMA as the spokesman for American medicine. Although the trustees could report to the Kansas City session of 1936 that no legislature had passed such a bill, the news failed to comfort an organization still perturbed by the California association's action.[42]

Perhaps less significant than the conduct of the California medical society, but hardly less irritating, was the work of other groups within the profession that either expressed favorable views on unorthodox plans of medical service or in other ways undermined the Association's leadership. At least one group clamored for a complete state system of medical care and another ventured forth to bring in disquieting facts about the number of physicians who favored some type of health insurance. In October, 1933, Joseph Slavit organized The Medical League for Socialized Medicine, with headquarters in Brooklyn, and announced the league's platform. This organization sought adequate medical care for all, with medical facilities and physicians' services provided at government expense.[43] Although no great number of physicians joined the league, the publication of Slavit's views in widely read periodicals embarrassed the AMA, along with the unorthodox remarks of other physicians that the popular press occasionally carried.

The work of the Medical Advisory Committee of the American Foundation in 1936 appears to have disturbed the Association more

[41] HD, *Proceedings* (86 Annual Session, June, 1935), pp. 16–17; T. Henshaw Kelly, HD, *Proceedings* (86 Annual Session, June, 1935), p. 48; Editorial, *JAMA*, 104 (April 6, 1935), 1243–44. For the AMA's criticism of the bill see Editorial, *JAMA*, 104 (May 11, 1935), 1757–58.

[42] HD, *Proceedings* (87 Annual Session, May, 1936), p. 16.

[43] Brown, *Physicians and Medical Care*, pp. 197–98; Joseph Slavit, "The Challenge of Socialized Medicine," *Survey Graphic*, 23 (December, 1934), 597.

than Slavit's activities. This committee, composed of over 100 prominent physicians, sponsored a survey of the views of 2,200 doctors about the social aspects of medical practice. From every state, both rural and urban, physicians submitted data that showed endorsement of ideas out of line with the AMA's policies. A surprising number expressed approval of the adoption of compulsory health insurance, many favored the idea of some form of health insurance, and a large number saw a need for greater public aid for medical education and public health services.[44] Not the least disastrous effect of this survey, from the AMA's point of view, was the organization of the Committee of Physicians for the Improvement of Medical Care, whose moderate proposals for greater federal, state, and local government co-operation in establishing adequate public health facilities appeared dangerous.[45]

Combating the Compulsory Insurance Movement

Whether agitation for a compulsory insurance system arose from within or without the profession, it met the Association's strong opposition. The AMA was especially severe in its criticism of prominent advocates of a national insurance program. The *Journal* looked skeptically upon the social scientists, who carried their investigations into the social and scientific fields of medicine, and generally questioned their competence to evaluate the significance of their findings. It leveled frequent criticisms at Michael M. Davis, whose doctoral degrees in social science left him unfit, according to the *Journal,* to deal with problems of medical economics. It also attacked the reputable authority, Nathan Sinai, whose doctoral degree in the field of public health, when combined with his advocacy of compulsory health insurance, became an unsatisfactory mixture. But a medical degree provided no protection against attack for Hugh Cabot of the Mayo Clinic, whose daring commitment to the same cause brought him in conflict with the Association. Never forgetting that private foundations financed the work of the Committee

[44] *American Medicine: Expert Testimony out of Court* (New York: The American Foundation, 1937), see evidence in Vol. 2, pp. 932–53, 976–1100, 1101–1294; Rorty, *American Medicine Mobilizes,* pp. 217–19.

[45] Harold Maslow, "The Background of the Wagner National Health Bill," *Law and Contemporary Problems,* 6 (Winter, 1939), 609; Editorial, *JAMA,* 109 (July 3, 1937), 32; Editorial, *JAMA,* 109 (October 16, 1937), 1280-81; Rorty, *American Medicine Mobilizes,* pp. 219–20.

on the Costs of Medical Care, the AMA also stood ready to oppose any that encouraged the adoption of compulsory health insurance.[46]

While attacking the sources of compulsory health insurance agitation, the Association also employed other means for combating the movement. Even before the New Deal era began, the AMA formulated plans for carrying its crusade against heretical schemes of medical care to the public. The newly created Bureau of Medical Economics produced materials that presented the Association's stand and strengthened the position of its spokesmen. Before the end of Roosevelt's first term, the bureau had issued a wide variety of pamphlets, and leaders of the Association had publicized throughout the nation their objections to compulsory insurance schemes and all general plans for state provided medical care.

The Association overlooked no method of getting its views before the public. In addition to the dissemination of millions of pamphlets, it found most of the nation's periodicals willing to print at least some of its attacks. Newspapers spread its views and occasionally ran syndicated articles prepared by the Bureau of Medical Economics. Occasionally the Association's spokesmen spread their message by radio, and at least once they met compulsory health insurance advocates in a radio debate on a national network. When the topic of socialized medicine became the high school debate subject during the school year of 1935–1936, the AMA set forth its position in the National University Extension Association Debate Committee's *Ninth Annual Debate Handbook* and supplied many debating teams with material against compulsory insurance schemes.[47]

The Association also overlooked no argument that showed promise of effectiveness in the battle against compulsory health insurance, or any general system of state provided medical service, and erected standards to which it felt no compulsory system could conform. It insisted on professional control of all features of the system and the noninterference of third parties in the relationship between physicians and patients. It also demanded the preservation of the patients' liberty to choose any legally qualified practitioner, and professional control over

[46] See Editorial, *JAMA,* 106 (January 11, 1936), 124; *JAMA,* 106 (May 16, 1936), 1737; *JAMA,* 104 (May 25, 1935), 1912.

[47] Morris Fishbein, *AMA Bulletin,* 31 (January, 1936), 16; HD, *Proceedings* (87 Annual Session, May, 1936), p. 23; Editorial, *JAMA,* 105 (October 19, 1935), 1273. The AMA made available 14 of its pamphlets dealing with problems of medical economics for use by high school debating teams.

all institutions giving medical service.[48] In advancing the Association's cause, its most adroit spokesman, Morris Fishbein, bitterly denounced the compulsory insurance threat. He described Russia's socialized plan as the "sovietized system of red medicine" and claimed to give a picture of the operation of any socialized medical plan in the United States from the viewpoint of American physicians.

> They see in the systems proposed the multiplication by hundreds of thousands of bureaucratic employees who idle through their six-hour days; they see them snooping into the intimacies of American family life, coming between the doctor and his patient, and waxing fat on the tax money extorted from wage earners and employers alike.[49]

The Bureau of Medical Economics repeatedly emphasized that medical service was no commodity, subject to political disposal by mass production methods, and stressed the personal element in medical care. The *Journal* attempted to provide reasons why the government should support public education, but divorce itself from the task of providing medical service.[50] Faced with the problem of explaining the expansion of compulsory health insurance schemes among foreign nations, the bureau replied:

> It would scarcely be maintained that the continuous increase almost from the beginning of the United States government, of the appropriations for "internal improvements" (the old "pork barrel bills"), or of the similar increase in military pensions indicates universal approval of all features of these systems.[51]

The bureau also discounted the claim for the popularity of compulsory health insurance systems abroad. It referred to a questionnaire, prepared by the International Association of Physicians, purporting to determine the popularity of these systems. According to this report only four of the 19 foreign medical associations that replied stated that the programs were "generally satisfactory" to both physicians and the insured.[52] From

[48] R. G. Leland and A. M. Simons, "Do We Need Compulsory Health Insurance? No," The American Academy of Political and Social Science, *Annals,* 170 (November, 1933), 126.

[49] *JAMA,* 102 (March 3, 1934), 699; "Health Security for the American People," *AMA Bulletin,* 31 (February, 1936), 41.

[50] HD, *Proceedings* (86 Annual Session, June, 1935), p. 59; *JAMA,* 107 (August 22, 1936), 591.

[51] Bureau of Medical Economics, "A Critical Analysis of Sickness Insurance" (Chicago: American Medical Association, 1934), p. 19.

[52] *Ibid.,* pp. 85–86. A year after this report, Simons and Sinai wrote "It may be said at once that a very thorough search of the available sources of information has failed to find a single condemnation of such systems with a request for a return to private practice." *The Way of Health Insurance,* p. 113.

the position that most foreign schemes had proved unsatisfactory, the AMA pressed the view that compulsory health insurance would not be popular in the United States. Fishbein charged that very few Americans wanted any compulsory medical plan and that any dissatisfaction with private medical care lay "among the 10 per cent of our people who, because of ignorance, stupidity or prejudice, prefer the by-ways of charlatanism and faith healing."[53]

Hopes of the Opposition

The AMA's increasing agitation against compulsory health insurance, toward the end of the first New Deal term, only convinced compulsory health insurance advocates of the vitality of the issue. Although disappointed that the Social Security Act made no provision for health insurance and that no state legislature had passed the Epstein bill, they saw no reason to give up the struggle. A survey of the National Resources Committee in 1935–1936, showing that one-third of the 39,000,000 American families and individual consumers had an annual income of less than $780 and had currently gone in debt one billion dollars in excess of earnings, gave strong support to the committee's contention that a large portion of the population could neither budget nor pay for normal medical services.[54] Compulsory health insurance advocates hoped to convince the public that the excessive selling costs of voluntary insurance could be saved in a compulsory scheme, and that the adoption of such a system resulted in no deterioration of medical service.[55] They hoped to show the nation that compulsory health insurance fitted into the framework of democratic institutions and promoted public interest. They found in American society in the thirties the prerequisites for the successful operation of a compulsory health insurance plan: industrialization, a large portion of the population with insufficient incomes for adequate medical care, a feeling of social responsibility, and an awareness of the social consequences of disease.[56]

[53] Fishbein, *AMA Bulletin,* 31 (February, 1936), 40.

[54] Davis, *America Organizes Medicine,* pp. 50–51; Simons and Sinai, *The Way of Health Insurance,* pp. 168–70.

[55] Simons and Sinai, *The Way of Health Insurance,* p. 176; Epstein, *Insecurity: A Challenge to America,* pp. 445–64, 851–58.

[56] Simons and Sinai, *The Way of Health Insurance,* pp. 167–95. See pp. 233–34 below for Simmons' record on the insurance issue.

Chapter 11 THE ROLE OF RESISTANCE

THE DARK SHADOWS OF THE GREAT DEPRESSION still stretched across the nation when the Roosevelt administration scored an overwhelming victory in November, 1936. Although much unemployment and destitution persisted, the administration's program had produced some generally desirable results while creating at the same time unwavering support and implacable opposition. Between extreme partisan reactions, the AMA steered a fairly moderate course although beginning to move more closely toward the side of the administration's enemies.

The Association had several reasons for showing no particular enthusiasm over the New Deal victory. It felt that the struggle against the depression demanded a moderation and caution that the victorious party might not provide and feared that the hasty enactment of legislation would create more problems than it corrected. Recognizing the appeal of the compulsory health insurance movement, the AMA doubted that a somewhat sympathetic administration would long resist its pressures. It also felt that the party might interpret the election results as a popular demand for more comprehensive social legislation which would prove menacing to the medical profession.

Association's Strategy

Interpreting the election as a renewal of the compulsory health insurance threat, the AMA devised its plans for battle. It developed a strategy that included three broad programs through which it hoped to defeat the proponents of compulsory insurance legislation. With the continuation of a direct campaign against all forms of compulsory health insurance it attempted to counteract the influence of the movement and prevent the development of public sentiment in favor of compulsory schemes.

By encouraging local societies to develop plans for providing the indigent with medical aid, it hoped to remove situations that seemed to justify the institution of comprehensive governmental plans of medical care. By resisting the threat of further federal control of state health activities, it attempted to arrest the progress of trends toward compulsory health insurance on the national level.

Revived Health Insurance Threat

Agitation for compulsory schemes showed no signs of abating as the AMA prepared to defend traditional patterns of medical care against alleged attack. The second New Deal term had just begun when Senator Arthur Capper of Kansas introduced a bill that provided for a federally subsidized system of state health insurance closely modeled after the Epstein bill.[1] In June, the trustees informed the House of Delegates at Atlantic City that the Social Security Board had undertaken a broad study of social insurance and predicted that it would give much attention to the compulsory insurance issue. The AMA also found disturbing the continued interest shown by several state legislatures in compulsory health insurance proposals. Although the trustees reported that the New York and Rhode Island legislatures had recently rejected compulsory measures, they found no reason to believe that the issue had lost its appeal.[2]

The Association not only noted agitation on the political scene for compulsory health insurance and extended federal programs of medical care, but showed even greater shock at the growth of this agitation within the profession. While attracting no sizable body of physicians, Joseph Slavit's Medical League for Socialized Medicine continued to press its views upon the profession. More dangerous to medical unity, however, was the work of the Committee of Physicians for the Improvement of Medical Care that grew out of the survey of medical opinion which the Medical Advisory Committee of the American Foundation conducted in 1936. The AMA felt that the committee that stemmed from this survey wore a mask of respectability that made its activities all the more dangerous. When the committee set forth its

[1] HD, *Proceedings* (87 Annual Session, June, 1937), p. 16. See also Davis, *America Organizes Medicine,* p. 254.

[2] HD, *Proceedings* (87 Annual Session, June, 1937), pp. 16–17.

principles in November, 1937, calling for greater federal and state co-operation in solving health problems, and larger public expenditures for medical education and hospitals, its opposition to some of the AMA's policies became quite pronounced. Its platform, which soon received the written endorsement of 430 physicians, convinced the AMA that sinister influences were at work within the profession.[3]

Resumption of Warfare

Against the forces that seemed to undermine the foundations of private medical practice, the AMA continued an attack that proved fairly effective during the first Roosevelt administration. The *Journal* repeatedly set the Association's position before an ever-growing membership and its editor stood ready to attack critics of the prevailing forms of medical care.[4] The Bureau of Medical Economics produced material supporting the Association's case and the *Bulletin* also participated in a fight that had begun to require an enormous expenditure of the AMA's time and effort.

Although the AMA feared that the decisive New Deal victory of 1936 would lead to an extension of social legislation at both the state and federal levels, unforeseen developments served to discredit the administration and retard its program. The Association, while never standing alone in outspoken opposition to some of the New Deal legislation, now witnessed the mushroom growth of such organizations as "Committee to Preserve Our Liberties" and "Associates for America" that formed

[3] Statement of Richard Smith, Subcommittee of Senate Committee on Education and Labor, Seventy-sixth Congress, first session, *Hearings on S. 1620 to Establish a National Health Program* (Government Printing Office, Washington, 1939), Part 1, p. 180. In April, 1937, the editor of the *Journal* cited an article by Esther Everett Lape, director of the foundation's study, which stated that "medical men" considered that compulsory health insurance degraded medical service. Although the committee's report actually showed considerable medical opinion in favor of various forms of health insurance, the editor concluded that the study revealed "the unlikelihood that sickness insurance, either voluntary or compulsory, will answer the problems of medical care suitably for the people of the United States." Editorial, *JAMA*, 108 (April 10, 1937), 1262.

[4] For an example of the editor's sensitivity to criticisms of medical practice see his attack on Archibald J. Cronin's *The Citadel*, and on Hugh Cabot, who endorsed it. *JAMA*, 109 (September 18, 1937), 957. In 1936 the membership of the AMA for the first time passed the 100,000 mark, reaching 100,591. It jumped to 103,755 in 1937 constituting 62.8 per cent of all the doctors in the United States. Garceau, *Political Life of AMA*, p. 132.

when Roosevelt announced his plan for the reorganization of the Supreme Court. Although the President's scheme actually upset no historical precedents, hostile critics seized upon the proposal to convince the public that tyranny and socialism threatened. The shock of the Supreme Court fight had not passed when the nation sank into the business recession of 1937–1938, convincing some that the New Deal had no real solutions for the problems of the depression.[5] While the congressional election of the latter year indicated that the President's popularity had not greatly decreased, the court fight and recession tended to weaken confidence in the New Deal program.

The Association's attack upon threatened political innovations appears to have made a greater impression on the medical profession than on the public. Its alarmist literature kindled an evangelistic fire among some physicians who were shaken by the government's alleged attack on human liberties. In order to shift some of the growing burden of the Association's political activities, but partially to prevent the government from classifying the AMA as a political organization and subject to the payment of taxes, several of its members organized the National Physicians' Committee for the Extension of Medical Service in 1939. Appealing to medical institutions, private physicians, and the drug trade for financial support, the committee sought public attention in national magazines, with advertisements extolling the virtues of individualism. Furthermore, the Association's indoctrination program made its membership more susceptible to financial appeals from the National Committee to Uphold Constitutional Government, organized in the same year by the violent New Deal critic and newspaper chain owner, Frank E. Gannett.[6]

Despite the AMA's attack upon unorthodox plans for meeting the costs of medical service, the agitation for compulsory health insurance did not diminish. Behind this agitation, as the AMA well knew, lay an uncomfortable amount of popular support. Of the nine constitutional amendments submitted to the voters of New York for ratification in 1938, the one authorizing the adoption of a compulsory health insurance system received the largest vote. Three state legislatures, including that of New York, considered but failed to enact compulsory health insurance bills that year. On the national level, the Capper bill hung as a perennial threat in the Senate, while similar measures vied for the atten-

[5] Wecter, *Age of Great Depression,* pp. 105, 151–52, 209.

[6] Davis, *America Organizes Medicine,* p. 175; Rorty, *American Medicine Mobilizes,* pp. 308–9.

tion of the House.[7] Although the AMA maintained close contact with the activities of state legislatures, it found difficulty in estimating the success of its crusade against compulsory health insurance at the end of the second New Deal term. Yet its spokesmen, who pressed the fight before lay groups throughout the nation, had less difficulty in deciding that the task of delivering the public from the impending threat of "politicalized medicine" rested largely on the AMA.[8]

Constructive Counteroffensive

While engaged in an impressive effort to defeat the movement for compulsory health insurance through a direct attack, the AMA also adopted a constructive plan for combating compulsory insurance agitation. Its second method called for the promotion of schemes adopted by local societies for administering medical care to the indigent. These plans proposed to put much of the enormous charity work that had already overburdened many physicians on a more orderly basis. After many medical societies prepared to provide this service, usually in conjunction with the federal relief program, the AMA believed that such arrangements provided a potential check to the threat of compulsory insurance. Although at first largely interested in preventing the incorporation of unethical professional practices in these programs, the second New Deal term found the AMA urging the widespread adoption of professionally sponsored programs of indigent medical care and preventive medicine.[9]

The method that medical societies developed in establishing headquarters to prorate the burden and meager remuneration of medical service to indigent classes demonstrated its advantages. While conforming to no precise pattern, all plans offered medical assistance to patients

[7] Statement of Robert F. Wagner, Subcommittee of the Senate Committee on Education and Labor, Seventy-sixth Congress, first session, *Hearings on S. 1620*, Part 1, p. 170; HD, *Proceedings* (90 Annual Session, May, 1939), pp. 24, 19; Davis, *America Organizes Medicine*, p. 254.

[8] HD, *Proceedings* (90 Annual Session, May, 1939), p. 23. For a schedule of the places where six leaders of the AMA spoke in December, 1939, see *JAMA*, 113 (December 2, 1939), 2065. The AMA preferred the terms "state managed medicine" or "politicalized medicine" to the use of the terms compulsory health insurance or socialized medicine. *JAMA*, 114 (April 6, 1940), 1364.

[9] For the very slow progress made by professionally sponsored plans up to 1935 see p. 185n above.

in dire need. For some physicians these programs provided a needed supplement to their small and uncertain incomes, and for the profession as a whole the schemes distributed the burden of medical care on a broader basis. As a by-product, such plans enhanced public respect for the medical profession. When from these programs medical-service bureaus developed, providing care to low-income groups usually on a reduced postpayment basis, the AMA also encouraged this movement as a deterrent to compulsory health insurance. In 1938, the trustees observed with satisfaction that at least 250 county medical societies had established plans for aiding indigents and low-income groups.[10]

When several state medical associations inaugurated similar programs on a state-wide basis, the AMA again approved. Initiated under professional guidance rather than lay leadership, the Association had little reason to fear their growth. It viewed the adoption of these plans as another justified attempt to weaken the case for compulsory health insurance. Although none had advanced far beyond the embryonic stage at the end of the second New Deal administration, 14 (including the District of Columbia) were in the early stages of development by June, 1940.[11]

Resisting Federal Encroachments

In addition to the Association's public crusade against the adoption of unorthodox schemes of meeting the cost of medical care, and its support of society plans for relieving the indigent and low-income classes, it followed a third course in safeguarding the profession's interests. It watched the development of federal programs for threats to private practice and resisted the extension of federal control over public medical service. Its opposition to governmental policies appeared more spectacular as the administration moved from the political triumph of 1936, more intent on enlarging the scope of social legislation and less inclined to tolerate interference.

[10] HD, *Proceedings* (89 Annual Session, June, 1938), p. 29. For a brief account of the development of these plans see HD, *Proceedings* (91 Annual Session, June, 1940), p. 29.

[11] HD, *Proceedings* (91 Annual Session, June, 1940), pp. 29–30. A state-wide program of preventive medicine initiated in Indiana by the state society was favorably received by the Reference Committee on Medical Education. It was considered as a deterrent to a compulsory health insurance system. HD, *Proceedings* (89 Annual Session, June, 1938), pp. 66–68.

The first major incident adding further strain to the relations between the AMA and the federal government grew out of the administration's response to the Dust Bowl crisis. Through the Resettlement Administration the government initiated a belated program of federal aid in 1937 for parts of a stricken area extending from the Dakotas to Oklahoma, where a recurrence of dust storms had reduced much of the region to wasteland and many of its inhabitants to poverty. Attempting to check the growing peril of human wreckage, the government arranged medical, surgical, nursing, hospital, and dental care on a group service basis. The Federal Security Administration, which soon replaced the Resettlement Administration, extended the program from the Dust Bowl region to include a third of a million people in 30 states by January, 1940. Eventually many destitute and low-income farm families of 881 counties received medical aid through group-service plans provided by liberal farm loans.[12]

This broad program of medical service, expanded to include even a few families above the low-income levels, met some opposition from the AMA. Although the program allowed professional responsibility for medical care and provided for the free choice of physicians and medical payment adjusted to family income, the AMA believed that it opened the way for many abuses. It watched the development of the program with much apprehension and urged all county medical societies to send copies of the agreements they made with the Federal Security Administration to its Bureau of Medical Economics. It noted that the plans as established in some areas only vaguely defined the classes eligible for medical benefits, while leaving the termination date for the programs in greater doubt. It also contended that the language of the agreements sometimes obscured the principle of the free choice of physicians upon which all plans actually rested.[13] The Association found particularly objectionable the administration's alleged attempts to induce physicians into arrangements for unlimited medical service at stipulated annual incomes. Warning that no practice inimical with the highest medical standards should be allowed, the Association charged that the FSA's

[12] Wecter, *Age of Great Depression,* pp. 173–75; Mitchell, *Depression Decade,* p. 215.

[13] HD, *Proceedings* (90 Annual Session, May, 1939), pp. 79, 86; HD, *Proceedings* (88 Annual Session, June, 1937), pp. 62, 18, 24; R. C. Williams, "The Medical Care Program for Farm Security Administration Borrowers," *Law and Contemporary Problems,* 6 (Autumn, 1939), 586.

medical program provided "an admirable setup for very objectionable practices in the direction of socialized medicine, so-call."[14]

National Health Survey

Although the AMA watched suspiciously the development of the emergency farm-medical program, it found the administration's plans for a broad national health system even more alarming. Behind the government's proposed attack upon the nation's principal health problems lay the challenging facts disclosed by the National Health Survey of 1935–1936. This government-sponsored undertaking, representing the most extensive survey of family health problems ever conducted, fell in line with earlier studies in revealing deplorable deficiencies in medical care.[15] It showed that about 40 per cent of 2,300,000 city dwellers, canvassed in a survey that reached nearly 740,000 families, belonged to families that had annual incomes under $1,000, and that half of these had received relief during 1935. It revealed that 57 per cent more disabling illnesses of at least a week in duration occurred among families on relief than among those on or above the $3,000 annual-income level. The survey provided conclusive proof that a large portion of the population had incomes that left little if any margin for meeting the expense of medical care.[16]

[14] HD, *Proceedings* (88 Annual Session, June, 1937), p. 62; HD, *Proceedings* (90 Annual Session, May, 1939), p. 86.

[15] Besides the extensive survey of the Committee on the Costs of Medical Care that was completed in 1931, the Public Health Service conducted a survey among 11,500 families of wage earners two years later. The National Health Survey, however, embraced over 2,500,000 people. Beulah Amidon, "Who Can Afford Health?" *Public Health Pamphlet No. 27* (Public Affairs Committee Incorporated, rev. ed., 1941), p. 11; J. Frederic Dewhurst and Associates, *America's Needs and Resources* (New York: The Twentieth Century Fund, 1955), p. 302. For accounts of the methods employed in conducting this survey and for additional findings see George St. J. Perrott, Clark Tibbitts, and Rollo H. Britten, "The National Health Survey: Scope and Method of Nation-wide Canvass of Sickness in Relation to Its Social and Economic Setting," Federal Security Agency, United States Public Health Service, *Public Health Reports,* 54 (September 15, 1939), 1664–65, and Rollo H. Britten, Selwyn D. Collins, and James S. Fitzgerald, "The National Health Survey: Some General Findings as to Disease, Accidents, and Impairments in Urban Areas," *ibid.,* 55 (March 15, 1940), 444–70 *passim.*

[16] Amidon, "Who Can Afford Health?" pp. 7, 10–11; Rollo H. Britten, "The National Health Survey: Receipt of Medical Service in Different Urban Population Groups," U. S. Public Health Service, *Public Health Reports,* 55 (November 29, 1940), 2199–200. Amidon says that the survey covered 776,000 families

AMA's Health Surveys

Anticipating that the administration would rely heavily upon the disclosures of this survey to justify an extension of federal control over medical affairs, the AMA decided to conduct one of its own. In December, 1937, the Board of Trustees authorized the profession to conduct an investigation of the adequacy and accessibility of medical care, and the Bureau of Medical Economics quickly arranged for the survey. The bureau provided the state societies with a special form for reporting on state-wide medical facilities and furnished the survey committees of local medical societies with abundant materials for the undertaking. Although the local committees appear to have proceeded cautiously with the assignment, by the middle of May, 1939, 502 county societies in 37 states had completed the task which many local societies in several other states had also undertaken.[17] By July 1, some 17,000 physicians had filed forms for this survey, in which 4,119 pharmacists, 1,256 hospitals, and 822 health departments and other agencies and institutions also participated. By this date the Association had also heard from 605 medical societies in 873 counties of 38 states.[18]

The AMA's criticism of the government's survey appeared long before its own had been completed. At the special session of 1938, President-elect Rock Sleyster referred to the "haphazard surveys of small sections of the population conducted by inexperienced relief workers. . . ." Such surveys, he maintained, ignored the fact that "the medical problem is coexistent with the need of food, clothing, shelter, heat, and light . . ." and that the medical profession gave millions of dollars in free medical service daily.[19] Only a few months earlier the AMA's Advisory Committee on Medical Care expressed the same feeling.

> We are not interested so much in the theoretic reforms of many of the so-called leaders of medicine, which in most cases are products of the noble thought and the library table. It is not of great importance to find

---

but Britten puts the figure at 739,893. For comments on the limitations and significance of the survey see George W. Bachman and Lewis Meriam, *The Issue of Compulsory Health Insurance* (Washington, D.C.: The Brookings Institution, 1948), pp. 153–73.

[17] HD, *Proceedings* (90 Annual Session, May, 1939), pp. 28, 84.

[18] "American Medical Association Study of Need and Supply of Medical Care," Subcommittee of Senate Committee on Education and Labor, Seventy-sixth Congress, first session, *Hearings on S. 1620,* Part 2, pp. 458–59. For additional information see HD, *Proceedings* (90 Annual Session, May, 1939), p. 84.

[19] HD, *Proceedings* (Special Session, September, 1938), p. 5.

out what those who are engaged in teaching or cloistered specialists and institutional doctors think about medical care, and we already know what governmental officials and social workers think. The facts of the situation must come from those who are in direct contact with the actual practice of medicine. We must find out from them to what extent reform in medical care is needed and get their opinions as to how it can best be accomplished.[20]

The Association's high esteem for its own survey stood in sharp contrast to its low regard for others. It felt that a careful investigation made under professional auspices outranked all surveys directed by amateurs and, by a loose mode of reckoning, indicated that its own survey embraced a population of over 43,000,000, a number far in excess of the modest estimates claimed for similar studies.[21] It used its own investigations to refute the alarming claims that wide segments of the population could not afford and did not receive adequate medical care. To charges of inadequacy, the Association replied that "Fully 90 per cent of all the sources consulted reported that they knew of no significant number of persons needing and seeking medical care who were unable to obtain it."[22] While the medical profession and related interests passed favorable judgment on the adequacy of their services, they also volunteered an opinion of the caliber of medical care rendered by government agencies. The survey, as interpreted by the AMA's Committee on Medical Care, showed the inferior character of service provided under governmental auspices and contended that the investigation showed no real public interest in compulsory health insurance.[23]

Whereas the AMA drew comforting conclusions from its survey of medical service, a supplementary study conducted by its Council on Medical Education and Hospitals proved equally consoling. Charged in 1938 with the responsibility of reporting on hospital and health facilities in the United States, the council quickly turned its attention to the situation in the state of Mississippi. It apparently assumed that if a survey revealed adequate medical facilities in this economically retarded

[20] HD, *Proceedings* (89 Annual Session, June, 1938), p. 72. W. F. Braasch was the chairman of this committee.

[21] HD, *Proceedings* (90 Annual Session, May, 1939), p. 84. The Committee on Medical Care stated that the population of all the counties reported on by medical societies was 43,790,068, according to the 1930 census. This, however, does not mean that a careful survey was taken of the health conditions of so large a portion of the population.

[22] *Ibid.*, p. 85. The committee further said that "The overwhelming majority of opinion from all sources agree that forty thousand and not forty million persons in the United States are denied needed medical service."

[23] *Ibid.*

state, few questions about the adequacy of such facilities in other states would be raised.

Although the study showed a ratio of physicians to population in Mississippi in 1938 of 1 to 1,353, compared with the national ratio of 1 to 762, and serious problems resulting from such matters as lack of highly trained hospital personnel and deficiencies in hospital accommodations for Negroes, the council did not consider the situation critical. It gave a rather favorable picture of medical services in a state where per capita income during the depression years reached only $202 as late as 1940. Although Mississippi portrayed a depth of poverty that would have overtaxed any charitable system the council reported that:

> Extensive inquiry among all classes of the population, including doctors, health officers, nurses and workers, elicited the almost uniform response that there is practically no one in Mississippi who cannot secure medical care regardless of his ability to pay.[24]

Despite the accumulation of evidence in the Association's files, reflecting most favorably upon the availability and adequacy of medical service, an increasing percentage of the population became harder to convince. From the ranks of the hard-pressed industrial workers and the burdened low-salaried professional classes came support for a movement to extend social insurance that found much of its leadership among the social scientists. Promoted also by a federal administration convinced of serious deficiencies in the social security system, agitation for an improved governmental health program reached new heights in 1938. Those attributing such agitation largely to an insignificant fringe of visionaries had their opinions shaken by the National Health conference that convened in July.

National Health Conference

This conference, called by the President upon the suggestion of his Interdepartmental Committee to Coordinate Health and Welfare Activi-

[24] A. G. Mezerik, *The Revolt of the South and West* (New York: Duell, Sloan, and Pearce, 1946), p. 31; HD, *Proceedings* (90 Annual Session, May, 1939), pp. 48, 64, quotation, pp. 71–72. In 1939, the total farm income from 57,696 of Mississippi's 287,841 farms fell in the classification that ranged from $100 to $249. *United States Sixteenth Census, 1940, Agriculture,* Vol. 3, p. 988. In 1935-1936, the average income of the lowest one-third of the families of the United States was only $471 which indicates that poverty was not localized. Lucy Sprague Mitchell, Eleanor Bowman, and Mary Phelps, *My Country 'Tis of Thee: The Use and Abuse of Natural Resources* (New York: The Macmillan Company, 1940), p. 298.

ties, brought together representatives of various groups to consider a revision and expansion of the nation's health program. In addition to the prominent physicians, public health authorities, and social workers who attended, women's clubs, farmers' organizations, and labor unions also sent representatives. Upon instruction from the House of Delegates, seven prominent figures within the AMA attended the conference, including President Irvin Abell and the editor of the *Journal,* still Morris Fishbein. Representatives also attended from several state medical societies.[25]

Before a conference that showed great enthusiasm for opening an attack upon the nation's unsolved health problems, the interdepartmental committee proposed an ambitious program. It presented the shocking picture of a nation woefully deficient in preventive medical services and adequate hospital facilities, with one-third of its population receiving either inadequate medical care or none at all. It asserted that an even larger portion of the population bore the economic burden of illness only with great difficulty. Its program called for an expansion of maternal and child health services, provided for by increased expenditures on a federal-state co-operative basis, within the framework of the social security system. It urged the expansion of hospital facilities and the provision of public medical care for the destitute, and for families whose marginal incomes barely removed them from this class. It also suggested the need for an insurance plan offering protection to the wage earner against temporary and permanent disability.[26]

While these recommendations proposed an extension of federal operations in the fields of health and social security, the committee advanced a much bolder idea. It shocked the Association's leaders with a proposal for a comprehensive medical care program financed by insurance payments or taxation, or by both of these methods. Although the committee

[25] Amidon, *Public Health Pamphlet No. 27,* p. 28; Irvin Abell, HD, *Proceedings* (Special Session, September, 1938), p. 3. The interdepartmental committee appointed in 1935 was made up of representatives from the Social Security Board, and the Departments of Labor, Agriculture, Treasury, and Interior. "A National Health Program," Social Security Board, *Social Security Bulletin,* 1 (August, 1938), 10.

[26] *Ibid.* One writer says that at the National Health Conference there "appeared for the first time—as far as I am aware—clear, unmistakable evidence that there were large bodies of people who clearly saw the need and firmly demanded that the Government take a hand in applying the remedy." Hugh Cabot, *The Patient's Dilemma: The Quest for Medical Security in America* (New York: Regnal & Hitchcock, 1940), p. 232. The AMA reported the details of the conference in *JAMA,* 111 (July 30, 1938), 432–54.

recommended the adoption of the plan on the state level and indicated that its cost would probably not exceed the amount annually spent for inadequate medical care, some at the conference found the recommendation no less objectionable.[27] Since this proposal actually embraced activities provided for in other of the committee's recommendations, it became a very important issue at the conference.

Developments at the assembly convinced the AMA that the medical profession still faced grave dangers. It believed that the administration had used the conference to advance a national health program not altogether desirable. It observed indications of an inadequate grasp of the scope and complexity of problems of medical care on the part of laymen who urged radical changes in the present system.[28] Overwhelmed by the spirit of the conference, and unable to commit the Association to any course of action, the organization's spokesmen returned from the assembly in considerable dismay.

An Emergency Session

Expecting the President to submit a national health program to the first session of the Seventy-sixth Congress, which would convene in January, 1939, the Association's leadership saw signs of a developing crisis. Aware that there would be no regular session of the House of Delegates before Congress met, the trustees authorized the speaker to call for an early special meeting.[29] When the third special session in the Association's history convened on September 16, the delegates faced problems similar to those that confronted the special assembly of 1935. While the earlier session had convened to appraise the proposed social security system, the latter met to consider recommendations dealing largely with its extension.

The September session prepared for a speedy consideration of the issues raised at the National Health Conference. Five subcommittees of the Reference Committee for the Consideration of a National Health Program studied different sections of the comprehensive plan advanced

[27] *Social Security Bulletin,* 1 (August, 1938), 10–11.

[28] See, for example, the address of Irvin Abell, HD, *Proceedings* (Special Session, September, 1938), p. 4.

[29] *Ibid.,* p. 6.

at the conference and offered appraisals.[30] These evaluations were substantially incorporated into the committee's final report to the session.

Although the subcommittees expressed approval of many portions of the program, they rejected some and amended others. The instances of the subcommittees' approval, however, seemed to overbalance their objections and tended to give a false impression of general agreement with the recommendations of the interdepartmental committee at the National Health Conference. Subcommittee reports endorsed the principle of compensation for wages lost through sickness, and favored the establishment of cash-indemnity plans administered by state societies for periods of prolonged illness. They recognized the existence of emergencies requiring federal assistance to the states in meeting the burden of indigency, and they endorsed the idea of nongovernmental hospital service insurance, partially or completely covering the expense of hospitalization. They also approved of the proposal for greater federal expenditures in expanding public health services, adding that allotments to states should be on the basis of population, special health problems, and financial needs.[31]

Close examination, however, reveals significant reservations that the subcommittees attached to their endorsement of some of the recommendations of the interdepartmental committee. They accepted the proposal for the expansion of federal public health work, but urged the consolidation of all public health activities into a federal department of public health, headed by a medical doctor holding a cabinet position. Approval of the proposal for federal aid to the states, in meeting the problems of indigency, rested on the view that such assistance was tolerable only when the burden of indigency exhausted state reserves. Subcommittee endorsement of the principle of group hospitalization carefully excluded approval of all plans that covered the costs of medical care. Likewise, approval of income-loss insurance

[30] The Reference Committee for the Consideration of a National Health Program was composed of the chairmen of the five subcommittees, who were Terry M. Townsend (N.Y.), William F. Braasch (Minn.), E. L. Henderson (Ky.), Samuel P. Mengel (Penn.), and C. W. Roberts (Ga.). The five subcommittees studied the following sections of the report submitted at the conference. Subcommittee 1, the recommendations for the extension of public health services; subcommittee 2, the recommendations for the expansion of hospital facilities; subcommittee 3, the recommendations on medical care for the medical needy; subcommittee 4, the recommendations on the general program of medical care; and subcommittee 5, recommendations on insurance against loss of wages during sickness. HD, *Proceedings* (Special Session, September, 1938), p. 30.

[31] *Ibid.*, pp. 52, 51, 49.

depended on the freedom of such plans from federal subsidization or "financial or administrative participation in their activities."[32]

The subcommittees could not endorse some of the conclusions and recommendations of the interdepartmental committee, even with reservations. They rejected completely the committee's proposal for a national program of medical care embodying compulsory health insurance. They considered such a system a "complicated, bureaucratic one which has no place in a democratic state" and lending itself inevitably to "political control and manipulation."[33] Although admittedly without sufficient evidence proving the contrary, the subcommittees threw grave doubt upon the accuracy of statistics submitted at the National Health Conference that indicated great deficiencies in the distribution of medical service. They also questioned the alleged need for the immediate addition of 180,000 beds to the nation's hospital facilities and doubted the necessity of a ratio of hospital beds to population as high as 4.5 to the thousand.[34]

Response to Administration's Program

While the subcommittee reports committed the House of Delegates to no official policy, they nevertheless indicated the temperament of a sizable portion of that body. They served also the immediate purpose of influencing the final decisions of the session. Embodied in the final report of the Committee for the Consideration of the National Health Program, which the House of Delegates accepted, appeared the principal recommendations of the subcommittees. This report represented the AMA's official reaction to the administration's proposed health program as outlined at the National Health Conference. Below in summary form appears the position of the House of Delegates.[35]

The September session of the House of Delegates did not content itself with an official declaration and reaffirmation of policies. It called for the establishment of a committee headed by President Irvin Abell and composed of not more than six other physicians, for consultation with the administration about the proposed national health legislation.[36] Its experience with the movement for a comprehensive health program also aroused greater appreciation for the need of medical surveys and pro-

[32] *Ibid.*, pp. 49, 51, quotation, p. 52.
[33] *Ibid.*, p. 52.
[34] *Ibid.*, p. 50.
[35] *Ibid.*, pp. 53–54.
[36] *Ibid.*, pp. 54–55.

fessionally sponsored plans for indigent medical care. It suggested that the work of the Bureau of Medical Economics be considerably expanded to include needed research projects and urged additional aid to local societies in developing plans for providing indigents with medical service.[37]

OFFICIAL POSITION OF THE HOUSE OF DELEGATES ADOPTED SEPTEMBER 16–17, 1938, ON THE RECOMMENDATIONS MADE BY THE INTERDEPARTMENTAL COMMITTEE TO COORDINATE HEALTH AND WELFARE ACTIVITIES TO THE NATIONAL HEALTH CONFERENCE OF 1938

Issue	*Position*	*Reservations*
1. Extension of public health service	Desire extension	(1) Through national health department headed by medical doctor with cabinet post (2) Expanded services not to include treatment of disease unless local agencies unable
2. Hospital construction	Expansion where need established	(1) Expansion only after existing facilities used; government aid implied
3. Medical care for medically needy	Need for government aid may arise in poorer communities	(1) Co-ordinated with programs for better food, clothing, etc. (2) Public welfare procedure simplified (3) Arranged by responsible local officials with local medical profession
4. Voluntary hospitalization insurance	Approves expansion	(1) Proceed along "sound" lines (2) Exclude coverage for all types of medical care
5. Compulsory health insurance	Opposes adoption	(1) Disapproves of the establishment of compulsory systems in any form
6. Cash-indemnity insurance	Approves expansion	(1) Agencies established to provide it to comply with state statutes (2) Agencies must meet approval of state and local medical societies
7. Income-loss insurance	Approves adoption	(1) Profession not responsible for disability certifications
8. Workmen's compensation	Approves extension	

Although the House of Delegates couched its views in tempered language, it actually surrendered little ground to the forces pressing for a national health program. It surrounded its approval of an extension of public health services with sufficient safeguards to protect private practice. Its recognition of the necessity of federal aid in meeting indigent needs constituted no repudiation of earlier views and its stand on volun-

[37] HD, *Proceedings* (Special Session, September, 1938), p. 55.

tary health insurance only emphasized a more favorable attitude that had been developing. In opposing compulsory health insurance the delegates upheld the Association's traditional policy. Their position suggested no necessity for governmental aid in hospital construction and only in their acceptance of the principle of income-loss and indemnity insurance did they appear to have taken a more indulgent position than before.

Having officially registered its objections to the proposals made by the interdepartmental committee at the National Health Conference, the AMA threw its weight against the passage of legislation enacting a national health program. Exactly four months after the special session of the House of Delegates convened, President Roosevelt submitted a message to Congress clearly showing the administration's intention of pressing for revisions in the social security legislation of 1935. In another congressional message of January 23, 1939, he spoke with greater insistency about the urgency of meeting the nation's health problems and submitted the findings and recommendations of the interdepartmental committee. When on February 1, the House Committee on Ways and Means began public hearings on social security legislation the AMA saw the approach of another major conflict with the administration.[38]

Opposition to National Health Bill

Although hearings on the social security system began on February 1, not until the last day of the month did a bill appear in Congress that embraced the administration's health program. This measure, introduced by Senator Wagner of New York, took the AMA by no surprise. Somewhat resentful that the government had never consulted the committee established by the special session for consultation with the administration on the proposed health program, the Association now prepared to defend its position at Congressional hearings. On May 5, Arthur W. Booth, chairman of the Board of Trustees, laid before the Senate subcommittee of the Committee on Education and Labor, that had also begun hearings on the measure, many of the AMA's objections to the Wagner bill.[39]

The subcommittee found that the Association's opposition passed beyond the point of compromise. The militant trustee cited alleged weak-

[38] *Social Security Bulletin,* 2 (February, 1939), 2.

[39] Seventy-sixth Congress, first session, *Hearings on S. 1620,* Part 1, p. 156. For the full text of the bill see *ibid.,* pp. 1–16. While the bill is generally called "The Wagner Bill," it was expected to bear the title "The National Health Act of 1939" if passed.

nesses in the bill which the AMA believed endangered both professional interests and public welfare. Criticizing the measure for making no provision for a national health department, he considered it just as deficient in safeguarding the rights of physicians in providing for the treatment of disease. Seeing a close approximation to a national system of compulsory health insurance, he objected to the provisions for federal control over federally subsidized state plans for indigent medical care and referred to the federal subsidization of temporary disability compensation schemes as dangerous. Although approving of the principle of disability compensation insurance partially covering the loss of wages, he objected to an additional provision that offered medical care in some cases.[40]

Perhaps the most impressive arguments that Booth presented touched on the extravagance of the proposed scheme. He saw no reason why all states must be embraced in a national health program when, in his opinion, only a few, if any, faced health problems that outweighed their resources. He contended that this bill definitely made federal aid to the states for medical care the rule and not the exception. He condemned the hospital expansion program that the bill proposed as the height of extravagance, when hospitals throughout the nation faced the embarrassing problem of many empty beds. He saw no indication that the people of the different states considered the inadequacies in medical care anything like as serious as did the principal supporters of this bill.[41]

Only ten days after Booth's appearance before the Senate subcommittee, the ninetieth annual session of the House of Delegates convened in St. Louis under an ominous political overcast. The threat of the inauguration of a national health program which had so greatly disturbed the profession became the principal topic of discussion. A committee appointed by the speaker drew up exhaustive criticisms of the Wagner bill in a report that the House of Delegates readily accepted.[42] Although repeating many objections already announced, this 22-point attack upon the bill provided a comprehensive statement of the Association's

[40] *Ibid.*, pp. 155–56.

[41] *Ibid.*, pp. 153–56. For another attack of the AMA on the Wagner bill that centered around its alleged extravagance and financial unsoundness, see the reply of the Bureau of Legal Medicine and Legislation to the favorable analysis made by J. N. Baker, an Alabama state health officer and member of the House of Delegates of the AMA. *JAMA,* 112 (April 22, 1939), 1597–98.

[42] For a brief summary of the process leading to the adoption of the report see HD, *Proceedings* (91 Annual Session, June, 1940), p. 54. HD, *Proceedings* (90 Annual Session, May, 1939), pp. 20–21, provides an analysis of the bill by the board.

position. The table below summarizes the AMA's criticisms of the bill and its own alternative proposal.[43]

SUMMARY OF OBJECTIONS OFFERED BY THE NINETEENTH SESSION OF THE HOUSE OF DELEGATES, MAY, 1939, TO THE WAGNER BILL ALONG WITH ALTERNATIVE PROPOSAL

Nature of Objections	*Position of the House of Delegates*
1. Infringement on medical profession	1. No safeguards for "continued existence of the private practitioners."
	2. "Insidiously promotes the development of a complete system of tax supported governmental medical care."
	3. Provides for medical service in addition to wage-loss compensation.
2. Infringement on states	1. Federal subsidies for medical care become the rule not the exception.
	2. Provision for "supreme federal control" as federal agents may approve or disapprove of state health plans.
	3. Need for federal assistance in one state should not bring federal control in all.
	4. Suggestions for such grants-in-aid programs usually represent pressure from federal officials and not from states.
3. Extravagant	1. No provision for use of existing vacant hospital beds.
	2. Federal aid to states in need does not necessitate federal aid to all.
4. Unsound and unscientific	1. Question of how and when to give federal aid to states unanswered.
	2. "inconsistent with the fundamental principles of medical care established by scientific medical experience. . . ."
	3. "prescribes no method for determining the nature and extent of the needs for preventive and other medical services. . . ."
	4. No recognition of factors as suitable food and housing to prevent disease.
Nature of Proposal	*Method Approved by the House of Delegates*
Encourage expansion of preventive medical service and medical care for indigent.	1. Through "local determination of needs and local control of administration. . . ."
	2. Possibly through federal agency or officials of existing agencies to which state in need may apply.
	3. Provision for singular action without involving disposal of aid to all states.

[43] HD, *Proceedings* (90 Annual Session, May, 1939), pp. 89–90.

Representatives of the AMA lost no time in informing the Senate Committee on Education and Labor of the Association's comprehensive attack upon the Wagner bill at the St. Louis session. Only eight days after the session closed, 17 prominent physicians and leaders of the Association gathered in Washington to supplement the testimony given by Booth on May 5. This number included Rock Sleyster, president of the AMA, Edward H. Cary, chairman of the Legislative Committee, R. G. Leland, director of the Bureau of Medical Economics, and Morris Fishbein.[44] While their attack followed authorized lines, subcommittee questioning brought out additional information. Whereas the Association had claimed that the St. Louis session unanimously endorsed the report against the Wagner bill, Fishbein confessed that complete unanimity did not exist. He conceded that although the vote was unanimous, about five delegates favored the bill with amendments, and that these delegates represented the views of betwen 5,000 and 10,000 physicians.[45]

Although the Association's Committee on Legislative Activities later indicated that the contacts established in Washington by this appearance had strengthened opposition to the measure, the testimony apparently had no great influence on the subcommittee. In August, it issued a report endorsed by the Committee on Education and Labor, which expressed approval of the basic objectives of the bill. The committee announced its intention to give the measure additional study, however, and to await a new session of Congress in January, 1940, before reporting out an amended bill.[46]

The Association's Platform

With the prospect of renewed agitation for the passage of a revised Wagner bill early in 1940, the Association dared not relax in its efforts to defeat the measure. In continuing its attack, the AMA saw the need for providing, in cogent language, a summary of its own position on current health issues. Although the Association's leaders and publications had spread its views throughout the nation, the AMA had prepared no simple digest of its position. On December 2, 1939, "The

[44] Editorial, *JAMA,* 112 (June 3, 1939), 2289; HD, *Proceedings* (91 Annual Session, June, 1940), p. 54.

[45] Seventy-sixth Congress, first session, *Hearings on S. 1620,* Part 2, pp. 428–29.

[46] HD, *Proceedings* (91 Annual Session, June, 1940), p. 54; Abel Wolman, "The National Health Program—Present Status," *American Journal of Public Health,* 30 (January, 1940), 3–5.

Platform of the American Medical Association" began to appear regularly in the *Journal* when the Association adopted a method of publicity based on simplicity and reiteration.[47]

THE PLATFORM OF THE AMERICAN MEDICAL ASSOCIATION

1. The establishment of an agency of the federal government under which shall be co-ordinated and administered all medical and health functions of the federal government exclusive of those of the Army and Navy.

2. The allotment of such funds as the Congress may make available to any state in actual need, for the prevention of disease, the promotion of health and the care of the sick on proof of such need.

3. The principle that the care of the public health and the provision of medical service to the sick is primarily a local responsibility.

4. The development of a mechanism for meeting the needs of expansion of preventive medical services with local determination of needs and local control of administration.

5. The extension of medical care for the indigent and the medically indigent with local determination of needs and local control of administration.

6. In the extension of medical services to all the people, the utmost utilization of qualified medical and hospital facilities already established.

7. The continued development of the private practice of medicine, subject to such changes as may be necessary to maintain the quality of medical services and to increase their availability.

8. Expansion of public health and medical services consistent with the American system of democracy.

Although the AMA expected the development of a serious crisis early in 1940 over the establishment of a national health program, it rejoiced when none occurred. The growing international tension largely diverted the administration's interest from broad attacks upon domestic problems to considerations of national security. The widening of the social security system in 1939, with the inclusion of coverage for survivors in the old-age insurance plan and larger appropriations for social welfare

[47] Editorial, *JAMA,* 113 (December 2, 1939), 2060.

programs, also reduced the urgency of establishing a more comprehensive system.[48]

Lessening of Tension

The opening of the new decade found the administration seeking the AMA's support of a modest federal hospital construction program. The gap of estrangement between the Association and the administration seemed to have narrowed when the President invited representatives of the AMA to attend a conference on January 10 to discuss the proposed program. Although the possibility of a rapprochement appeared doubtful, since the House of Delegates had recently expressed fears that even the release of surplus veterans' hospitals for public use might lead to "socialized medicine," ten representatives of the AMA attended the conference.[49] This medical group noticed, however, that the President now spoke disapprovingly of the Wagner bill and that his proposal for constructing 50 hospitals, where the need seemed most acute and where the public agreed to maintain them, carried a denial of any intention to provide federal subsidization for maintenance. While sympathetic with the President's objectives and agreeing that none should be constructed except where the actual need existed and where the public would maintain them, the Association's representatives contended also that existing facilities should first be used, and that hospitals must meet the standards set by the AMA and the American College of Surgeons.[50]

Soon after the conference, the Wagner-George bill, embodying the President's proposal, was introduced in the Senate. Leaders of the AMA appeared before the Senate Committee on Education and Labor, suggesting changes that later the proposed Taft amendment to the bill partially incorporated. Although the amended Wagner-George bill passed the Senate on May 30, the Association saw the need for further changes. The AMA wanted approval by the proposed National Advisory Hospital

[48] For these changes see Earl E. Muntz, *Growth and Trends in Social Security* (Studies in Individual and Collective Security [New York: National Industrial Conference Board, Inc., 1949]), pp. 176, 150, 169, 171.

[49] HD, *Proceedings* (91 Annual Session, June, 1940), p. 55; HD, *Proceedings* (90 Annual Session, May, 1939), p. 85.

[50] Editorial, *JAMA,* 114 (January 20, 1940), 250–51. Here are also found a few other requirements desired by the medical group. Representatives of the AMA worked with representatives of the American, the Protestant, and the Catholic Hospital Associations in drawing up these requirements.

Council of all construction projects; elimination of osteopathic representation on the council; a reconsideration of the method for electing representatives to the council; and a definition of a hospital that would exclude all diagnostic, health, and treatment centers.[51]

When this measure, to which the Association sought only minor amendments, died with the expiration of the Seventy-sixth Congress, the AMA showed no regret. The trustees reported to the Cleveland session of 1941 that the less popular Mead hospital construction measure had met the same fate, and that the threat of the enactment of the Wagner National Health bill and the Capper-Epstein health insurance measure had also temporarily passed.[52] From the viewpoint of the American Medical Association, the Seventy-sixth Congress had resisted pressures for the passage of legislation that seemed objectionable.

The trustees' report also showed the Association's growing interest in political affairs. It announced that the Association had established a federal legislative bulletin service at the beginning of the Seventy-seventh Congress to supply state societies with information about congressional activities that concerned the medical profession.[53] By this time, however, the growing seriousness of the international crisis had pushed most domestic issues into the background.

The Association's attitude toward the New Deal program during Roosevelt's second administration appeared less favorable than during the first. It could make few concessions to the administration after the second term began without abandoning its historic views. When the administration seemed to be moving toward compulsory health insurance, almost total estrangement developed. Yet experience with the depression and the New Deal programs led the AMA to accept a few governmental measures related to health and medical care that marked some retreat from earlier positions.

[51] HD, *Proceedings* (91 Annual Session, June, 1940), p. 55.
[52] *JAMA,* 116 (April 19, 1941), 1796.
[53] *Ibid.*

Chapter 12 THE VOLUNTARY HEALTH INSURANCE ISSUE

THE AMA NEVER ALLOWED the dramatic character of the New Deal program which so quickly captured the nation's interest to divert its attention from nonpolitical and less spectacular developments affecting medical practice. Since World War I it had witnessed the ominous spread of group and contract practice and, more recently, the rapid growth of voluntary group health insurance schemes. While still believing that newer forms of medical practice often imperiled the profession's standards, it saw additional dangers in the rising popularity of group hospitalization insurance.[1]

Spread of Voluntary Health Insurance

The rapid growth of the voluntary health insurance movement in the New Deal era resulted in a large measure from the same conditions that produced the New Deal itself. The depression, which brought its legacy of poverty, hunger, and disease awakened a poor and embittered population to the need of economic security during periods of sickness. The self-respecting citizenry of the nation that had experienced the humiliation of destitution and charity now looked for systematic means of meeting the cost of illness, a fruitful mother of poverty. Likewise, the impetus that the depression gave to collective experiments, whether to organizations of consumers established for the cheaper purchase of goods or to tenant farmers' unions created to resist the oppression of landlords, all

[1] Refer to chap. 9 for an account of the AMA's attitude toward group and contract practice and group hospitalization insurance in the period before the New Deal.

types provided useful precedents in the development of collective experiments for meeting the costs of hospital care.[2]

Although the unsettled economic conditions of the early years of the depression provided convincing proof of the need for some form of sickness insurance, the very character of voluntary plans contributed to their popularity. Well in line with historic patterns of social action, the voluntary principle found favor among many who opposed the adoption of any compulsory system. In fact, the movement drew support from some who preferred compulsory insurance. Convinced of the futility of any direct effort to secure the establishment of a compulsory plan, some proponents of the idea advised the Fabian tactics of attrition and indirection. They saw little hope for the successful operation of voluntary schemes and believed that a nation once conditioned to the idea of applying the insurance principle to sickness problems would ultimately initiate a compulsory system. Although some of the backers accepted voluntary insurance only as an expedient, most of them opposed any compulsory form.

Prestige of the Movement

The forces promoting group hospitalization insurance in the early New Deal era not only increased in numerical strength but gained in prestige as well. Widespread demonstration of the advantages of such insurance had attracted the attention of a number of reputable organizations. In February, 1933, the American Hospital Association officially endorsed the voluntary principle after a seven-year study of methods of providing hospitalization.[3] The American College of Surgeons, which began its study of group hospitalization in 1933, shocked portions of the medical world a year later with an official endorsement of voluntary group insurance. By the middle of 1934, leaders of the Michigan State Medical Society had expressed approval, and in August the American Dental Association laid down principles to which it expected any voluntary plans to conform that covered the costs of dental care.[4]

[2] For observations on some co-operative enterprises see Wecter, *Age of Great Depression,* pp. 276–77; Sherwood Eddy, *Eighty Adventurous Years* (New York: Harper & Brothers Publishers, 1955), p. 156.

[3] Brown, *Physicians and Medical Care,* p. 168; Richardson, *Origin and Development of Group Hospitalization,* p. 22.

[4] Richardson, *Origin and Development of Group Hospitalization,* pp. 23–24; *The Literary Digest* (October 27, 1934), p. 19; Cabot, *The Doctor's Bill,* p. 229;

While the backing of these professional organizations contributed immeasurably to the appeal of group health insurance, substantial support also came from a number of private philanthropic foundations. The generous aid that foundations gave to the studies of the Committee on the Costs of Medical Care only encouraged other philanthropic grants for the promotion of health insurance programs. After a careful study of hospital care in England, the Duke Endowment appropriated $25,000 in April, 1935, for the establishment of a state-wide voluntary group hospitalization plan in North Carolina. A year later the Commonwealth Fund established a similar service in Kingsport, Tennessee, at about the time that the trustees of the Julius Rosenwald Fund pledged $100,000 to the American Hospital Association for the promotion of the idea.[5]

AMA's Resistance

The growing support that the movement secured in the years from 1933 to 1936 brought prompt reactions from the AMA. It had not given up its attack upon the majority report of the Committee on the Costs of Medical Care when the new administration was installed on March 4, 1933. While watching carefully the course of developments at the nation's capital, it showed as much concern about the apparent vitality of the health insurance issue. Only three weeks after the new administration began, the editor of the *Journal* explained the Association's hesitancy to approve any voluntary plans. He charged that their failure to include the services of all doctors and hospitals in an area promoted strife within the profession and among hospitals. He also contended that when plans restricted the choice of physicians and hospitals they repudiated a sacred maxim in medical care. Another writer in the same issue summarized the majority and minority reports of the Committee on the Costs of Medical Care, asserting that those who signed the majority report admitted that the voluntary idea opened the way for the adoption of a compulsory system.[6]

Mary Ross, "The Issue of Health," *Survey Graphic,* 23 (December, 1934), 586. For an account of the activities of a group within the American Dental Association that worked for the inclusion of dental care in insurance plans see *The Literary Digest* (March 16, 1935), p. 14.

[5] Richardson, *Origin and Development of Group Hospitalization,* pp. 24–28.

[6] Editorial, *JAMA,* 100 (March 25, 1933), 973; Lewellyn F. Barker, "Investigations and Conclusions of the Committee on the Costs of Medical Care," *JAMA,* 100 (March 25, 1933), 868. The same issue of the *Journal* also contained an article referred to on p. 184 above.

The issue that so greatly disturbed the *Journal* in the early spring of 1933 naturally received attention from the House of Delegates that convened at Milwaukee in June. President Edward H. Cary's address on the first day provided a reliable forecast of the Association's action, as he informed the body that their "official family" had already endorsed the principal minority report of the Committee on the Costs of Medical Care. The House of Delegates soon received the report of the Reference Committee on Legislation and Public Relations that severely criticized the majority's recommendations and urged endorsement of the minority report. The house readily obliged, approving a resolution which declared that the minority report was "expressive, in principle, of the collective opinion of the medical profession."[7]

Endorsement of the principal minority report represented no departure from the AMA's traditional opposition. While the report recommended an expansion of governmental aid for indigent medical care which would reduce the burden that the medical profession had assumed, it called for the elimination of government competition in the practice of medicine. It also denounced corporate medical practice financed by intermediate agencies and only vaguely suggested the idea of experimentation within existing institutions of methods that harmonized with medical standards.[8] It raised no objections to proposals for the establishment of plans for distributing the costs of medical care when set up by county medical societies, but listed eight principles to which these plans must conform. While denouncing the idea of compulsory health insurance, the minority report referred to the futility of further expanding any voluntary plans except those initiated by local societies.[9]

The same session not only took an official position upon the widely publicized reports of the Committee on the Costs of Medical Care, but also attempted to create a united voice within the organization. Long troubled by the well-known and unorthodox views of some medical groups on important political and economic questions, the Association

[7] HD, *Proceedings* (84 Annual Session, June, 1933), pp. 3, 58.

[8] Barker, *JAMA,* 100 (March 25, 1933), 868; The Committee on the Costs of Medical Care, *Medical Care for the American People: Final Report,* pp. 163–83. The proposal suggesting experimentation with methods that harmonized with the profession's traditional standards is almost too vague to be meaningful. The report does refer, however, to plans of either prepayment or postpayment as a desirable arrangement for victims of chronic illness. *Ibid.,* pp. 176–79.

[9] *Ibid.* pp. 179–81, 163–64. Signers of the minority report referred to plans adopted by ten county societies in Iowa as appearing to be satisfactory. Yet these examples were not voluntary insurance plans at all but cases of local governmental subsidization of medical care for the aged through payments to local societies. The report cited no cases of voluntary plans of which the signers approved. See p. 74.

strove to establish at least an appearance of internal unity. The organs of many state societies had already felt the impact of the *Journal's* attack on novel methods for meeting the costs of medical care and had hastily taken its position. The trustees pushed along the movement toward conformity by submitting to the Milwaukee session a resolution which they had endorsed in February calling upon all national medical organizations, whose admission requirements included membership in the AMA, to register their opinions upon issues affecting medical practice only through channels that met the Association's approval.[10]

Contrary to the view that spokesmen for the AMA later expressed, abundant evidence supports the position that by the end of 1933 the Association had not clearly differentiated between the theory and practice of voluntary group hospitalization schemes and followed a policy that militated against both. The contention "that the American Medical Association in 1933 was opposed only to those voluntary plans which involved certain harmful features. . . ." is hardly supported by the Association's actions.[11] While the AMA might find in the realm of fancy an impractical plan that met its approval, it detected intolerable corruption in all of those that touched the earth. The Milwaukee session provided a splendid opportunity that the delegates missed for clearly favoring the voluntary principle, while opposing objectionable features of many plans. The session took pains to re-emphasize the difference between contract practice per se, which it did not oppose, and certain objectionable features that sometimes accompanied it.[12] The AMA had offered more criticism of group hospitalization schemes than of cases of

[10] Bridgman, "The American Medical Association and the Great Depression," p. 212; "Report of Board of Trustees," HD, *Proceedings* (84 Annual Session, June, 1933), pp. 20, 55. For the Trustees' action on this resolution submitted by the Pennsylvania state society see *JAMA,* 100 (March 4, 1933), 668.

[11] Dickinson, "History of Attitude of AMA toward Voluntary Health Insurance," p. 19.

[12] The Reference Committee on Medical Legislation came the nearest to drawing a distinction between the theory and practice of voluntary insurance. This committee condemned "any plan which incorporates principles contrary to the remarks on contract practice." HD, *Proceedings* (84 Annual Session, June, 1933), p. 58. Yet the AMA had several other reasons for condemning voluntary insurance. Point seven of its criticisms of certain forms of contract practice stated that such practice was objectionable if "its provisions or practical results is contrary to sound public policy." This standard was broad and vague enough to condemn any plan of either contract practice or group hospitalization that the AMA wished to destroy. For the Association's attitude toward contract practice see pp. 173–76 above and HD, *Proceedings* (84 Annual Session, June, 1933), p. 26.

contract practice, yet the delegates left no indication at all that they approved of even the theory of group insurance.[13]

The evidence indicates that they held the view expressed by the *Journal* on January 21 that commercialism, competition, and lay influence appeared as almost inherent evils within voluntary schemes. They seemed in full agreement with the views of President Dean Lewis, who told the body, "It is well known that voluntary health insurance has not been successful and that when started it has soon become compulsory."[14] In attacking plans so inextricably bound up in alleged abuses, the AMA made no distinction between theory and practice. Much evidence indicates that the weaknesses detected in voluntary schemes convinced the Association that no practical voluntary group plan would be free from highly objectionable features. Probably no plan that it later supported would have met its approval at this time. Its endorsement of the principal minority report of the Committee on the Costs of Medical Care reflected basic hostility toward voluntary group insurance.

The attitude reflected by the Association toward voluntary health insurance for many months after the Milwaukee meeting harmonized perfectly with the spirit displayed by this session. It continued to publicize the evils of these plans, frequently attacking voluntary health insurance in a general way. Nor did it ignore the forces that agitated the medical profession about the adoption of voluntary insurance or more radical schemes. Through its own organs, as well as through popular publications and scholarly journals of other professional organizations, it carried its views to the nation.

Much of the Association's fight against voluntary schemes lay in its offensive against the Committee on the Costs of Medical Care. While the AMA had largely confined its earliest criticism to its own publications, in November, 1933, a nonmedical scholarly journal published its attack. In *The Annals of the American Academy of Political and Social Science,* Roscoe G. Leland, director of the Bureau of Medical Eco-

[13] Dickinson cites a *Journal* editorial of December 3, 1932, that seemed to approve of the idea of individuals carrying insurance to cover the costs incurred by "a major illness or operation," and which stated that insurance companies might offer such policies if the demand was sufficient. "History of Attitude of AMA toward Voluntary Health Insurance," p. 17. This editorial, however, does not show that the AMA approved of any practical plans to meet the nation's needs, for characteristics that would have made them effective, would have also made them objectionable to the AMA.

[14] *JAMA,* 100 (January 21, 1933), 193–94; quotation, *JAMA,* 100 (June 17, 1933), 1909.

nomics, and his colleague, Algie M. Simons, a former prominent Socialist and a recent proselyte from the compulsory health insurance forces, denied the reliability of much of the evidence that the committee had amassed.[15] After challenging the definition of illness set forth in one of the committee's publications, they argued that it had established no method for accurately determining variations of morbidity in different income groups. They also charged that it "failed to establish any statistical measure of the amount of neglected illness," and that any use of its materials that indicated statistical accuracy was "almost wholly misleading."[16]

Leland and Simons seemed just as critical of any proposals for voluntary health insurance as of the studies of the Committee on the Costs of Medical Care. They saw the multiplication of difficulties in the operation of voluntary schemes.

> It is always easy in the voluntary stage to find examples of fairly satisfactory schemes and by carefully omitting all mention of the unsatisfactory ones, to build up an argument for extension of insurance. But experience shows not only that the unsatisfactory features show a tendency to aggravation with expansion, but also that time and growth tend to introduce new and even more undesirable features.[17]

While openly suspicious of the future for voluntary health insurance, they listed four standards to which any plans of medical care must conform. They affirmed the necessity of the profession's control over all features of medical service as well as control over all institutions providing medical care. They also contended that no third party must be allowed to intervene between physician and patient "in any of the relations connected with medical service," and that the patient's free choice of a physician must be maintained.[18]

[15] Simon's opposition to compulsory health insurance is difficult to explain after he wrote, with Nathan Sinai, *The Way of Health Insurance,* a volume very favorable to compulsory insurance, which appeared in 1932. Soon after the publication of this book he accepted a position with the Bureau of Medical Economics, presumably after rejecting the idea of compulsory health insurance. An account of his contributions to the Socialist movement, which deals mostly with the first two decades of the twentieth century, is found in John J. Harmon, "Algie Martin Simons, 1870– ," (unpublished senior thesis, Princeton University, 1947).

[16] Leland and Simmons, "Do We Need Compulsory Public Health Insurance? No," The American Academy of Political and Social Science, *Annals,* 170 (November, 1933), 121. For a reply to some of the arguments that the AMA advanced against the findings of the Committee on the Costs of Medical Care, see Rorty, *American Medicine Mobilizes,* pp. 205–7.

[17] Leland and Simmons, *Annals,* 170 (November, 1933), 122.

[18] *Ibid.,* p. 126.

Although by published attacks the AMA obstructed the progress of the voluntary health insurance movement, it did not confine its opposition to the printed page. In advancing the movement on the local level, Michael M. Davis encountered opposition from the Association. In Nashville, Tennessee, the Davidson County Medical Society allowed him to present a voluntary plan that it failed to endorse only after an official of the AMA had exerted pressure to prevent its adoption. When an executive committee of the Michigan State Medical Society called upon officials of the AMA for information about a method of providing medical care for the state's families of low income, it secured no aid and aroused antagonism. According to Davis, the Association tried to dissuade the American Hospital Association from officially endorsing voluntary health insurance.[19]

Despite the resistance the Association offered to the spread of health insurance, the popularity of prepayment hospitalization plans increased in the middle thirties. The endorsement of the voluntary insurance principle by the American College of Surgeons and the Michigan State Medical Society in 1934, and the friendliness that the American Dental Association displayed added immeasurably to the strength of the movement. When in the same year the New York legislature pioneered in passing enabling legislation for the establishment of voluntary plans, the health insurance advocates achieved another important victory.[20]

The agitation for voluntary insurance that the Association dared not ignore at the Milwaukee session of 1933 required even more attention at the annual meeting a year later. The delegates who gathered at Cleveland in June, 1934, soon learned that the position of the Board of Trustees had not substantially changed. At a closed session the trustees presented an account of the Association's historic attitude toward the health insurance controversy, carrying their discussion back to the inauguration of the British compulsory system in 1912. They reminded the delegates of powerful forces at work to establish some "foreign" plan of health insurance in the United States, and of the growing popularity of comprehensive systems of social security. They found voluntary health insurance the opening wedge toward the adoption of a compulsory scheme repeating the argument that "voluntary insurance has always

[19] Michael M. Davis, "Change Comes to the Doctor," *Survey Graphic,* 23 (April, 1934), 164; Cabot, *The Doctor's Bill,* p. 229. For information about the plans worked out by the Michigan society see Frederick C. Warnshuis, "Michigan Makes Ready," *Survey Graphic,* 23 (December, 1934), 639–40; Bridgman, "The American Medical Association and the Great Depression," p. 247.

[20] Richardson, *Origin and Development of Group Hospitalization,* p. 36.

been the forerunner of compulsory insurance, and even the most ardent advocates of voluntary insurance admit that fact."[21]

Association's Platform

Although the Cleveland session offered no commendation of voluntary health insurance, the delegates appeared a little more favorable to the idea. They adopted a health insurance platform recommended by the Board of Trustees, which indicated that even these officials had somewhat tempered their attitude on the voluntary insurance issue. While in no way succumbing to the health insurance agitation, the Association officially accepted a platform including standards specific enough to prevent rejection of voluntary schemes on vague and general grounds. The platform reflected the Association's more extensive study of the issue and its formulation of a more rational method for assessing the merits of any plan.[22]

Position of the American Medical Association in 1934 on Voluntary Health Insurance Plans

1. All features of medical service in any method of medical practice should be under the control of the medical profession. No other body or individual is legally or educationally equipped to exercise such control.

2. No third party must be permitted to come between the patient and his physician in any medical relation. All responsibility for the character of medical service must be borne by the profession.

3. Patients must have absolute freedom to choose a legally qualified doctor of medicine who will serve them from among all those qualified to practice and who are willing to give service.

4. The method of giving the service must retain a permanent, confidential relation between the patient and a "family physician." This relation must be the fundamental and dominating feature of any system.

5. All medical phases of all institutions involved in the medical service should be under professional control, it being understood that hospital service and medical service should be considered separately. These insti-

[21] HD, *Proceedings* (85 Annual Session, June, 1934), p. 43.

[22] HD, *Proceedings* (85 Annual Session, June, 1934), p. 55. Before the House adopted this platform the Bureau of Medical Economics submitted 12 principles to which it thought voluntary plans should conform. The delegates, however, reduced this platform to ten points. HD, *Proceedings* (85 Annual Session, June, 1934), p. 43. While these points are listed in ordinal sequence in the *Proceedings,* the cardinal method is here employed.

tutions are but expansions of the equipment of the physician. He is the only one whom the law of all nations recognizes as competent to use them in the delivery of service. The medical profession alone can determine the adequacy and character of such institutions. Their value depends on their operation according to medical standards.

6. However the cost of medical service may be distributed, the immediate cost should be borne by the patient if able to pay at the time the service is rendered.

7. Medical services must have no connection with any cash benefits.

8. Any form of medical service should include within its scope all legally qualified doctors of medicine of the locality covered by its operation who wish to give service under the conditions established.

9. Systems for the relief of low income classes should be limited strictly to those below the "comfort level" standard of incomes.

10. There should be no restriction on treatment or prescribing not formulated and enforced by the organized medical profession.

Although the platform adopted by the House of Delegates in 1934 largely embodied principles that the *Journal* had already expressed, its action marked an advance toward the acceptance of voluntary insurance schemes. Just as important as what the decalogue included are the points it omitted. It made no reference to "foreign" innovations in medical care, and it excluded the Association's contention that voluntary health insurance opened the way for the introduction of compulsory plans. Nor did it refer to the argument that voluntary schemes worked as a divisive force within the profession and among hospitals and weakened professional control over the administration of medical service. Although many plans still combined features that the *Journal* had long condemned, the Association now adopted a more favorable attitude toward the idea of voluntary health insurance. Partially accounting for the development of a more friendly spirit appears to have been the growing unpopularity of the *Journal's* policy within the profession, and particularly among the vocal elements of the Michigan State Medical Society.[23]

[23] HD, *Proceedings* (85 Annual Session, June, 1934), p. 54. The Michigan State Medical Society had already sent representatives to England to determine the success of the British medical system. While opposing the adoption in the United States of any foreign compulsory schemes, they reported that the British system had worked successfully in the interest of the profession and the public and had produced no deterioration in medical service. Warnshuis, *Survey Graphic,* 23 (December, 1934), 614.

While the Cleveland session appeared more sympathetic toward the idea of voluntary health insurance, it seemed less disposed to tolerate the alleged abuses of contract practice. Despite the Association's discouragement of such plans in the 1920's, contract schemes had multiplied as poorly paid physicians sought desperately to replenish their exhausting resources with a stable income.[24] Yet the House of Delegates surrounded contract schemes with stronger restrictions that threatened the very foundations on which many had been established. In addition to making a slight change in the definition of contract practice, the delegates adopted an amendment to the standard of ethics that stated:

> It is unprofessional for a physician to dispose of his professional attainments or services to any lay body, organization, group, or individual, by whatever name called, or however organized, under terms or conditions which permit a direct profit from the fees, salary, or compensation received to accrue to the lay body or individual employing him. Such a procedure is beneath the dignity of professional practice, is unfair competition with the profession at large, is harmful alike to the profession of medicine and the welfare of the people, and is against sound public policy.[25]

Platform Breeds Confusion

Although the delegates dealt at length with the voluntary health insurance question at the Cleveland session, they failed to speak decisively upon this troublesome issue. As the Association's legislative body wavered, the profession had no clear idea of official policy. Neither did a platform that failed to ease the minds of some physicians satisfy

[24] The trustees told the Milwaukee session in June, 1933 that "more than 250 hospitals are either engaged in or are considering furnishing hospital care under some form of contract" and added that "This new phase of contract practice has been stimulated by the urgency of the present financial stress and is being vigorously promoted for profit by lay corporations and individuals, who are capitalizing to their own advantage on the present hospital situation and the popular appeal for medical care at low rates." HD, *Proceedings,* (84 Annual Session, June, 1933), p. 13. See also Brown, *Physicians and Medical Care,* p. 166.

[25] "Principles of Medical Ethics," chap. iii, Art. IV, sec. 5, *American Medical Directory* (1938), 5th ed., p. 15, quoted in Joseph Laufer, "Ethics and Legal Restrictions on Contract and Corporate Practice of Medicine," *Law and Contemporary Problems,* 6 (Autumn, 1939), 519. For the *Journal's* comments on the significance of this amendment see *JAMA,* 103 (July 28, 1934), 263–64. See p. 175 above for the earlier definition of contract practice.

a growing number of interested laymen who had difficulty in interpreting the Association's action.

Following the Cleveland session observers searched for the location of old landmarks. Some announced with noticeable uncertainty that the Association had staked its claims inside the hinterland of an area pre-empted by the voluntary insurance movement. Mary Ross, who surveyed the scene, made her way out of the confusion only with the aid of an official guide, Morris Fishbein. While classifying the sixth point of the Association's platform as obscure and hardly subject to a literal interpretation, she found the Association more favorably disposed to voluntary insurance. This opinion was reached, however, only after Fishbein had announced in an address after the June session that the AMA had never opposed the voluntary insurance principle.[26]

In February, 1935, the *Literary Digest* also found a need for Fishbein's help as it searched for the Association's position. Sensing that the attitude of the AMA toward voluntary health insurance had undergone some change, it remarked:

> In an editorial published two weeks ago *The Journal* stated its position in a way which indicated that medical leaders have changed their point of view. The former attitude seemed to be one of uncompromising opposition to any form of health insurance. Now it appears that some forms of sickness insurance will be acceptable, provided organized medicine initiates and controls them.[27]

Despite Fishbein's strong insistence that the Association's policy had not changed, he failed to convince some prominent members of the organization who even long afterward contended otherwise.

Position in Retrospect

Writing 14 years after the historic Cleveland session, Louis H. Bauer, a member of the Board of Trustees and president of the Medical Society of the State of New York, referred to the minority report of the Committee on the Costs of Medical Care and said:

> This report has frequently been used to show that the American Medical Association was formerly opposed to voluntary medical insurance. No other attitude could have been taken at that time. The only experience

[26] Ross, *Survey Graphic,* 23 (December, 1934), 586.
[27] *The Literary Digest* (February 9, 1935), p. 17.

> in the matter of voluntary health insurance was in Europe, where these experiments failed, and did lead to compulsory health insurance. It will be noted, however, that this report did recommend the development by state or county medical societies of plans for medical care.[28]

Bauer's statement, indeed, brought no reply from Fishbein, who two years earlier had stated:

> In 1932 the Committee on the Costs of Medical Care offered its proposals for change in the nature of the practice of medicine. These too were officially opposed by the medical profession, which at that time also opposed voluntary sickness insurance as well as voluntary hospitalization insurance. Perhaps a word is necessary now to indicate the reason for this attitude. The medical profession is scientifically trained. Before any new method of treatment is accepted, the value must be demonstrated and the safety of the method must be assured. Medicine as a profession demands equally that social experiments in the field of medical practice prove their value and their safety before they are acceptable and before they are extended to the public.[29]

As the special session of the House of Delegates convened in February, 1935, to consider the impending threat of a political program hostile to its interests, it had no time to deal further with the voluntary insurance issue. Less than four months later, however, the regular session in Atlantic City turned its attention to this disturbing question. Although the tempered stand of the House of Delegates in 1934 had left the Association's position in considerable doubt, the Atlantic City session offered no explanation for its earlier moderate action. In fact, considerable evidence showed that although the governing body had verged on approval of voluntary schemes in 1934, it had retreated from this position a year later.

Abiding Fears of Voluntary Health Insurance

The attitude of the Bureau of Medical Economics seems to have represented the sentiment of the body. In its report the bureau warned that "sane progress" came by evolutionary means and not by "sudden jumps." It sought to ease whatever minds were tortured by the thought of wide-

[28] Louis Hopewell Bauer, *Private Enterprise or Government in Medicine* (Springfield, Illinois: Charles C. Thomas, Publisher, 1948), p. 65.

[29] *JAMA*, 130 (February 23, 1946), 511. See also *JAMA*, 128 (June 30, 1945), 672–74.

spread, unmet medical needs with the assurance that the actual situation bore little relation to exaggerated claims. It charged that the exclusion of minor cases of sickness from consideration

> . . . leaves only from 10 to 15 per cent of the low income class whose medical expenses each year constitute a heavy burden or so-called catastrophe. Some of these are capable of meeting even these expenses without any special arrangements. They do undertake and meet such expenditures far less imperatively needed than medical care for serious illnesses without requiring the establishment of any special social machinery.[30]

While the bureau aimed its report partially against the establishment of unsound political experiments, its communication served the additional purpose of encouraging satisfaction with the existing situation.

The bureau got substantial backing from some committees. The Reference Committee on Medical Economics commended its studies on group hospitalization and expressed its conviction that "the natural development of such schemes would lead sooner or later to an inclusion of medical service in one form or another with inevitable deterioration in the quality of service."[31] The Reference Committee on Medical Research listed ten dangers it found in such schemes, one of which was "The almost inevitable transition of voluntary plans into sickness insurance operated by the state." The Board of Trustees also endorsed the committee's views, offering several objections to most forms of group health insurance.[32]

Although the Atlantic City meeting adopted reports that showed decided fear of voluntary insurance, Fishbein continued to inform the public that, with certain restrictions, the AMA did not oppose such schemes.[33] Yet, it became increasingly difficult to reconcile the Association's actions with this pronouncement. The AMA's determined move against an Oklahoma physician who operated a group payment hospital clinic seemed to confirm charges of its consistent hostility to voluntary programs.

Since 1929, Michael A. Shadid had attracted considerable publicity with his successful plan that provided adequate and inexpensive medical care for the people in and near Elk City, Oklahoma. Ostracized by the

[30] HD, *Proceedings* (86 Annual Session, June, 1935), p. 59; quoted sentences p. 57.

[31] HD, *Proceedings* (86 Annual Session, June, 1935), p. 46.

[32] HD, *Proceedings* (86 Annual Session, June, 1935), pp. 63, 13.

[33] Fishbein, *AMA Bulletin,* 31 (February, 1936), 41.

local medical society, he finally encountered opposition from the AMA. When the Association heard that several local residents were negotiating for a government loan to buy stock in his co-operative institution it issued a vigorous protest. In an effort to stop the negotiations, the House of Delegates in 1936 authorized the trustees to communicate their disapproval to the President of the United States and other high-ranking political officials. The Association insisted that "federal aid for this or any other hospital similarly situated . . . is contrary to public policy and to the interests of the medical profession. . . ." Apparently the AMA's effort was unsuccessful, as the hospital added a three-story addition in 1936 and continued to operate with remarkable success.[34]

The Association's leadership recognized the existence of growing internal pressures before the Kansas City session opened in 1936. It had already denied the request of five state medical societies for a special session to be held early in that year to consider problems of medical economics.[35] When the delegates convened in May, President-elect J. Tate Mason confessed that numbers of physicians thought that some changes in the administration of and payment for medical care were imperative. Yet he said the experience of other nations convinced them that

> . . . voluntary prepayment and insurance schemes in the hands of the profession at the outset, drift inevitably, as do all plans initiated by private groups, into bureaucratically administered compulsory insurance under governmental control. They felt that the most certain method of hastening state medicine is for the medical profession to institute radical changes in medical practice in the form of some experiment of this kind.[36]

He added, however, that while most physicians disapproved of the establishment of any insurance plan for the population as a whole, they did not object to experiments approved and carried on by local societies.

Although Mason's address had introduced the voluntary insurance issue, the trustees' reference to the subject was more significant. Their report showed surprising friendliness toward the idea, which

[34] Quotation, HD, *Proceedings* (87 Annual Session, May, 1935), p. 68; Garceau, *Political Life of AMA*, p. 104. For comments on the successful operation of this hospital at mid-century see statement of Michael V. Shadid, Subcommittee of Senate Committee on Labor and Public Welfare, Eighty-first Congress, second session, *Hearings on S. 1805* (Government Printing Office, Washington, 1950), pp. 213, 215, 217.

[35] HD, *Proceedings* (87 Annual Session, May, 1936), p. 27.

[36] HD, *Proceedings* (87 Annual Session, May, 1936), p. 5.

indicated that pressures at work within the organization had somewhat tempered their attitude. Harsh criticisms of inherent weaknesses in voluntary insurance found no place in the report, as the trustees denied earlier opposition to the idea. Aware of attacks made upon the Association's position, they stated that:

> The protagonists of group hospitalization have created the erroneous impression that the medical profession opposes all group hospitalization plans. Those plans offered by community-wide, noncommercial associations of hospitals designed to offer hospital facilities to low-income groups in a manner and at a cost commensurate with knowledge gained from experience and sound advice, which have a representation of the local medical profession in the administration to assure the exclusion of features objectionable to the practice of medicine, have encountered no serious obstruction on the part of medical societies. The most encouraging progress in group hospitalization has been made by these plans.[37]

Recognition of Great Unmet Medical Needs

The trustees' report constituted an admission that voluntary plans could successfully operate without impairment of professional standards, and that a serious problem of unmet medical needs existed that justified their adoption. This report represented some advance over the Association's earlier view that practically all could afford adequate medical care and that compulsory schemes almost inevitably resulted from voluntary experiments. While the Association had begun to recognize the incapacity of a sizable part of the population to afford the expense of medical service, it still resisted the idea that the supply of physicians was inadequate. The Committee on Legislative Activities informed the Kansas City meeting of the preliminary findings of a survey it had not yet completed. Basing its conclusions on reports from 16 states, it asserted that "localities lacking medical services are extremely elusive."[38]

Despite the conciliatory attitude that the Kansas City session manifested toward voluntary insurance, the AMA opposed the efforts of ambitious physicians who worked independently in developing plans for meeting the costs of medical care. While somewhat unsure about its own course of action, it nevertheless discouraged the efforts of more

[37] HD, *Proceedings* (87 Annual Session, May, 1936), p. 22.
[38] HD, *Proceedings* (87 Annual Session, May, 1936), p. 57.

confident groups. When the Cooperative League of the United States established the Bureau of Cooperative Medicine in 1936 to formulate plans for budgeting medical costs, the AMA soon showed considerable resentment. Although the two physicians who headed the bureau were in good standing with the Association and sought the co-operation of its leadership, they met only rebuffs. In April, 1937, the *Journal* assailed one of their proposals as a revival of the principles of lodge practice and no different from currently operating radical schemes. The editor remarked, "A man who is both a sincere co-operator and a competent physician finds his intellect in a civil war. . . ." The editor showed no sympathy for the unauthorized work of independent groups.[39]

Since the movement for voluntary insurance had increased in strength and showed every sign of permanence, the AMA exerted greater effort to control a tide that had risen without its direction. Indeed, it began to show sympathy for struggling hospitals caught in the crisis of the depression. The trustees noted in their annual report of 1937 that the income of hospitals from contributions and endowments had fallen by approximately two-thirds, but that the charity load had almost quadrupled.[40] This report constituted another admission that many sick people could not afford the costs of medical care. It also showed considerable sympathy for struggling hospitals, without referring to their search for "any port in a storm."[41]

Statement on Voluntary Insurance Plans

Nevertheless, the Association recognized that the spread of voluntary schemes multiplied opportunities for the development of abuses. In 1937, the House of Delegates at Atlantic City showed particular concern about the inclusion of medical services in hospitalization contracts, when

[39] Rorty, *American Medicine Mobilizes,* pp. 280–81; Editorial, *JAMA,* 108 (April 3, 1937), 1181.

[40] HD, *Proceedings* (88 Annual Session, June, 1937), p. 20.

[41] See p. 183 above. Although the AMA's attitude toward voluntary health insurance was undergoing some change, the evolution was imperceptible to some observers. Writing in 1937, Louis B. Reed said, "The American Medical Association . . . probably fearing that hospitalization insurance will become a precedent for more comprehensive forms of health insurance, has been lukewarm, to say the least, in its attitude toward the development." *Health Insurance: The Next Step in Social Security* (New York: Harper & Brothers Publishers, 1937), pp. 188–89.

the trustees warned that hospitalization and medical services were difficult to separate. The delegates adopted another set of principles to govern the operation of group hospitalization plans.[42]

The principles approved in 1937 considerably enlarged the platform that the delegates adopted three years earlier. While the Association seemed chiefly interested in safeguarding the basic principles of private practice in 1934, these fundamentals were less imperiled by voluntary schemes in 1937. Its last set of principles dealt principally with points that less directly affected the profession's interests and were more closely related to the mechanical operation of voluntary plans. Only the first, fifth, sixth, and seventh points were incorporated into the later list. These emphasized that the medical profession should have complete control over medical service under all plans, and that these services should have no connection with the cash benefits the plans provided. Standing out among the new points added by the Association in 1937 were the ones that urged the confinement of voluntary schemes to the low-income classes, and that itemized the services which hospital plans might cover. This list included only board, bed, medicines, operating room, nursing care, and surgical dressings.[43]

The problem of what services should be included in voluntary schemes became more pressing as the plans continued to spread. The Association's opposition to the inclusion of any medical services led to serious difficulties. Having broadened its viewpoint on the value of voluntary schemes, it made still further concessions. Although the fourth point of the 1937 platform carefully excluded all medical services, the San Francisco session a year later modified this position. It enlarged this point by adding:

> If for any reason it is found desirable or necessary to include special medical service such as anesthesis, radiology, pathology, or medical services provided by outpatient departments, these services may be included only on the condition that specified cash payments be made by the hospitalization organization directly to subscribers for the cost of such service.[44]

[42] See Appendix, pp. 408–9 for a statement of these principles.

[43] See Appendix, pp. 408–9, and pp. 236–37 above.

[44] The AMA's position in 1937 and the modification a year later is summarized in HD, *Proceedings* (90 Annual Session, May, 1939), p. 29. In 1938 the trustees reported that 21 state societies had voted against the inclusion of medical services in hospitalization contracts and that only one state society seemed favorable to the idea. HD, *Proceedings* (89 Annual Session, June, 1938), p. 32.

Although the Association surrounded this concession with several restrictions, it showed some willingness to regard its platform as less than unalterable.

This session also revealed that the AMA still had some misgivings, however, about the spread of voluntary schemes. The trustees called attention to what appeared to be inevitable weaknesses in voluntary plans. They referred to the administration costs (that were often excessive), and to the impossibility of calculating premium rates that would allow for the costs of applying new scientific processes. They also noted the natural tendency of subscribers to secure services covered by their insurance whether needed or not, but failed to note that they could be admitted into hospitals only on physicians' orders.[45]

Changing Temper of AMA

Although the special session of September, 1938, had been called to consider the political problems raised by the administration's proposed national health program, it did not ignore the voluntary insurance question. At the opening of this session, Harrison H. Shoulders, the speaker of the house, repeated the familiar claim that "The House of Delegates has never displayed an attitude of opposition to study and experimentation with plans for the financing of medical care by individuals or by the government."[46] In line with the more conciliatory spirit that the Association had already manifested, the delegates endorsed the principle of voluntary insurance and considered other economic issues related to illness. While reaffirming its well-known opposition to compulsory schemes, it endorsed the idea of cash-indemnity insurance as a supplementary method for alleviating the economic strains of sickness. With surprising haste, it also gave assent to the idea of protection from the loss of income resulting from illness, but largely left to the inquirer's imagination its views on how this was to be accomplished.[47]

[45] HD, *Proceedings* (89 Annual Session, June, 1938), p. 30.

[46] HD, *Proceedings* (Special Session, September, 1938), p. 2.

[47] *Ibid.*, p. 54; Editorial, *JAMA,* 111 (September 24, 1938), 1188. The House of Delegates did not make clear how the income-loss plan, which it endorsed, should operate, giving approval only to the idea. It endorsed cash-indemnity insurance as a means of protection against the cost of "emergency or prolonged illness."

When the special session considered various phases of health insurance in 1938, it seemed unaware that the movement for prepaid group insurance had already entered a new stage of development. The idea of group insurance for the public finally found its counterpart on the administrative level when hospitals over wide areas grouped together under similar or identical plans to provide their services. While hospitals in some localities had operated under uniform plans for several years, not until the inception of the Blue Cross Plans in 1937 did the movement truly enter a national phase. Supported by the American Hospital Association that created the Council on Blue Cross Plans a year later, this development showed great promise of respectability and permanence. The movement also started about the time that a number of state medical societies had registered their approval of the voluntary principle.[48] Yet, when the AMA's weight on the side of voluntary insurance might have added much encouragement, it became involved in a widely-publicized legal action brought by the federal government, that caused many to discount its professed friendliness toward voluntary insurance.

Federal Prosecution

On July 31, 1938, Thurman W. Arnold, assistant attorney general of the Department of Justice, announced his intention of pressing charges against the American Medical Association and several affiliated societies for alleged violation of the restraint-of-trade provision of the Sherman Anti-Trust Act.[49] The government claimed that the AMA and the Medical Society of the District of Columbia had attempted to crush a plan launched by the nonprofit, co-operative Group Health Association, Inc., that provided hospitalization and medical service for employees of the Home Owners' Loan Corporation and their dependents. It charged that officials of both medical organizations had threatened to expel any physician who served on the staff of the Group Health Association or who entered into medical consultations with physicians employed by this agency. The government also contended that these organizations had at-

[48] Richardson, *Origin and Development of Group Hospitalization,* pp. 18, 31, 84–86.

[49] Arnold's action was against the Academy of Surgery of Washington, D.C., the Harris County Medical Society of Texas, and 21 individuals, as well as the AMA. *JAMA,* 111 (December 24, 1938), 2397.

tempted to close the Washington hospitals to physicians on the staff of the Group Health Association.[50]

The AMA was greatly disturbed by the government's action. The *Journal* deplored the fact that the government had started on a course that was "inclined to cast public discredit on a great profession and to impugn the motives of workers in that profession." It looked upon the government's move as more persecution than prosecution and frequently cited newspapers that sided with its position.[51]

The first stage of what became an extended battle, however, went in favor of the Association. Along with the other medical societies and defendants, the AMA demurred to the government's indictment, and Judge James M. Proctor of the federal district court of Washington, D.C. sustained the demurrer. He maintained that many of the government's charges were too vague for consideration and denied that the practice of medicine was a trade under the Sherman Act.[52]

The stubborn Arnold refused to accept Proctor's decision as final and carried the case to the United States circuit court of appeals. This court on March 4, 1940, reversed the decision of the district judge and declared that the practice of medicine constituted a trade.[53] Six weeks later, the American Medical Association filed a writ of certiorari with the Supreme Court for a review of the decision. The writ was denied, however, and the Supreme Court declined to hear the case before the defendants had actually stood a jury trial in the Federal district court. While the jury that soon heard the case acquitted all of the individual defendants, the Harris County Medical Society and the Washington Academy of Surgery, it found the American Medical Association and the

[50] Benjamin D. Raub, Jr., "The Anti-Trust Prosecution against the American Medical Association," *Law and Contemporary Problems,* 6 (Autumn, 1939), 595–96; Paul A. Dodd and E. F. Penrose, *Economic Aspects of Medical Services* (Washington, D.C.: Graphic Arts Press, 1939), 278–79. The AMA gives this indictment in full in *JAMA,* 111 (December 31, 1938), 2495–500. The Department of Justice secured an indictment after it failed to obtain a consent decree. *JAMA,* 113 (August 5, 1939), 502.

[51] Quotation, *JAMA,* 112 (January 7, 1939), 51; Editorial, *JAMA,* 113 (August 5, 1939), 502; Editorial, *JAMA,* 111 (August 6, 1938), 539–40; *JAMA,* 112 (January 7, 1939), 53–58; *JAMA,* 113 (August 5, 1939), 507–11.

[52] Raub, "The Anti-Trust Prosecution against the AMA," pp. 596–98; *JAMA,* 113 (August 5, 1939), 502, 505–6.

[53] *JAMA,* 113 (September 16, 1939), 1134; *JAMA,* 113 (October 28, 1939), 1646; *JAMA,* 114 (March 9, 1940), 874; *JAMA,* 113 (October 16, 1940), 965–71. Arnold wanted to carry the case directly from the district court to the Supreme Court but this request was not granted.

Medical Society of the District of Columbia guilty of violating the Sherman Act.[54]

The final stage of the litigation was just as disappointing to the AMA as the decision in the district court. The Supreme Court granted the Association's petition for a writ of certiorari and agreed to review the case. Confining its consideration to the questions of whether medical practice was a trade under section 3 of the Sherman Act; whether the evidence proved restraint of trade; and whether the Clayton and Norris-LaGuardia Acts exempted the Association from prosecution under the Sherman Act, it upheld the decision of the district court. The highest tribunal announced its decision on January 18, 1943, and a few days later the Association sent the government a check for $2,500 in payment of fines.[55] Far more important to the Association than the penalties assessed, however, was the loss in prestige it had suffered by the litigation.

Medical Society Plans

The long contest with the federal government did not diminish the Association's interest in the voluntary health insurance issue. In fact, it became more strongly convinced that professional initiative in organizing voluntary plans not only provided the most reliable safeguard against the incorporation of objectionable features, but also served as the best deterrent to the introduction of a compulsory system. In 1939, the trustees noted with considerable pride that medical society plans which had numbered only 150 in 1934 had grown to more than 450 in five years and added that:

> . . . medical societies throughout the United States have in operation more experiments with new plans for the distribution of medical services than all the proponents of group payment plans have ever proposed.[56]

The trustees referred to the two types of plans, one of which prorated whatever funds were available for medical service to physicians who agreed to administer medical services on this basis, and the other that incorporated the cash-indemnity principle and paid a designated sum

[54] Editorial, *JAMA,* 114 (June 8, 1940), 2308; Editorial, *JAMA,* 116 (April 12, 1941), 1646.

[55] Editorial, *JAMA,* 120 (October 24, 1942), 624; *JAMA,* 121 (April 10, 1943), 1228.

[56] HD, *Proceedings* (90 Annual Session, May, 1939), p. 28.

for medical care. They followed the example set by an earlier session in showing preference for the latter type. They also cited the excessive burdens that a part of the population bore in having to resort to personal finance companies for loans to cover sickness bills and suggested the idea of developing special finance plans under the direction of local societies.[57]

While the AMA had showed little sympathy for the unauthorized efforts of member physicians to form groups for combating the threat of compulsory health insurance, it nevertheless supported one that was organized late in 1939, after the Association's approval had been secured. When influential leaders within the organization, at a meeting in Chicago on November 18, established the National Physicians' Committee for the Extension of Medical Service, the Association had a vigorous ally in the struggle. Standing out among the officers of the new organization were Edward H. Cary, a former president of the AMA, and Nathan S. Davis III, whose very name added an element of reverence to the movement. The appointment of Charles W. Mayo of Rochester, Minnesota, to the central committee further enhanced the prestige of the organization.[58]

This new group readily announced its purposes. While asserting independence of the AMA, it planned to join the Association's crusade against compulsory health insurance and other political threats to the medical profession. It expressed interest in promoting the development of society plans for meeting the needs of low-income classes and admitted the existence of serious unmet medical needs. In addition, the organization called attention to the threat of "government paternalism" which it hoped to oppose with a nation-wide campaign to present the medical profession in a better light.[59]

The organization of the physicians' committee did not result in a relaxation of the AMA's efforts to control the development of voluntary-insurance schemes. The Bureau of Medical Economics gave an extended account of health insurance developments to the New York session in 1940 and summarized its own activities. It reported on the completion of several research projects on the economic aspects of medical service as well as the revision of a study that had appeared in pamphlet form as "Factual Data on Medical Economics." Among other things, this pamphlet combined an account of the various plans that lay organiza-

[57] *Ibid.*, pp. 29, 32.

[58] *JAMA*, 113 (December 2, 1939), 2063.

[59] *Ibid.*

tions had developed for administering medical care with a study of schemes initiated by many local medical societies.[60] The bureau seemed somewhat disturbed by the recent inclusion in some hospitalization plans of ward benefits covering services that physicians normally performed. Although admitting that a few voluntary schemes "may conform to the principles adopted by the House of Delegates," it added that the AMA had given "No approval, endorsement or recommendation . . . to individual group hospitalization plans."[61]

Although the AMA's interest in the development of voluntary insurance continued, its attention was largely diverted to more pressing issues. As the European war raised many grave problems of national security, most of the Association's energies went into the program of military preparedness. The Cleveland session of 1941 had little time for the insurance question, although the trustees did refer to the subject, indicating that they had no objection to reasonably priced insurance plans launched by reliable companies when the benefits were paid directly to the insured.[62]

Summary of Position

The AMA considerably changed its position on the voluntary health insurance issue in the period from 1933 to 1941. Its attitude evolved from pronounced hostility to suspicious friendliness.[63] It began to feel that group hospitalization as well as medical society plans held promise of checking the threat of compulsory health insurance and of meeting a great public need. As this view matured, the Association made a serious effort to control the direction of the voluntary insurance movement.

[60] HD, *Proceedings* (91 Annual Session, June, 1940), p. 1907.

[61] *Ibid.*, p. 1910, quotation, p. 1909. This session adopted a resolution introduced by an Oregon physician that expressed disapproval of the conduct of some insurance companies in trying to set physicians' fees and in demanding reports on diagnosis and treatment that had not been authorized by the insured. HD, *Proceedings* (91 Annual Session, June, 1940), p. 62.

[62] *JAMA,* 116 (April 19, 1941), 1808.

[63] One writer sets 1942 as the date when the AMA "definitely aligns with group hospitalization." Richardson, *Origin and Development of Group Hospitalization,* p. 84. Another speaks of the Association's cautious acceptance of voluntary insurance in February, 1935, but he is referring to experimentation under the control of medical societies. Edwin E. Witte, with a foreword by Frances Perkins, *The Development of the Social Security Act* (Madison: The University of Wisconsin Press, 1962), p. 183. As this chapter shows the process was one of gradual accommodation to the general voluntary health insurance movement.

Chapter 13 PROTECTING THE NATION'S HEALTH, 1921–1941

WHILE THE AMERICAN MEDICAL ASSOCIATION frequently opposed the extension of federal authority over the nation's health and medical problems in the two decades that followed the Republican triumph of 1920, it nevertheless championed the idea of stronger federal power for curbing many public health abuses. Fourteen years of experience with the feeble enforcement of the weak food and drugs legislation of 1906 led the Association to urge a more vigorous attack upon medical charlatans and nostrum promoters.[1] It knew that the reforms the act had procured in the manufacturing and advertising of food and drugs had been in a large measure offset by the discovery of newer and more subtle ways of exploiting the public.

Broadening Fields of Exploitation

The period that fell between the close of World War I and the beginning of World War II offered medical charlatanry more liberties than it imposed restraints. As the frontiers of scientific medicine extended, quackery found even broader fields of operation. Scientific explorations into the mysteries of vitamins, hormones, and antibiotics not only provided better medical care for the public, but also opened up new sources of gain for the unscrupulous.[2] While scientific research

[1] See pp. 84–92 above for the AMA's appraisal of the original act and its experience with enforcement problems.

[2] Edwin E. Slosson discusses some of the new areas of scientific research in "Science, Mistress and Handmaid" (In Preston William Slosson, *The Great Crusade and after, 1914–1918,* Vol. 12 of *A History of American Life,* Arthur M. Schlesinger and Dixon Ryan Fox, eds.; New York: The Macmillan Company,

kindled the imagination of crafty promoters who sought easy ways to riches, its failure to discover cures for various major ailments made the boastful claims of pretending healers all the more impressive.

Promotion of Fads and Quackery

The impetus that quackery indirectly received from the discovery of new fields of scientific investigation only partially accounted for its popularity. Largely instrumental in its spread was the expenditure of enormous sums in extravagant advertising and publicity. Virtually free from the hampering effects of any restrictive legislation, the "unholy alliance" between quackery and advertising agencies flooded the nation with fraudulent nostrum claims and misleading propaganda. As the market swelled with competitive products, the desperate battle for survival drove aggressive firms to even greater extremes in promotional advertising.[3]

The early postwar era not only left the advertising efforts of unscrupulous firms almost unfettered, but also multiplied the opportunities for deception and fraud through clever methods of publicity. The great growth in newspaper circulation and the astonishing increase in the amount of space allotted to advertisements served well the interests of disreputable proprietary enterprises. Although newspapers at the beginning of the century usually limited advertisements to one-third of the total space, by 1924, 110 dailies in 63 cities had surrendered more than 45 per cent of available space to advertisers. In addition to newspaper publicity, however, exploiters resorted to other media of communication.

1931), pp. 377–78. He states that "The American public, as usual, was quick to try to catch and utilize every new discovery, sometimes indeed before the scientists themselves were agreed upon it or had worked out its bearings and limitations." *Ibid.*, p. 380, used with permission. One writer states that technological forces that had so often given consumers superior products nevertheless left them poorly prepared in the market place to distinguish "the better from the worse." Reed Dickerson, *Products Liability and the Consumer* (Boston: Little, Brown and Company, 1951), p. 3. Some of the advances of medical science during this period are treated in C. D. Haagensen and Wyndham E. B. Lloyd, *A Hundred Years of Medicine* (New York: Sheridan House, 1943), pp. 122–31, and Morris Fishbein, *Frontiers of Medicine* (Baltimore: The Williams and Wilkins Company in co-operation with the Century of Progress Exposition, 1933), pp. 182–83.

[3] Arthur J. Cramp, *Nostrums and Quackery and Pseudo-Medicine* (Chicago: American Medical Association, 1936), III, 78, cites the medical mail-order business as showing the close connection between advertising agencies and medical quacks.

By the time that sales of radios and accessories had jumped from $66,000,000 in 1922 to $842,548,000 seven years later, charlatans of the healing world had learned the effectiveness of radio publicity.[4]

Besides the sweeping technological improvements in mass communications that served the ulterior purposes of quackery, the unstable character of the national temperament also abetted its growth. A restless generation, in revolt against many social traditions, became in turn a ready market for a multiplying number of novelties and fads. The raising of the hemline of skirts lowered public appreciation of uncomely females and drove many wretched victims of obesity to the nostrum counters for the latest dietary fads. Receding hairlines that left denuded scalps above and depressed spirit below encouraged the sale of hair-restoring frauds. Surplus stretches of unwanted hair provided a ready market among many sensitive females for hair-removing nostrums, while others in search of lost youth or imaginary beauty found dyeing compounds particularly helpful. Manufacturers of skin preparations promised to give the coarsened faces and calloused hands of toiling women the touch of the sheltered beauties along New York's Park Avenue. Mail-order optical concerns, with their crude methods of distant diagnosis, promised better sight even to the hopeless, while manufacturers of hearing aids offered assistance in ushering in a utopia where the deaf could hear and the blind could see. Many deodorant manufacturers befriended growing numbers increasingly sensitive to the haunting thoughts of personal offense and made enormous sums exploiting the sense of smell.

The insatiate thirst for easy profits impelled exploiters of the credulous public to find a "fake for every ache," and more than one for most.[5] Innumerable compounds of varying value promised to quiet the turbulent storms in gaseous stomachs, while others claimed superior power in purging sluggish colons. Respiratory ailments provided a lucrative field for exploitation, and ghouls of human misery continued to market consumption and cancer cures. Nostrums sold as diabetic remedies flooded the market, as the enfeebled number afflicted with this malady

[4] Slosson, *Great Crusade and after,* pp. 347, 352; Frederick Lewis Allen, *Only Yesterday: An Informal History of the Nineteen-Twenties* (New York: Harper & Brothers Publishers, 1931), p. 165. See Editorial, *JAMA,* 94 (April 12, 1930), 1146, for the AMA's description of the depths to which radio advertising sank in the twenties.

[5] W. W. Bauer, *Health, Hygiene and Hooey* (Indianapolis: The Bobbs-Merrill Company, Publishers, 1938), 168.

showed a sharp increase. The nostrum market for female ailments flourished, as sensitive and prudish women concealed their gynecological symptoms from understanding physicians and chose instead the impersonal ways of quackery. Cures for venereal diseases were promised through secret, self-applied remedies, without fear of exposure to social disgrace or demands of abstinence, and reached a market that cut across the boundaries of sex.

Other factors favoring the growth of a lucrative nostrum industry in the early postwar era were the greater prosperity that portions of the population enjoyed, and the greater skill exercised in the marketing of worthless compounds. Although agriculture and a few industries did not share in the unstable prosperity, the average real per capita income rose from $336 in 1914 to $396 twelve years later, an increase of 28.7 per cent.[6] While producers for every need and fancy competed for a larger share of the temporarily growing income, none did so more successfully than the exploiters of frauds and fads. Without loosening their hold on the most gullible classes, many worked their way into the better newspapers with a type of toned-down advertising that the AMA described as "falsehood by implication."[7] Instead of announcing their products as "sure cures" for incurable diseases, they chose rather to advertise their nostrums as cures for the symptoms of these maladies.

AMA Takes Action

As a new era of scientific technology brought its exploitative opportunities as well as benefits, the AMA's aggressive war on quackery did not await the federal government's retarded efforts to deal effectively with the problem. Before most crusading organizations became much impressed by the magnitude of the nostrum menace, and long before the public rose up again in alarm, the AMA carried on the fight with characteristic vigor.[8] Apparently without hope of immediate and effec-

[6] Slosson, *Great Crusade and after*, p. 165.

[7] Cramp, *Nostrums and Quackery*, III, 21.

[8] One writer states that with the beginning of the twenties, better business bureaus that operated in 31 major cities by 1921 had carried on their own disciplinary movement with only minor setbacks. Kenner, *Fight for Truth in Advertising*, pp. 99, 240. Yet the writer produces little evidence to show that better business bureaus had done much more than ignore frauds and fakery in the field of health or that they had offered much protest against the extortions of the cosmetic industry. See pp. 183–85; 186–87.

tive governmental action, the Association pressed a campaign that consisted largely of independent exposures of frauds and fads. Through the work of the Propaganda Department, which became the Bureau of Investigation in 1925, the Association acquired an inexhaustible store of damaging evidence against nostrum industries. Through its own regular publications, the *Journal* and the newly established *Hygeia,* as well as through bulletins and pamphlets, the Association exposed the way of quackery and attempted to inform the unwary public about the extent of the nostrum menace.[9] Local better business bureaus throughout the nation relied extensively upon the Association's services in their feeble efforts to check some of the crudest forms of medical exploitation, and social agencies of almost every type sought its assistance.[10]

Fully aware that the success of proprietary medical enterprises depended largely upon extravagant advertisements, the AMA continued its efforts to purge the nostrum from the columns of the lay and secular press. Although the general level of advertising had risen considerably in the first two decades of the century, much room for progress remained.[11] Always denying that a selfish motive prompted its attack upon proprietary medical advertising, the Association contended that it stood to profit from the extravagant efforts of proprietary concerns. As late as 1936, Arthur J. Cramp, recent director of the Bureau of Investigation, wrote:

> . . . if the medical profession looked at the "patent medicine" business from a dollar-and-cents viewpoint it would raise no objection to it. . . . Every piece of advertising devised to convince the public that a pain in the lower part of the back means kidney disease will send, probably, as many people to the family physician as it will send to the drug counter.[12]

[9] Besides collaborating closely with the Association's Chemical Laboratory, the Bureau of Investigation secured information from three other sources: federal, state, and local governments; various journals; and from various special commissions. Arthur J. Cramp, "The Work of the Bureau of Investigation," *Law and Contemporary Problems,* 1 (December, 1933), 54. *Hygeia* began a crusade against nostrums with the first issue published in April, 1923. See Arthur J. Cramp, "Patent Medicines: What Is a 'Patent Medicine' and Why?" *Hygeia,* 1 (April, 1923, Chicago: American Medical Association, 1923), pp. 43–45. The work of the Bureau of Investigation is discussed by Bliss O. Halling, in Fishbein, *History of AMA,* pp. 1034–38.

[10] Cramp, *Nostrums and Quackery,* III, p. vi.

[11] George H. Simmons, in *ibid.,* p. iii.

[12] Cramp, in *ibid.,* p. vi.

Exposures of Medical Fakery

Despite the Association's long warfare on medical quackery, the postwar era thrust upon the organization some of its hardest battles. It found that several medical pretenders had survived its attacks earlier in the century and had devised even more subtle methods of reaching the public. One of these was the notorious Albert Abrams, who until his death in 1924 held undisputed title as "dean of twentieth century charlatans."[13] Having abandoned the ranks of conventional practitioners in 1910, he started a movement based upon his novel teachings of "Spondylotherapy," combining several features of osteopathy and chiropractic.

As profits from this form of quackery declined, he appealed to the public with another scheme that he described as electronic reactions. Through two instruments sent in separate wrappers that were not to be opened, Abrams promised a diagnosis and treatment of a prospective patient's ailments. A drop of blood or an autograph of a remote patient constituted another part of his scheme and allowed him to discover in the patient "areas of dullness," by placing a healthy party before an electronic device at the San Francisco office. Areas of dullness supposedly revealed to Abrams not only the disease and cure, but disclosed also the patient's religion. He claimed to be able to separate Jew, Catholic, and Protestant, and to differentiate several variations in the latter. The AMA exposed his lucrative activities and noted that upon his death he left an estate of about $2,000,000. It also watched the competition Abrams created among numerous osteopaths and chiropractors who began to interest the public in weird devices called "Neurocalometers" and "Oscilloclasts."[14]

Although Abrams's death removed a notorious figure from the realm of medical swindlers, other charlatans soon proved probably more effective in exploiting vast areas of national credulity. The Association's

[13] *Ibid.*, p. 112. Although Abrams engaged extensively in quackery before the end of World War I and was occasionally attacked by the *Journal*, he is not exposed in the AMA's first two volumes on nostrums and quackery. He developed his most sensational schemes in the latter part of his exploitative career, although as early as 1911 he had given the AMA some trouble. Fishbein, *History of AMA*, p. 116; Nathan Flaxman, "A Cardiology Anomaly Albert Abrams (1863–1924)," *Bulletin of the History of Medicine*, 27 (May–June, 1953), 260.

[14] Cramp, *Nostrums and Quackery*, III, 112, 116; Martin Gardiner, *Fads and Fallacies in the Name of Science* (New York: Dover Publications, Inc., 1957), pp. 204–7.

relentless war on cancer quackery had proved only partially successful, and clever promoters still found lucrative rewards in this form of exploitation. The year of Abrams's death was also the year when Harry M. Hoxsey and two others established the ephemeral "National Cancer Research Institute and Clinic" in Chicago.[15] When for undisclosed reasons this triumvirate broke up, the persistent Hoxsey, long trained in the art of cancer quackery, transferred his operations to a small Illinois town.

Capitalizing upon a combination of civic pride and popular credulity that no urban area monopolized, he singled out Taylorville, in the central part of the state, as a promising center for further exploitative adventures. An intensive advertising campaign, conducted by a skillful promoter, informed the local residents that "All the world will soon be beating a path to Taylorville, site of the Hoxide Cancer Sanitarium." Businessmen were told that persons will "come from far and near and each of them will spend money here."[16] Hoxsey secured sufficient support for the launching of his scheme and resurrected a defunct local chamber of commerce to serve his purpose.

The widespread publicity campaign that drew a number of cancer victims to the Hoxsey establishment quickly aroused the wrath of the AMA. The Association did not wait for deceived supporters and victims of the Hoxsey swindle to discover for themselves the fraudulency of the enterprise. The first issue of the *Journal* in 1926 not only carried an account of Harry Hoxsey's exploits in cancer quackery, but also exposed several of his past associates, as well as his father's indulgence in cancer curing, veterinary medicine, faith healing, and blackmailing. The *Journal* identified the "Hoxide cure" as "Essentially the escharotic treatment with arsenic as the base," and remarked that the arsenic, when applied to malignant tissue, often ate into blood vessels causing patients to bleed to death. It deplored the fact that Hoxsey would reap "a rich harvest from gullibility and suffering" before the fraudulency of his operations was widely known.[17]

When the sanitarium in Taylorville failed early in 1928, Hoxsey still had difficulty in eluding the *Journal's* vigil and avoiding its exposures. This publication cited his brief exploits in the nearby towns of Jacksonville and Girard, before the hunger for other prey drove him

[15] Cramp, *Nostrums and Quackery,* III, 14.

[16] *JAMA,* 86 (January 2, 1926), 56.

[17] *Ibid.,* p. 57.

to larger cities. The *Journal* followed his activities from Muscatine, Iowa, to Atlantic City and did not lose the trail that ran through Detroit and Wheeling, not always missing penal institutions.[18] But the harassed Hoxsey continued his work, and the *Journal* noted in 1941 that a court in Dallas, Texas, had rendered a decision which Hoxsey planned to appeal, finding him guilty of practicing medicine without a license and assessing a fine of $25,000 and a five-month prison sentence.[19]

While no graduated scale of ethics can serve in classifying charlatans of the healing world, some did exceed others in their capacity for deception. With unusual skill a few employed the most modern means of publicity and acquired an influence which surpassed that of Abrams even in his most successful years. The rapid rise of Norman Baker to a top position among medical promoters illustrates the success achieved by one who readily saw how the radio as well as the press could be subverted to serve the purposes of quackery.

Although Baker's formal education was less than two years in high school, he brought to his new adventure an unusual degree of effrontery and considerable experience as a salesman and vaudeville entertainer. At Muscatine, Iowa, he established the "Baker Hospital" and a radio station, and from there he issued a magazine bearing the title "TNT" (The Naked Truth). To his citadel came hordes of cancer sufferers who had heard his bold assurance that "Cancer is Conquered." Even Hoxsey, during an interruption in independent activities, worked for a time with Baker, only to discover that one of his own cures was being used extensively by the Iowa promoter.[20]

Despite the fact that Baker's methods bore all the marks of fraud, his Muscatine experiment proved highly rewarding. Monthly receipts that amounted to $1,000 in October, 1929, rose to over $75,000 in June, 1930. Such astonishing success not only increased the exploiter's

[18] Cramp, *Nostrums and Quackery,* III, 15. See *JAMA,* 87 (July 31, 1926), 331, for some of Hoxsey's troubles in Taylorville. In 1931, he was sentenced in Detroit to serve six months in a local house of correction for practicing medicine without a license. Fishbein, *History of AMA,* p. 501.

[19] Hoxsey's exploitations have extended far beyond the bounds of this chapter. In 1955 he engineered the establishment of a branch hospital at Portage, Pennsylvania, that grossed $241,000 during the first year of operation. *Life,* 80 (April 16, 1956), 125–28. Not until 1960, however, did the federal government appear to have brought Hoxsey's exploitations at both his Dallas and Portage institutions under control. Young, *Toadstool Millionaires,* pp. 260–61.

[20] Alvin Winston, *The Throttle: A Fact Story of Norman Baker* (Muscatine, Iowa: Baker Sales Co., 1934), pp. 29–30; Cramp, *Nostrums and Quackery,* III, 15, quoted slogan, p. 9.

temerity, but also left him unwilling to ignore exposures of his practices that were soon forthcoming.[21] In April, 1930, the *Journal* launched an attack upon his daring enterprise that reached a wider lay audience through the pages of *Hygeia.* These publications offered abundant proof of the falsity of his claims and publicized his preposterous assertion that the AMA had offered a million dollars for his cancer cure. To the *Journal's* exposure, Baker responded with a counterattack on the Association, attempting even to blacken the reputation of a former editor of the *Journal,* George H. Simmons.[22]

Faced with the problem of dwindling profits following the Association's exposure, and hurt by the action of the federal government in revoking his broadcasting license in 1931, Baker filed a libel suit for $500,000 against the AMA. In a trial at Davenport beginning in early February, 1932, the Association had the rare opportunity of exposing the claims of quackery in a legal battle. Having little difficulty in convincing the jury of the truthfulness of its charges, it secured a favorable verdict on March 3.[23]

Although Baker operated a powerful station at Nuevo Laredo, Mexico, after the revocation of his license at Davenport, he never overcame the blow administered by the American Medical Association. The Federal Communications Commission denied his application to open another station at Muscatine in 1935, and the next year the state supreme court enjoined him from engaging in further medical exploitation in Iowa. But even these obstructions did not completely discourage the defiant promoter. In 1937, he was sentenced to four months in prison and fined $2,000 in a federal district court in Texas for relaying messages to a foreign station to be broadcast to the American public. Despite a desperate attempt to evade governmental regulations and survive the attacks of the AMA, Baker's efforts to resurrect his lost empire were futile.[24]

[21] Cramp, *Nostrums and Quackery,* III, 9.

[22] Editorial, *JAMA,* 94 (April 12, 1930), 1147; Editorial, *Hygeia,* 8 (May, 1930), 419. Baker's attack on Simmons appears in *TNT,* 2 (June, 1930), 12–16, where he brings in evidence which he claims was gathered in 1913 by Sam H. Clark, editor of a Bismarck, North Dakota, publication that appeared to identify Simmons with quackery and illegal medical practice during his early medical career in Lincoln, Nebraska. (Copy in Baker File, AMA, DI.)

[23] Arthur J. Cramp, *Hygeia,* 10 (May, 1932), 432–33.

[24] *JAMA,* 109 (July 31, 1937), 375. For a later four-year federal prison sentence that Baker served and his death September 9, 1958, see *JAMA,* 125 (August 5, 1944), 890, and also *Racine* [Wisconsin] *Journal-Times,* September 11, 1958. Baker File, AMA, DI.

While the exploitations of Baker and Hoxsey made them strong contenders for the title Abrams had held as "dean of twentieth century charlatans," the realm of quackery produced an even more adroit figure. Nearly three decades of sensational chicanery gave the AMA justification for branding John R. Brinkley "as the greatest charlatan in medical history." Combining astuteness and a total disregard for ethics with a diploma from an irregular medical school (allegedly a diploma mill), Brinkley held an advantage over contemporary quacks who had to practice without either a medical diploma or license.[25]

Although Brinkley had a long history as a specialist in venereal disease quackery, bootlegging, the issuance of bad checks, debt evasion, and in the receipt of large quantities of subpoenas and court orders, not until after his descent upon the little town of Milford, Kansas, late in 1917, did he begin to acquire a national reputation.[26] In penetrating the less-exploited field of sexual rejuvenation, Brinkley promised to restore to aging and impotent males the lost balance between sexual vitality and unbounded imagination. From his radio station in Milford, he urged a potential market of humiliated men to capture the sexual strength of youthful years by an operation that supposedly transplanted portions of goats' testicles into the human scrotum. He also found radio a profitable way to prescribe his own compounds for victims of many maladies who wrote about their ailments and saw no need of visiting Brinkley's establishment. But an apparent sincerity that succeeded in drawing large numbers to Milford also seemed to have charmed local residents as well. The gift of a new church building to the Methodists, bearing a tablet that read "Erected to God and His Son Jesus in appreciation of the many blessings conferred on me, By John R. Brinkley," indicated not only the profitableness of his exploits, but also how he found a heavenly sanction for his mission.[27]

The financial rewards of medical quackery allowed the goat-gland doctor to try his skills at political demagoguery. Although pushing into a more crowded field, he found the citizens of Kansas well prepared

[25] Fishbein, *History of AMA*, p. 503. For an account of how Brinkley's claims to medical education combined both reality and fiction see Gerald Carson, *The Roguish World of Doctor Brinkley* (New York: Rinehart & Company, 1960), pp. 15–26, which is a thorough study of Brinkley's whole career.

[26] Fishbein, *History of AMA*, pp. 504–7; *JAMA*, 90 (January 14, 1928), 133–35.

[27] *JAMA*, 94 (April 26, 1930), 1339; quotation, Fishbein, *History of AMA*, pp. 507–8. See Carson, *Roguish World of Brinkley*, pp. 151–52 for a description of this operation.

for his type of diet and highly appreciative of whatever variations he had to offer. Brinkley entered the governor's race in 1930 too late for his name to appear on the ballot, but nevertheless conducted a sensational campaign. Promising to build a lake in every county of Kansas and urging free textbooks, low-priced licenses for most vehicles, and better roads, he polled 183,278 votes in an election in which probably enough votes to secure victory were thrown out because his supporters failed to spell his name simply, John R. Brinkley. Although defeated as an Independent in his second race two years later, he polled 244,607 votes against 278,581 for the winning Republican candidate, Alfred M. Landon.[28]

Several years before a course of quackery vaulted Brinkley into a position of considerable prominence, the AMA became aware of his presence. As early as 1924, the *Journal* called attention to his disreputable practices, but in no such way as to distinguish his expoitative ability from that of many other medical pretenders. The Association soon learned, however, that he combined unscrupulousness with an unusual measure of ingenuity and resourcefulness, and that his exploitation constituted a serious menace to the public and profession. In January, 1928, the *Journal* alerted the profession to Brinkley's activities in a stinging survey of his work.[29]

Not until 1930, however, did the movement develop against the Milford practitioner that hastened the end of his Kansas career. When the *Kansas City Star,* the Kansas Board of Medical Registration and Examination, the Kansas State Board of Health, and the state medical society launched a concurrent attack on the Brinkley fakery, they received the Association's full support. The AMA strengthened the attack in Kansas by supplying information from its own files and supported the Federal Trade Commission's investigation that led to a revocation of the license of his radio station.[30] In addition, the Associa-

[28] Fishbein, *History of AMA,* pp. 510–11; Secretary of State (Kansas), *Twenty-Seventh Biennial Report* (1929–1930), p. 103; Secretary of State (Kansas), *Twenty-Eighth Biennial Report* (1931–1932), p. 131. In 1930 Harry H. Woodring, Democrat, was elected governor with 217,171 votes, and the next candidate, Frank Houcke, Republican, received 216,920 votes. It is reported that Brinkley polled 20,000 votes in the gubernatorial election in Oklahoma where he was not even a candidate. In the 1932 race Brinkley ran third, following Woodring, who polled 272,944 votes.

[29] *JAMA,* 82 (January 12, 1924), 132; *JAMA,* 90 (January 14, 1928), 134–37.

[30] For examples of the AMA's assistance see A. B. MacDonald, the *Kansas City Star,* to Morris Fishbein, April 30, 1930; Arthur J. Cramp to MacDonald,

tion launched its own campaign against the embattled doctor through the *Journal*. The struggle in which Brinkley also lost his Kansas license to practice medicine drove the harassed practitioner to establish his headquarters at Del Rio, Texas, closer to the Mexican radio station that he established in 1931.[31]

Wherever Brinkley went, however, he failed to escape the notice of the AMA. Turning from his goat-gland specialty to other forms of medical exploitation, he lost none of his power to ensnare the public. In 1937, the *Journal* publicized the chemical analysis of one of his compounds, "Formula No. 1020," which was sold at a price as high as $100 for six ampules. The Association's Chemical Laboratory reported that this formula could be duplicated "by dissolving one part of indigo in 100,000 parts of water," and the *Journal* remarked:

> The kind of genius capable of taking a body of water like Lake Erie, coloring it with a dash of bluing and then selling the stuff at $100 for six ampules represents a type which all the world up to now has never been able to equal. John R. Brinkley is the absolute apotheosis in his field. Centuries to come may never produce again such blatancy, such fertility of imagination or such ego.[32]

Despite the *Journal's* exposures, the Brinkley business experienced astonishing prosperity, and an income of over $1,300,000 in 1937 tempted him to risk a legal battle with the AMA. Following an attack in *Hygeia* upon his practices in 1938, Brinkley filed a libel suit against its editor, Morris Fishbein, seeking damages of $250,000. The editor had little trouble in substantiating his charges, and the close of the trial marked a decided turn in Brinkley's fortunes. In 1941, he found himself confronted with litigation in a federal court over claims amounting to more than $1,600,000. Countering with a statement of bankruptcy, he listed his property as worth less than $49,000 and itemized it to include among other possessions, 90 head of cattle, six head of horses, a few

---

April 22, 1930; A. S. Ross, Board of Medical Registration and Examination, to N. P. Colwell, March 20, 1930; Colwell to Ross, March 27, 1930; Earle G. Brown, Kansas State Board of Health, to Morris Fishbein, February 12, 1930; Cramp to Brown, February 18, 1930; J. F. Hassig, Kansas State Medical Society, to Olin West, March 19, 1930, April 2, 1930; Cramp to Hassig, April 7, 1930; Frank H. Lovette, Federal Trade Commission, to *Journal of American Medical Association*, April 21, 1930; Cramp to Lovette, April 24, 1930. (Brinkley File, AMA, DI.)

[31] *JAMA*, 94 (April 26, 1930), 1339–41; Carson, *Roguish World of Brinkley*, pp. 187–92, 167–68.

[32] *JAMA*, 108 (April 3, 1937), 1197.

geese, but no surviving goats. Suffering now from serious physical frailties, death a year later closed the checkered life of the fallen king of quackery.[33]

While the AMA exposed many other medical charlatans in the period between the two World Wars, its struggles with these pretenders illustrate the nature of its fight. Yet the Association's warfare against commercial exploitation at the expense of health extended far beyond this narrow range. The AMA kept ever alert to the multiplying number of frauds and fads and equipped itself to meet the problems they presented. In addition to the Council on Pharmacy and Chemistry that had long carried on the nostrum fight, the Association used other councils and committees to supplement its work. The Council on Medical Education and Hospitals not only served as a rating agency for hospitals and colleges, but also brought many laboratories that made "diagnostic tests for roentgen-ray laboratories" under its inspection. The Association established the Council on Physical Therapy to examine devices perfected in that realm, and in 1929 organized the Committee on Foods to protect the public against the extravagant claims of many food manufacturers.[34]

As the Association established more elaborate machinery for combating the forces that imperiled the nation's health, it noticed an encouraging revival of public interest in the problem of protecting health against commercial exploitation. In fact a redeeming feature of an era that allowed widespread commercial exploitation was its capacity to produce and tolerate critics that assessed its own guilt. Toward the end of the twenties, the severe indictments of a few social prophets announced the rise of a new protest movement closely resembling that of the earlier muckrakers. Showing little disposition to attack the structure of the economic order itself, and supporting their protests with ready reserves of evidence, the crusaders of the later era got a favorable reception even among that portion of the business world that had grown tired of the strenuous activity required in competitive plunder.

[33] Fishbein, *History of AMA,* pp. 514–61; Carson, *Roguish World of Brinkley,* pp. 237–46.

[34] Morris Fishbein, "The American Medical Association's Work for Consumer Protection," *Law and Contemporary Problems,* 1 (December, 1933), 50–51; Fishbein, *History of AMA,* pp. 375, 379; Raymond Hertwig, "The Work of the Committee on Foods," *Law and Contemporary Problems,* 1 (December, 1933), 55, 58.

Revival of Muckraking

In an iconoclastic spirit shared with the contemporary writers of the "Lost Generation," the critics turned up the seamy side of business practice to public view. Stuart Chase and F. J. Schlink shocked the nation with the publication of *Your Money's Worth* in 1927, showing the heavy toll consumers paid the business world for the exploitation of their credulity. Schlink's organization of Consumer's Research Inc. two years later and the subsequent establishment of the National Consumers' League gave the nation assurance that other exposures would be forthcoming. These organizations, which sometimes based their conclusions on too hastily examined evidence, nevertheless supplied the public with much useful information. They turned out a number of books exposing business practices, among which was the sensational *100,000,000 Guinea Pigs* written by Arthur Kallet and F. J. Schlink, which appeared in 1933. This startling exposure, that excited the public and irritated much of the business world, served as a fitting complement for T. Swann Harding's *The Joy of Ignorance,* published a year earlier.[35]

The public had not forgotten these attacks upon devious business practices when the press brought out more critical accounts. James Rorty revealed much of the sordid side of advertising in *Our Master's Voice,* published in 1934. In 1936, Ruth deForest Lamb, in *American Chamber of Horrors,* substantiated many earlier exposures and supplied others, as well as revealing how forces were at work to prevent the strengthening of food and drugs legislation. During the same year, J. B. Matthews, in *Guinea Pigs No More,* pointed out much business deception and urged as a partial solution the creation of a national department of consumers with cabinet status.[36] Peter Morell strengthened the

[35] David F. Cavers, "The Food, Drug and Cosmetic Act of 1938: Its Legislative History and Its Substantive Provisions," *Law and Contemporary Problems,* 6 (Winter, 1939), 5–6; James F. Corbett, "The Activities of Consumer Organizations," *ibid.,* 1 (December, 1933), 61, 65; Arthur Kallet and F. J. Schlink, *100,000,000 Guinea Pigs* (New York: Grosset & Dunlap, Publishers, 1933); T. Swann Harding, *The Joy of Ignorance* (New York: William Godwin, Inc., Publishers, 1932). For a feeble attack upon these organizations that publicized business corruption see G. L. Eskew, *Guinea Pigs and Bugbears* (Chicago: Research Press, 1938). Eskew accused them of publishing "rot" provided by persons whose names they never made known. See p. 49.

[36] Ruth deForest Lamb, *American Chamber of Horrors* (New York: Farrar & Rinehart, Incorporated, Publishers, 1936), pp. 278–327; J. B. Matthews with appendix by Oscar S. Cox, *Guinea Pigs No More* (Covici, Friede Publishers, 1936), pp. 259–64.

list of critical reviews of business practices the next year with the publication of *Poisons, Potions and Profits,* and in 1938, a medical professor, Charles Solomon, in *The Traffic in Health,* severely exposed many practices of the drug and cosmetic industries. W. W. Bauer also brought to his writing the benefit of medical training and published *Health, Hygiene and Hooey* in the same year.

Exposures calling public attention to exploitative practices in the sale of foods, drugs, and cosmetics quickly awakened the interest of several civic organizations and added strength to the Association's crusade against nostrums, frauds, and many fads.[37] While exposing medical charlatans who found ingenious methods of deluding the public, it did not ignore the activities of many commercial firms whose practices were hardly less reprehensible. Although the Association's work in protecting the health and financial resources of the public from exploitation was quite extensive, the scope of this survey admits consideration of only a few.

Objections and Exposures

The AMA's attack on the objectionable practices of some business firms centered principally around a few abuses. None appeared more often than the fraudulent or deceptive claims made by manufacturers for their products. Even after making due allowance for some meaningless and perhaps innocent extravagance in sales promotion, the AMA found much advertising that adversely affected public interest. It also condemned some products as being actually or potentially harmful, even when consumed as the manufacturer's instructions authorized, and observed that others, while producing no harmful effects, were actually worthless. Not least among the Association's criticisms were those attacking the excessive price at which some firms sold their products. Through its own investigations and by publicizing the findings of other organizations and government agencies, the Association called the public's attention to these abuses.

[37] The General Federation of Women's Clubs was one of the organizations supporting the Association's struggle. Corbett, *Law and Contemporary Problems,* 1 (December, 1933), 65. Several trade journals also showed some aggressiveness in fighting fraudulent advertising in this period. Prominent among these were *Printers' Ink, Advertising and Selling, Sales Management,* and *Advertising Age.* Kenner, *Fight for Truth in Advertising,* pp. 187–89.

Deceptive advertising remained one of the greatest temptations for many establishments manufacturing medical compounds and other health products in the postwar era. Among the firms that the Association charged with this practice was the Histeen Corporation of Chicago, which exploited a nostrum that supposedly counteracted histamine poisons in relieving victims of hay fever and pollen asthma. Although the company claimed that its product was not habit forming, the analysis of the AMA's Chemical Laboratory proved otherwise. It showed that the recommended dosage would have supplied the user daily with "forty-eight grains of antipyrine, nearly two and one-half grains of phenobarbital and nearly one and one-half grains of ephedrine hydrochloride. . . ." About a year after the Association's exposure, federal authorities found the product misbranded because it was labeled as "non-habit forming" and was sold under misleading therapeutic claims.[38]

The Association found in the promotion of "Jack Sprat's Bread," widely heralded as "the enemy of fat," another example of deceptive advertising. In 1924 when the Carl Sulzer & Co. of Chicago had advertised the alleged merits of its product in many sections of the nation, the *Journal* brought out its exposure. It publicized the findings of independent sources which showed that the carbohydrate content of this product ranged from 36 to 40 per cent, compared with the upper limit of about 45 per cent in ordinary bread, and that its caloric content stood at 1,139 a pound, compared with 1,140 for ordinary whole wheat bread.[39] During the same year, the Association exposed the exploitation of Alfred W. Lowrie, a medical and religious quack of Hartford, Connecticut, who advertised on a more limited scale his "Sun and Moon Sacred Oil." Claiming that his compound contained "vibrations of life from the radio-activity of electricity, magnetism, electrons and atoms," Lowrie offered his mixture as a source of quick relief for sufferers from neuritis, rheumatism, influenza, hardening of the arteries, and sunburn. Unimpressed by his promotional extravagance, however, the AMA's Chemical Laboratory reported that Lowrie's product could be duplicated "by melting together 80 parts of cup grease, 15 parts of suet, 4 parts of oil of wintergreen, 1 part of oil of sassafras, a sprinkling of street dirt, and stir until cool."[40]

[38] Cramp, *Nostrums and Quackery*, III, 3.
[39] *Ibid.*, pp. 54–56, 178.
[40] *Ibid.*, p. 134.

Although misleading publicity entered into the promotion of Alka-Seltzer, the AMA primarily attacked this product as one that was actually or potentially dangerous. Expensive advertisements of the Dr. Miles Laboratories of Elkhart, Indiana, described the product as an "effervescent alkaline tablet" valuable for "common ailments." Having exposed firms exploiting much less popular compounds, the AMA did not allow the advertising of this establishment to go unchallenged. The Association's Chemical Laboratory found that a purchaser who followed the company's directions "would consume over seventy grains of aspirin and over six grains of salicylic acid" in one day, as well as small quantities of baking soda and citric acid. It attributed the widespread sale of this product largely to the public's lack of knowledge about the potential harmfulness of some of these ingredients. The AMA noted that whereas aspirin had no adverse effect upon some people, in others it produced swelling, nausea, and hives, and other harmful reactions. It also observed that after an early exposure of this product, the company had begun "incidently and vaguely" to mention that it contained an analgesic, acetylsalicylate.[41]

The Association's crusade against nostrums that uncovered many injurious products, also brought out that a number were relatively harmless. Into this class fell many yeast compounds, skin preparations, and some weird devices that promoters advertised as useful in the treatment of goiters and as height increasers. Although the manufacturers of Ironized Yeast appear to have found a ready market for their product, the AMA pointed out that the average diet of Americans was rich in iron and vitamin B that this compound supplied. The AMA also observed that purchasers ran little risk in buying many face creams, face powders, and cold creams, but that these articles when represented as "flesh foods" and "skin foods" were falsely advertised. It marveled at the public's credulity that enriched the exploiters of height-increasing devices and at the blunderings of the United States Patent Office in granting a patent to the manufacturers of the fraudulent Galvano Necklace, advertised as valuable in treating goiters. While the Association classified all of these devices and compounds as either useless or nearly so, it regretted that the public's money had been so unwisely spent.[42]

The Association also pointed out examples of incredible charges in the sale of many products. Aware that the retail price of most pro-

[41] *Ibid.*, pp. 120–22.

[42] *Ibid.*, pp. 127, 29–31, 90, 88–89.

prietaries bore no relation to their production costs or therapeutic value, the AMA did note a few firms that showed unusual exploitative powers. Enormous advertising expenditures, that jumped from almost nothing in 1920 to about $5,000,000 in 1930, brought a net profit (after taxes) of over $7,132,000 to the Lambert Company and lodged one of its products, Listerine, securely in the public mind.[43] Also aware that the extent of advertising and volume of business frequently bore no relation to the quality of a product, the AMA appraised the merits of this mixture. In 1925, Torald Sollmann of the Association's Council on Pharmacy and Chemistry described it as composed of thymol with small added quantities of benzoic and boric acid that sold for a dollar a bottle. Noting that bacteria did not accept the standard set by the nose for determining a good antiseptic, he added: "according to the bacteriologic test, as quoted by Wood, four hundred and ninety-five dollars worth of Listerine has the antiseptic action of a cent's worth of corrosive sublimate; or fifteen dollars' worth of Listerine equals a cent's worth of carbolic."[44]

While widely advertised articles often sold at exorbitant prices, the cost of advertising does not satisfactorily account for the extortionate prices of some products. The AMA found in the cosmetic business numerous examples of this type. Its examination of many "beauty clays" revealed that they were essentially mixtures of clay, water, and perfume. Although they ranged in price from $2 to $10 a pound, the Association noted that for ten cents any druggist would supply a purchaser with a pound of dry powdered clay "equal in beautifying power to, and purer than" the products it had examined. It found that the little-known "Seeqit," a compound sold for the relief of female ailments and costing $4.50 for a hundred tablets, consisted essentially of amidopyrine and caffeine, with fillers. The AMA observed that 100 five-grain tablets of amidopyrine sold for $1.50 a hundred, and that "Seeqit could produce no effect that could not be produced equally well by a plain tablet of amidopyrine U.S.P."[45]

Upon whatever ground the AMA condemned the exploitation of specific proprietaries, it leveled a general indictment against almost all. The proprietary industry, by its very nature, encouraged self-diagnosis by ailing masses, untrained in medical science, of illnesses that proprietary medicines purported to relieve or cure. Nor did the advice that manu-

[43] Harding, *The Joy of Ignorance,* p. 23.

[44] Cited in *ibid.,* p. 19.

[45] Cramp, *Nostrums and Quackery,* III, 36, 62–63.

facturers sometimes offered consumers to consult a physician if illness persisted placate the AMA, which saw in the use of such products perhaps even fatal delay in the initiation of effective treatment. Time and again the AMA cited the dangers that inhered in self-diagnosis and cited numerous examples of fatalities that resulted from the practice. *Hygeia* reported that in 1926 over 11,500 people died from the use of laxatives for acute abdominal pains resulting from appendicitis.[46] The AMA condemned the advertisement of "Tums" that promised relief for upset stomachs troubled by belching, "burning sourness," and nausea, showing that a stomach ulcer or cancer might produce these symptoms.

Weak Enforcement of Act of 1906

The great number of proprietary products exposed by the Association in the postwar era left it more firmly convinced that existing federal food and drugs statutes did not adequately safeguard public health, and that state laws failed to make up for the deficiencies. It well knew that what revisions had been made in the basic act of 1906 had done little to strengthen this measure, and that enforcement of the Pure Food and Drugs Act had been palpably weak. While aware of the Federal Trade Commission's efforts to curb business exploitation through the issuance of cease and desist orders, the AMA recognized that the commission's power to secure compliance was inadequate. It did not share the view of contemporary apologists for the current general level of business practices who found the situation almost beyond reproach. The Association believed that neither governmental restraint nor business ethics served as adequate guarantees against public exploitation.[47]

The history of the lax enforcement of the federal pure food and drugs legislation provided abundant justification for the Association's attitude. Nearly 30 years after the passage of the act of 1906, and despite thousands of violations, only two prison sentences had ever been imposed upon offenders, and the average fines levied amounted to only $67. Some manufacturers had learned to consider the fines as the license fee for

[46] John O. Bower, *Hygeia,* 8 (April, 1930), 325.

[47] From 1906 to 1930 there were five acts passed that revised legislation of 1906, some of which are discussed in chap. 5. For an account of each see Cavers, *Law and Contemporary Problems,* 6 (Winter, 1939), 5; Wilson, *Food & Drug Regulation,* p. 80. For a favorable picture of business practice see Kenner, *Fight for Truth in Advertising,* p. 165.

engaging in illegitimate activities. Although the estimated advertising expenditures of patent-medicine manufacturers reached $70,000,000 in 1929, as late as the middle thirties, the government had allotted only $163,329 in one year to the patent-medicine division of the Pure Food and Drugs Administration for its enforcement work. Acquaintance with the weak enforcement of the act led the National Civil Service Reform League to declare in 1925 that *"Actual regulatory inspection by the Federal Government seems to be almost negligible except in the case of meat. . . ."*[48]

Criticism of Food and Drugs Legislation

Although the Association saw little prospect during the twenties for a major overhauling of the federal pure food and drugs legislation, it nevertheless called the public's attention to deficiencies in the initial act and its amendments. Arthur J. Cramp, of the Association's Bureau of Investigation, who in the preceding decade had raised strong objections to the legislation, continued to cite its weaknesses.[49] In 1923, through the pages of *Hygeia* he repeated his criticisms, which were probably read by many laymen. Noting that proprietary manufacturers most effectively used newspapers, circulars, and billboards in advertising their products, he showed that federal legislation controlled only advertisements and labels on or surrounding the trade package. He observed that the laws required the listing of only 11 dangerous drugs used in proprietaries while "Such deadly poisons as strychnine, aconite, prussic acid, carbolic acid, arsenic . . ." and many others equally dangerous could be put in patent medicines without the public's knowledge.[50]

Cramp cited as a principal reason for the ineffective enforcement of the Pure Food and Drugs Act and its amendments the need of having to prove charges of both false and fraudulent misrepresentation to secure conviction. The necessity of establishing fraud required positive evidence that the manufacturers had deliberately and knowingly intended to defraud. He also noted that federal control of food and drugs did not

[48] Peter Morell, *Poisons, Potions and Profits* (New York: Knight Publishers, Inc., 1937), pp. 255–56; quotation, Kallet and Schlink, *100,000,000 Guinea Pigs,* p. 14.

[49] See p. 92 above.

[50] "Patent Medicines: What Protection Does the National Food and Drugs Act Give?" *Hygeia,* 1 (May, 1923), 106.

extend to products moving in intrastate traffic. Through another publication of the AMA, Cramp later called attention to the fact that federal legislation did not touch the cosmetics industry in which many dangerous drugs were used.[51]

New Legislation Proposed

Although the AMA frequently pointed to the need for a thorough revision of the federal food and drugs legislation and found its position supported by a growing number of outspoken organizations and laymen, not until the beginning of the New Deal era did prospects appear bright for this reform. Hardly had the Democratic administration taken control, when the new chief executive announced that his broad program of domestic reform included the enactment of an effective law. The earnestness of his intentions was readily revealed when the Department of Agriculture undertook the careful preparation of a more adequate measure and soon had it ready for introduction into the first session of the Seventy-third Congress.[52]

When on June 12, 1933, Senator Royal S. Copeland introduced the "Tugwell" or, properly called the "Copeland Bill" (S. 1944) that the Department of Agriculture had prepared, the administration quickly learned that its enactment would entail a long and bitter struggle. Opponents of the bill, more united than friends of the measure, fought furiously to prevent its passage, employing almost any strategy that showed promise of accomplishing this objective. Upon Rexford Tugwell, the Assistant Secretary of Agriculture, who had greatly aided in formulating the bill, came down torrents of abuse. His enemies exploited to the fullest extent a visit he had made to Russia and charged that Bolshevism had infested the Department of Agriculture and that the assistant secretary sought to become czar over the food and drugs industries. Finding in the measure the taint of Tugwell, Lawrence V. Burton,

[51] *Ibid.*, pp. 104–5; Cramp, *Nostrums and Quackery,* III, p. xii. The federal food and drugs legislation applied to cosmetics only when medicinal claims appeared on the labels. Lamb, *American Chamber of Horrors,* p. viii. For other accounts of the weaknesses of pure food and drugs legislation see Stuart Chase and F. J. Schlink, *Your Money's Worth* (New York: The Macmillan Company, 1927), 143–44; Kallet and Schlink, *100,000,000 Guinea Pigs,* pp. 206–16; and Lauffer T. Hayes and Frank J. Ruff, "The Administration of the Federal Food and Drugs Act," *Law and Contemporary Problems,* 1 (December, 1933), 16–18.

[52] Lamb, *American Chamber of Horrors,* pp. vii, 329; Mitchell Salem Fisher, "The Proposed Food and Drugs Act: A Legal Critique," *Law and Contemporary Problems,* 1 (December, 1933), 74.

the editor of *Food Industries,* emphatically declared that "No food manufacturer will accept this piece of legislation, no matter how little it will apparently affect him, without the most vigorous opposition that he can put up."[53]

Objections to "Copeland Bill"

The aggressive campaign that powerful food and drugs manufacturers conducted against the Copeland bill stood in sharp contrast to the feeble support it received. Although the measure represented a vast improvement over the original act, and for the first time would have brought cosmetic industries under federal control, it failed to inspire much enthusiasm among traditional proponents of more effective regulation. As early as June 14, the trustees of the AMA had pledged their support of efforts to secure adequate legislation and the Association had previously offered Tugwell assistance in preparing the bill.[54] But when the Senate subcommittee of the Committee on Commerce conducted hearings on the measure on December 6 and 7, at which a number of spokesmen for public health agencies and consumer organizations offered favorable testimony, the American Medical Association sent no official representative. The brief it filed showed considerable disappointment with the bill and emphasized the idea that it entrusted too much power to the Secretary of Agriculture.[55] Nearly two years later a spokesman of the Association declared that the AMA did not approve of the "Tugwell Bill" and had no part in drafting it.[56] Although the AMA wanted the enactment of adequate food and drugs legislation, it nevertheless left the impression that it endorsed the views of inveterate enemies of effective controls.

[53] Lamb, *American Chamber of Horrors,* p. 290; quotation, Lawrence V. Burton, "What the Food Manufacturers Think of S. 1944," *Law and Contemporary Problems,"* 1 (December, 1933), 122. Enemies of the measure began referring to it as the "Tugwell Bill." Although Tugwell had assisted in drafting the measure, it was introduced into the Senate by Copeland and should correctly bear his name. Lamb, *American Chamber of Horrors,* p. 290.

[54] HD, *Proceedings* (85 Annual Session, June, 1934), pp. 17–18.

[55] *Ibid.,* pp. 17–18; Cavers, *Law and Contemporary Problems,* 6 (Winter, 1939), 9; Seventy-third Congress, first session, *Hearings on S. 1944: Food, Drugs, and Cosmetics* (Washington; Government Printing Office, 1934), pp. 461–65.

[56] Statement of William C. Woodward, Subcommittee of House Committee on Interstate and Foreign Commerce, Seventy-fourth Congress, first session, *Hearings on H. R. 6906, H. R. 8805, H. R. 8941, and S. 5: Foods, Drugs, and Cosmetics* (Washington; Government Printing Office, 1935), p. 300.

Confronted with the problems of mounting opposition and unstable support, Senator Copeland, attempting to make the measure more palatable to the industries affected, introduced on January 4, 1934, S. 2000, embodying less objectionable provisions. When this measure failed to satisfy forces potentially capable of preventing its passage, on February 19 he introduced another bill, S. 2800.[57] Although the *Journal* on March 3 boldly expressed interest in effective food and drugs legislation, at the congressional hearings that had just occurred on S. 2800, the Association's spokesman denied that the AMA was pressing for the enactment of this measure and showed little interest in the bill.[58]

When the Senate failed to pass the Copeland bill (S. 2800) in 1934, the champion of the measure in the upper house introduced another bill (S. 5) on January 4, 1935. Like its predecessors this measure also proved disappointing to the AMA. Yet the vigorous struggle over the enactment of pure food and drugs legislation that had lasted for over 18 months allowed the Association time to state its position more clearly on what a new bill should include. Only a few days after the introduction of Copeland's last revised bill, the *Journal* carried recommendations prepared by the Council on Pharmacy and Chemistry and the Committee on Foods and endorsed by the Board of Trustees.[59]

AMA's Demands

This impressive list showed the Association's familiarity with virtually all the weaknesses of federal food and drugs legislation, and its awareness of the difficulty of drafting an effective measure. Among the Association's numerous demands a few especially deserve notice. It called for the regulation of all forms of advertising and defined advertising as "all ways and means of bringing articles to the attention of the public for commercial purposes." It sought to place responsibility for advertis-

[57] HD, *Proceedings* (85 Annual Session, June, 1934), p. 18. For charges that Copeland had become a tool of food and drugs manufacturers when he agreed to many changes in the first bill, see Morell, *Poisons, Potions, and Profits,* p. 250, and Matthews, *Guinea Pigs No More,* p. 251.

[58] *JAMA,* 102 (March 3, 1934), 696; Cavers, *Law and Contemporary Problems,* 6 (Winter, 1939), 12. This issue of the *Journal* even urged physicians to send telegrams to their senators and representatives expressing "the wish of the people for the successful passage of Senate Bill No. 2800. . . ."

[59] Cavers, *Law and Contemporary Problems,* 6 (Winter, 1939), 8; Lamb, *American Chamber of Horrors,* p. 330; *JAMA,* 104 (January 12, 1935), 125–26. The recommendations discussed below come from *ibid.*

ing on the firm or individual issuing it, or upon the "guarantor" who stood amenable under the requirements of the act. It demanded that testimonials used in the advertisement of drugs and drug preparations be accompanied by the names and addresses of the writers and that these testimonials be considered by the law as the claims of the advertiser. It sought to ban the use of testimonials of "a health, medicinal or therapeutic nature" in the advertisement of food products "by persons unqualified to express a scientific authoritative opinion. . . ." The AMA also asked that "suitable declarations" be required on the labels of all habit-forming drugs and that the government prohibit the sale of all drugs and drug preparations that failed to meet the standards set in official compendiums.

Particularly significant among the recommendations was one urging the regulation of the cosmetics industry. The AMA proposed to bring the advertisement of all cosmetics sold in interstate commerce under federal control and defined cosmetics as "all substances and preparations intended for cleansing, altering the appearance, or promoting the attractiveness of the person, unmedicated soaps excepted." It also called for close restrictions on the use of artificial colors in foods and recommended that the advertisement of "Special Purpose Foods" be carefully regulated. Upon all violators of the proposed legislation, the Association urged adequate penalties.

The AMA hoped that the Senate would strengthen the Copeland bill, but the measure as passed on April 28, 1935, fell far short of its demands. Nevertheless, the Association did not despair in its attempt to secure revisions, and sent William C. Woodward to testify before the House subcommittee of the Committee on Interstate and Foreign Commerce, when the lower body opened hearings on the bill. Woodward's appearance left no doubt of the Association's position and its disappointment with the proposed legislation. He declared that the AMA strongly favored more effective food and drugs legislation, but asserted that the measure under consideration offered inadequate protection. While contending that the "medical profession provisions" of the bill were weaker than those in existing legislation, he considered that since the proposed bill brought "devices, cosmetics, and advertising" under control, it was superior to the act of 1906.[60]

[60] Statement of William C. Woodward, Seventy-fourth Congress, first session, *Hearings on H. R. 6906, H. R. 8805, H. R. 8941, and S. 5: Foods, Drugs, and Cosmetics,* pp. 299, 320–21. Late in the year the *Journal* remarked that "On its face, the bill may appear to be materially more rigid in its requirements than the

No overwhelming pressures forced the House to consider promptly the measure that the Senate had passed, and the bill was not reported out of committee until May, 1936. Yet, opponents of effective regulation correctly suspected that only the enactment of a new measure would cause the agitation for more stringent legislation to subside. They decided that the best chances for both dismissing the issue and preserving their own interests lay in securing the enactment of as weak a measure as the nation would tolerate.[61] Their efforts to weaken the original Copeland bill had already been in a large measure successful.

Point of Despair

Although the early months of 1936 brought a temporary lull in Congress over the pure food and drugs issue, the AMA kept the profession informed about the deficiencies of the Copeland bill and the renewed efforts of opponents to weaken the measure. In May, the trustees told the Kansas City session that the bill as passed by the Senate was in general little better than the act of 1906, and in its provisions for the regulation of drugs, distinctly weaker.[62] Later in the month the *Journal* showed a spirit of defeatism and despair, declaring that "The bill, so far from the ideal, might much better be scrapped and a new beginning be made when a more favorable opportunity offers." Describing the emasculated measure it added:

> The bill first introduced has been subject to a sort of plastic surgery in the legislative operating rooms which has resulted in a specimen not even resembling the original model and utterly deficient in many particulars. Altogether the result is an asthenic, chinless and impotent monstrosity.[63]

Food and Drugs Act of 1906. It does cover cosmetics and therapeutic devices, which existing law does not cover at all. It is more rigorous in its requirements on the labeling of foods and drugs and in covering advertising as well as labeling. A careful study, however, discloses loopholes and evidences of weakness in its administrative provisions, particularly with reference to drugs, including 'patent' and proprietary medicine and prophylactic and therapeutic devices. These should be corrected before the bill is enacted." Editorial, *JAMA,* 105 (December 21, 1935), 2076.

[61] Cavers says that as opponents of more effective legislation knew that some bill would be enacted their strategy was "to restrict the measure narrowly enough to avoid the risk of embarrassing changes in merchandising and industrial practices while at the same time establishing in the public mind the belief that an acceptable law had been passed." Cavers, *Law and Contemporary Problems,* 6 (Winter, 1939), 4–5.

[62] HD, *Proceedings* (87 Annual Session, May, 1936), p. 15.

[63] *JAMA,* 106 (May 30, 1936), 1902.

The AMA showed neither surprise nor disappointment when the House passed the bill on June 19, but then voted it down when referred back by a conference committee.[64]

The final stage in the battle opened in 1937 when Senator Copeland introduced his bill that had undergone still further changes. This measure, like its immediate predecessor commanded the support of many food and drugs manufacturers who found its provisions innocuous. Unobstructed by any very formidable opposition, the measure passed the Senate on March 8.[65] The House made no serious attempt to act promptly, and many months dragged by in which it showed little concern. Only a tragic national episode that began in October sufficed to arouse a belated interest.

The Sulfanilamide Tragedy

The S. E. Massengill Company of Bristol, Tennessee (with branch plants in other cities), offered the public its new product, "Elixir Sulfanilamide," which combined in liquid form the new powerful drug sulfanilamide with diethylene glycol as a solvent. While sulfanilamide had proved very effective in the treatment of numerous ailments, if mixed with diethylene glycol it became a deadly compound.[66] When by November 11, 73 deaths had resulted from the use of the mixture, the public was startled. This shocking incident showed the nation that existing legislation did not require the testing of new medicines on laboratory animals before the compounds were sold to consumers, and that the government under the prevailing food and drugs legislation would have been powerless to act had the firm labeled its product a "solution" rather than an "elixir." The *Journal* remarked that the spectacle of the federal Food and Drugs Administration, attempting to handle this case with existing legislation, resembled "a hunter pursuing a tiger with a fly swatter."[67]

[64] Wilson, *Food & Drug Regulation,* pp. 125–26; Cavers, *Law and Contemporary Problems,* 6 (Winter, 1939), 17.

[65] *Ibid.,* p. 18.

[66] *Ibid.;* Wilson, *Food & Drug Regulation,* pp. 130–31. The company made no experiments to test the effectiveness or toxicity of the compound. It was tested only for "appearance, flavor, and fragrance." The elixir was developed by the company's chief chemist and pharmacist. *Ibid.,* p. 130.

[67] Editorial, *JAMA,* 109 (November 20, 1937), 1727; Helen Dallas and Maxine Enlow, "Read Your Labels," Institute for Consumer Education, *Consumer Series No. 2, Public Affairs Pamphlet No. 51* (rev., 1943), p. 3; quoted phrase, Editorial, *JAMA,* 109 (November 6, 1937), 1544. Eventually the death toll in this tragedy went well over 100.

Passage of New Legislation

The rapidity with which Congress moved to deal with the food, drugs, and cosmetics issue in 1938 stood in sharp contrast to the previous five years characterized by inactivity and delay. Although little pressure came from the press that found its interests closely tied to that of advertisers likely to be offended by effective legislation, Congress remembered the embarrassing disclosures following the sulfanilamide incident.[68] Hurriedly it passed the Wheeler-Lea bill, signed by the President on March 21, which brought under federal regulation types of advertising not covered by the act of 1906. It extended government regulation to forms of advertising aside from that on the trade package, including radio, newspapers, and simply the spoken word. Supplementing this measure was the Food, Drug, and Cosmetic Act that the President signed on June 25. This measure continued the government's control over advertising accompanying the trade package, and its authority to require the disclosure of contents on labels. In addition, it restricted any new drugs from entry into interstate commerce unless the manufacturer had filed an effective application with the Food and Drugs Administration.[69]

Reaction from the Sidelines

From the sidelines the AMA had watched with considerable suspicion the hurried efforts of Congress to enact this legislation. While the scientific character of the organization required that it demand a great deal along the lines of comprehensive and precise legislation, its experience on the political battlefronts had taught it to expect but little. The knowledge that Congress had again brought up the matter of food, drugs, and cosmetic legislation for consideration early in 1938 did not excite the AMA.

[68] The *New York Times* practically ignored the long legislative history of the Copeland Bill. Magazines with the widest circulations were either unfriendly toward effective legislation or silent on the matter. The principal newspapers giving support were the *St. Louis Post-Dispatch,* the *Christian Science Monitor,* and William Allen White's *Emporia Gazette.* Cavers, *Law and Contemporary Problems,* 6 (Winter, 1939), 3.

[69] HD, *Proceedings* (90 Annual Session, May, 1939), pp. 13, 20; *JAMA,* 110 (April 2, 1938), 1112–13; Wilson, *Food & Drug Regulation,* p. 145. The trustees seem to have mistaken in their report the provisions regulating new drug compounds in interstate commerce for a separate act and not as a part of the Food, Drug, and Cosmetic Act of 1938.

When the Association turned to consider the newly passed legislation, however, it was agreeably surprised. While it found numerous weaknesses in the measures, it considered the laws a forward step. The *Journal* cited reasons for appraising the acts as stronger than earlier legislation. It claimed that "the most noteworthy advance" of the Federal Food, Drug, and Cosmetic Act in the realm of drug control lay in the requirement that no new drugs could enter into interstate commerce unless the manufacturer first secured the consent of the Secretary of Agriculture. It considered this measure also stronger than the old legislation in lengthening the list of potentially dangerous drugs that the manufacturer must describe by "name, quantity, and proportion" on the label of the product. The *Journal* cited the new regulations governing "instruments, apparatus, and contrivances intended for use in the diagnosis, cure, mitigation, treatment or prevention of disease," as superior to the old. It seemed particularly pleased that the new legislation imposed stronger penalties on offenders, and that the cosmetic industry had at last passed under federal regulation.[70]

The *Journal's* appraisal of the new legislation, however, was not altogether favorable. It readily recognized that Congress had not enacted ideal laws. It showed considerable displeasure over the division of regulatory and executive power between the Federal Trade Commission and the Department of Agriculture. Some of the definitions of terms in the acts left much to be desired. The *Journal* also pointed out that the provisions dealing with the purity and labeling of cosmetics were too general. The government's failure to secure effective control under the Wheeler-Lea Act of the extravagant advertising of drugs sold exclusively to the medical profession, it also considered regrettable.[71]

Urges Federal Health Department

While the AMA pledged full support of the government's effort to administer the new legislation, it nevertheless indicated its intention of pressing for structural reforms in the organization of federal health activities. In June, the House of Delegates at Atlantic City adopted a resolution urging the establishment of a "federal executive department of health" headed by a physician.[72] Since the trustees had adopted a

[70] Editorial, *JAMA,* 111 (July 23, 1938), 324–25.
[71] *Ibid.;* Editorial, *JAMA,* 110 (May 28, 1938), 1840.
[72] HD, *Proceedings* (89 Annual Session, June, 1938), pp. 76, 77.

similar resolution the year before, which the House of Delegates had endorsed, the Association appeared to have attached great importance to this objective. Although the AMA preferred the direct and immediate establishment of a national health department, it nevertheless approved of the President's reorganization plan that fell short of this objective. When the administration transferred the United States Public Health Service and the Food and Drugs Administration to the Federal Security Agency, the AMA considered this action as a step toward the establishment of a federal department of health.[73] The Association had learned through many years of political experience that generally major objectives by democratic means are only slowly reached. President-elect Nathan B. Van Etten told the New York session in 1940 that this objective, like all worthy goals, could "only be effected by time and patience, by rational inquiry and enlightened persistence."[74]

[73] HD, *Proceedings* (88 Annual Session, June, 1937), pp. 29, 70; *JAMA,* 114 (May 25, 1940), 2119.

[74] HD, *Proceedings* (91 Annual Session, June, 1940), p. 6.

Chapter 14

THE AMA AND WORLD WAR II

THE AMERICAN MEDICAL ASSOCIATION quickly became aware of the responsibilities that World War II thrust upon the medical profession when the Pearl Harbor attack of December 7, 1941, snapped the last strands that bound the United States to a policy of nominal neutrality. As the stunned nation staggered before the demands of its extensive commitments, the AMA contemplated its own responsibilities in the struggle. When Germany and Italy hastened to join Japan in war against the United States, the Association saw developing a conflict of global magnitude, that eventually stretched a large part of the nation's medical resources over battlefronts spreading from Pacific jungles through African wasteland to the heart of Europe. Besides the medical requirements of an armed force that numbered at peak strength some 12,350,000 members, there remained the mounting problem of medical care for a civilian population increasingly uprooted and shifting.[1]

Major Wartime Problems

While the Association's wartime problems were fraught with infinite complexity, its general responsibilities in the great emergency became increasingly clear. Upon the AMA lay much of the responsibility for maintaining the delicate balance between the medical resources devoted

[1] Robert R. Palmer, Bell I. Wiley, and William R. Keast, *The Army Ground Forces: The Procurement and Training of Ground Combat Troops* (Washington, D.C.: Historical Division, Department of the Army, 1948), p. 1. The impact of the war upon the medical profession is well treated in the first chapters of Morris Fishbein, ed., *Doctors at War* (New York: E. P. Dutton & Company, Inc., 1945).

to military use and withheld for civilian needs. In addition, it sought to maintain an equitable balance in medical personnel among civilian areas. It likewise became concerned with the problem of protecting future physician supply as the national draft cut dangerously into the ranks of medical school enrollments.

Recruitment of Physicians

A brief comment must suffice in summarizing the Association's heroic effort to provide adequate medical care for the Armed Forces without imperiling the health of the civilian population. Opposing the idea of a physicians' draft, it sought to procure an adequate supply of physicians through voluntary enlistment. Eighteen months before the Japanese attack, it organized the Committee on Medical Preparedness in response to the government's appeal for a professional survey of the nation's medical resources. Despite the enormous task of canvassing some 184,000 physicians, the committee had almost completed its survey when the United States entered the war. Less than a year later the Association joined federal authorities in urging the creation of a professional recruitment agency which the President established October 30, 1942, as the Procurement and Assignment Service for Physicians, Dentists, and Veterinarians. This body headed by Frank Lahey, president of the AMA, and consisting of three other physicians and one dentist, maintained close contact with the Association's headquarters, designating the AMA's Bureau of Medical Economics as the Consultant Office of the Service.[2]

The Association never relaxed in its efforts to encourage the enlistment of physicians. It did not object when Army and Navy recruiting teams held before some reluctant doctors the threat of being drafted into the lowest ranks of the Services when its own efforts to encourage enlistment proved inadequate. Nor did it hesitate to call attention to particular centers where physicians had been most reluctant to enlist. The *Journal* blamed the shortage of March, 1943, "unquestionably on the failure of young available physicians in the large cities of the country,

[2] Irvin Abell, Annual Congress on Medical Education and Licensure, 1942, *Papers and Discussions* (Chicago: American Medical Association), pp. 17, 19, referred to hereafter as ACMEL with title and date; HD, *Proceedings* (94 Annual Session, June, 1943), p. 9.

particularly those of the eastern seaboard, to volunteer."[3] Despite the Association's efforts, however, the problem of military medical care often stood perilously close to the crisis stage. The draft that expanded the army alone from 267,000 in 1940 to nearly 7,000,000 in 1943 and to over 8,266,000 in 1945 largely offset the strides of voluntary enlistment.[4]

Civilian Medical Needs

Not only did the Association hear the incessant demands of the Armed Forces for larger quotas of physicians, but also the complaints of civilian areas dangerously divested of medical personnel. When the Procurement and Assignment Service based recruitment policies on a civilian physician-population ratio of 1 to 1500, the rapid approximation of this ratio only increased the volume of outcries.[5] From localities congested by an unprecedented flow of defense workers came appeals of greatest urgency for additional physicians and medical facilities. Portland, Maine, serves to illustrate a city that found itself in desperate need. Defense activity largely explained its wartime population growth of 50 per cent by early 1943, but this congested city of 120,000 had lost 45 physicians to the Armed Forces, retaining only 18 able to engage in general practice. Describing the city's plight a prominent local physician complained:

> We are absolutely unable to cope satisfactorily with the situation, and it will be most disastrous if an epidemic comes our way. Our hospitals are full to overflowing, and this is true throughout the state.[6]

Confronted by a crisis that threatened to undermine health and obstruct essential industrial production, the government moved hurriedly to deal with the problem, but with measures of only limited effectiveness. Late in 1941, the Public Health Service sought to establish contact with all physicians desiring to relocate in defense areas, and

[3] *JAMA,* 121 (April 3, 1943), 1161; quotation, Editorial, *JAMA,* 121 (March 27, 1943), 1092.

[4] R. Elberton Smith, *The War Department: The Army and Economic Mobilization in World War II* (Washington, D.C.: Office of Chief of Military History, Department of the Army, 1959), p. 122; Harold S. Diehl, *JAMA,* 124 (January 8, 1944), 109.

[5] Harvey B. Stone, ACMEL, 1944, *Papers and Discussions,* pp. 25–26.

[6] Adam P. Leighton, ACMEL, 1943, *Papers and Discussions,* p. 48. Leighton attributed the medical crisis in Maine largely to a "disjointed procurement policy."

by February of the next year had compiled a list of about 300 that expressed a willingness to move.[7] The Procurement and Assignment Service also attacked the problem by urging a shift among physicians to areas of acute shortage and reported that of the 587 relocations in 1942, it had encouraged the resettlement of 340. This agency also urged state legislatures to issue temporary licenses during the emergency to qualified physicians, but with little success. Congress responded late in 1943 with the enactment of Public Law 216, which provided moving expenses and a temporary subsidy for physicians and dentists relocating in areas classified as eligible for this type of federal assistance. The law, however, proved largely ineffective and resulted in only nine relocations.[8]

By the fall of 1944, however, agencies concerned with the resettlement of physicians had experienced substantial success in securing relocations. More than 4,000 physicians had accepted work in new localities, and less than 300 communities in the nation appeared to be in acute need of medical care. The Congressional Committee on Congested Production Areas reported on August 15, 1944, that a survey of 14 crowded areas revealed no inadequacy of medical service.[9]

Protecting Student Supply

While calling for the most efficient allocation of the nation's medical resources, the AMA also moved to protect future physician supply from the erosive effect of draft legislation. Partially through its insistence, the government agreed in 1941 to commission junior and senior medical students in either the Army or Navy and postpone their call to active duty until they had completed a year's internship. Later the War and Navy Departments authorized the extension of commissions to eligible freshmen and sophomore students as well, and also deferred medical students who failed to qualify for commissions. Although the Association believed in 1942 that governmental regulations guaranteed the supply

[7] Thomas Parran, ACMEL, 1942, *Papers and Discussions,* p. 16.

[8] *JAMA,* 121 (April 3, 1943), 1162; Mott and Roemer, *Rural Health and Medical Care,* pp. 381–82; Thomas Parran, ACMEL, 1944, *Papers and Discussions,* p. 25. See also HD, *Proceedings* (94 Annual Session, June, 1944), p. 25.

[9] Statement of Harvey B. Stone, Subcommittee of Senate Committee on Education and Labor, Seventy-eighth Congress, second session, *Hearings on S. Res. 74.* (Washington: Government Printing Office, 1944), Part 6, p. 1899. Stone was a member of the AMA's Council on Medical Service and Public Relations.

of physicians for three years, it had some fears about future student supply even though no immediate shortage appeared. In fact, the reserve of eligible premedical students from the Armed Services in 1943 exceeded the accommodations of the medical schools.[10]

Officials of the AMA seemed gratified when the government finally instituted a definite plan of recruitment for medical training, but nevertheless were displeased over the small allocations given to civilian sources. This program provided that the Army Specialized Training Program would supply 55 per cent of the freshman classes; the Navy V–12 Program, 25 per cent; leaving 20 per cent to be drawn from the civilian population. Since the government supplied 80 per cent of the students and assumed their expenses as well, medical schools found some relief from the perplexing problem of high operational costs and the threat of empty classrooms. From May, 1943, to October, 1945, the ASTP alone furnished the schools with 20,336 students.[11]

The Association raised strong objection to changes in the government's policy in 1944 that allowed no more deferments for medical students after July 1. The *Journal* absolved the profession of all future responsibility for physician shortage, and the AMA waged a vigorous fight for a bill (S. 637) introduced by Senator Allen J. Ellender, February 26, 1945, that called for deferment of substantial numbers of medical and premedical students. Although the Association failed in its effort, the ending of the war in Europe a few months later brought some prospect of relief.[12]

The Association supported other methods for maintaining an adequate physician reserve while dealing with student deferment issues. Its Council on Medical Education and Hospitals endorsed the principle of an accelerated wartime medical program, and its Bureau of Legal Medicine and Legislation worked effectively for a modification of medical practice laws in states that required 36 months of medical training for licensure. Somewhat reluctantly the AMA also accepted a two-year premedical

[10] HD, *Proceedings* (93 Annual Session, June, 1942), p. 44; HD, *Proceedings* (94 Annual Session, June, 1943), p. 59.

[11] James E. Paullin, HD, *Proceedings* (94 Annual Session, June, 1944), p. 4; Francis M. Fitts, ACMEL, 1946, *Papers and Discussions,* p. 20.

[12] Editorial, *JAMA,* 125 (July 8, 1944), 708; HD, *Proceedings* (94 Annual Session, December, 1945), p. 26; Editorial, *JAMA,* 127 (March 10, 1945), 592; AMA, Council on Medical Service and Public Relations, *News Letter* (March 22, 1945), p. 3, referred to hereafter as CMSPR with title. A companion bill sponsored in the House by Walter Judd of Minnesota did not get beyond the Committee on Military Affairs.

training standard for admission to medical schools during the emergency, instead of the normal three-year requirement.[13] It did not oppose shortening the period of internship and residency and made no great issue of the fact that medical schools whose teaching staffs had suffered serious wartime depletions had sometimes unwisely extended freshman enrollments beyond the ten per cent authorized by the Executive Council of the Association of American Medical Colleges in 1941.[14] Nor did it object to the government's appropriation in 1942 of $5,000,000 for student loans in various accelerated programs, from which medical students in 64 institutions borrowed $1,063,573 by the end of June, 1943.[15]

Position on New Medical Schools

While becoming reconciled to the slackening of standards of training during the war, the AMA nevertheless set itself against proposals for a considerable expansion in the number of medical schools. This agitation largely grew out of the wartime physician shortage, and from the realization that 19 states were without institutions for training physicians. Believing that a considerable increase in the number of medical schools was unnecessary and actually impossible under wartime conditions, the Council on Medical Education and Hospitals did no more than support proposals for a very modest expansion. It did, however, consult with officials of two schools who hoped to expand their programs to a four-year level, and placed on the approved list one newly created medical

[13] E. M. MacEwen, ACMEL, 1944, *Papers and Discussions,* p. 34; HD, *Proceedings* (93 Annual Session, June, 1942), pp. 44, 48; J. W. Holloway, Jr., ACMEL, 1943, *Papers and Discussions,* p. 34; *JAMA,* 118 (February 28, 1942), 751; "Forty-third Annual Presentation of Licensure Statistics," *JAMA,* 128 (May 12, 1945), 115. The military premedical program actually did not require two years of training but included during each term more than the normal course load. A study of the effects of the accelerated program in 67 schools showed that 63 per cent of the institutions believed that the program had hurt their academic standards. C. C. Carpenter, ACMEL, 1945, *Papers and Discussions,* pp. 37–38.

[14] The Council on Medical Education and Hospitals considered the accelerated internship program initiated January 1, 1944, as "educationally highly undesirable" but "the best available under prevailing conditions." HD, *Proceedings* (94 Annual Session, June, 1944), p. 51. For an account of the inadequacies of the internship program see Jean A. Curran, ACMEL, 1944, *Papers and Discussions,* pp. 36–39. For problems created by expanded enrollments and depleted faculties see HD, *Proceedings* (94 Annual Session, June, 1944), p. 50, and E. M. MacEwen, ACMEL, 1944, *Papers and Discussions,* pp. 34–36.

[15] *JAMA,* 122 (August 14, 1943), 1109; HD, *Proceedings* (Annual Session, June, 1943), p. 26.

school and two other institutions that had inaugurated a four-year program. Since the council felt that the inadequacy of medical care largely stemmed from the inequitable distribution of physicians, it did not believe that the establishment of medical schools would solve the problem.[16]

Position on Hospital Construction

Closely allied with the wartime problem of physician shortage was the generally recognized inadequacy of hospital facilities in many parts of the nation. The great demands of the military establishment, however, largely diverted the government's attention from civilian needs and allowed an attack upon the problem only with piecemeal legislation. Appropriations for construction through the Works Projects Administration and under the Lanham Act of 1943 lessened the crisis, but accomplished little more.[17] Not until near the end of the war did the AMA show much interest in federal measures supporting hospital construction. On February 28, 1945, however, R. L. Sensenich of the Board of Trustees appeared at a Senate hearing to voice the Association's approval of a hospital construction measure (S. 191), later known as the Hill-Burton Act. Maintaining that the bill "appears to provide a maximum of flexible adaptation to local conditions; with a minimum of undesirable uniformity and regimentation," he raised no more than minor objections to the measure. Prominent figures advocating the legislation felt the strength of the AMA's assistance, and the Surgeon-General of the United States Public Health Service later commented that the AMA's support "contributed unquestionably to the ready acceptance of the bill."[18]

[16] HD, *Proceedings* (94 Annual Session, June, 1944), p. 52; *JAMA,* 125 (May 13, 1944), 129; *JAMA,* 125 (August 19, 1944), 1144. The newly established school was Southwestern Medical College in Dallas and the two that developed four-year programs were Bowman Gray School of Medicine of Wake Forest College, Winston-Salem, North Carolina, and the University of Utah School of Medicine in Salt Lake City. For problems involved in using physicians who were war refugees see pp. 325–26 below.

[17] Oscar N. Serbein, Jr., *Paying for Medical Care in the United States* (New York: Columbia University Press, 1953), p. 275; HD, *Proceedings* (92 Annual Session, June, 1942), pp. 23–24.

[18] Senate Committee on Education and Labor, Seventy-ninth Congress, first session, *Hearings on S. 191 to Amend the Public Health Service Act . . .* (Washington: Government Printing Office, 1946), p. 139; Thomas Parran, ACMEL, *Papers and Discussions,* 1947, p. 19.

Support of Voluntary Hospitalization Programs

On no domestic front did the Association push more aggressively during the war years than in areas related to the payment for medical care. Though economic revival had replaced more than a decade of depression, many groups shared only remotely in the prosperity. The income of an unfortunate portion of the population still lingered on or below the subsistence level. Another sizable class normally survived in precarious comfort, but stood helpless before the spiraling costs of serious illness. Many in this low-income group not only needed a prepayment insurance program, but plans that adjusted professional charges to meager incomes as well. Then a substantial part of the population required no more than the assistance of voluntary plans for meeting medical costs, while still other groups found their use only convenient.

While recognizing that the burden of medical care for a part of the population must be borne by taxation, by the profession and private organizations, the AMA accepted the prepayment principle for spreading the cost of medical care for several income groups. During the war years it manifested a growing friendliness toward voluntary hospitalization plans for meeting the needs of classes with moderate incomes, abandoning an earlier idea that these schemes should be employed only among some of the lower income groups. The growth of these plans that enrolled 9.3 per cent of the population in 1940, and 22.8 in 1945, left the AMA with rather convincing proof of their popularity and permanence.[19]

Growth of Medical Society Plans

Even during the depression decade the AMA had also recognized the usefulness of professionally sponsored medical plans in meeting the needs of some lower income groups. Throughout the war years the Association took considerable interest in promoting their growth, as both a deterrent to lay influences over medical plans and to the adoption of a compulsory insurance system. Despite the AMA's insistence only on the adoption of cash indemnity plans, many societies launched nonprofit physicians' service schemes that had made some progress before the war. When the AMA decided in 1942 to endorse a movement

[19] Serbein, *Paying for Medical Care,* p. 383.

that it had never accepted and could no longer ignore, the future of physicians' service plans seemed more secure.[20]

No statistics adequately reveal the extent to which professionally sponsored plans met the wartime needs of low income families, but their growth was impressive. By the end of 1946 the Association's records showed 31 organizations offering straight cash indemnity benefits. Although the editor of the *Journal* disregarded the AMA's endorsement of physicians' service plans in reporting in November, 1943, that the Association approved of "prepayment plans on a cash indemnity basis" the service plan movement made substantial progress.[21] Only a month earlier the Michigan Medical Service reported an enrollment of 600,000 subscribers, and the California Physicians' Service, approximately 88,000, and by February, 1944, statewide Blue Shield plans operated in eight states. By the end of 1946, enrollment in the Michigan plan had climbed to 840,961, in the California plan to 419,672, while the Massachusetts Medical Service reported 460,514 subscribers. In addition to these plans the programs in Oregon and Washington that combined hospital,

[20] Resolution, Charles W. Morgan, HD, *Proceedings* (93 Annual Session, June, 1942), pp. 55, 68. See also pp. 249–51 above. There was a fundamental difference between cash indemnity and physicians' service plans, although the programs had many similar features. Strict cash indemnity plans provided stipulated payments for specified services physicians rendered, while in no way restricting the total charge for these services. Service plans, on the other hand, involved contracts with both consumer and physician groups, providing full physicians' services for specified illnesses from funds collected on a prepayment basis. In cases where available funds proved insufficient to meet the cost of physicians' services, proration of funds among participating doctors provided a basis for solvency. Ultimately, all plans that allowed unlimited medical services found it necessary to place restrictive clauses in their contracts. Both types of professionally sponsored plans were nonprofit and provided for professional control, group enrollment and limited medical coverage. Gradually cash indemnity plans incorporated a feature of service plans in which participating physicians agreed to accept the cash indemnity as full payment for subscribers with incomes below designated levels. For descriptions of these plans see Franz Goldmann, *Voluntary Medical Care Insurance in the United States* (New York: Columbia University Press, 1948), pp. 9–12, 83–92, 114–26, and Robert S. Young, *JAMA,* 127 (January 20, 1945), 165.

[21] Goldmann, *Voluntary Medical Care Insurance,* p. 85; quotation, Editorial, *JAMA,* 123 (November 20, 1943), 770. For comments on the editor's remarks see James C. McCann, "Medical Society Prepayment Program," *JAMA,* 126 (October 6, 1944), 342. As late as June, 1944, the Council on Medical Service and Public Relations stated that the medical profession had "approved prepayment plans on a cash indemnity basis for meeting the costs of medical care," without referring at all to service contracts. HD, *Proceedings* (94 Annual Session, June, 1944), p. 59.

medical, and other services had experienced remarkable growth.[22]

Enrollment statistics, however, provide no adequate measurement of the wartime success of professionally sponsored service schemes. Serious limitations impaired their usefulness and threatened to prevent widespread adoption. Generally providing for only group enrollment and confining recruitment to employed personnel and their dependents, the plans offered no coverage to wide segments of the population in need of prepaid medical care. Restrictive features that placed considerable limitations upon available services also discounted their usefulness. High operational costs that stood at 11.5 per cent in the Massachusetts plan and 14.1 in the Michigan program in 1945 appeared excessive. The separate organizational facilities frequently brought into existence for the administration of hospitalization and professionally sponsored plans added considerably to administrative cost and confusion. Adding to these limitations was the fact that they gave little encouragement to the growth of preventive and psychosomatic medicine.[23] Nor did a large part of the profession show much interest in promoting their development. In November, 1943, Louis H. Bauer of the Council on Medical Service and Public Relations (an agency of the AMA largely responsible for promoting the movement) complained of the profession's negligence in supporting professional plans, while the following June, Sidney R. Garfield, a California physician associated with the medical care program of the Kaiser industries, charged with perhaps some exaggeration that the medical society plans were "miserable failures."[24]

Agrarian Medical Problem

While encouraging the growth of medical society plans primarily designed for low-income groups, the AMA continued to support the medical program conducted by the Farm Security Administration for rural families of meager income. This program which allowed needy farm families to borrow federal funds for the payment of medical service

[22] John R. Mannix, "Voluntary Nonprofit Prepayment for Health Care," *JAMA*, 124 (February 26, 1944), 573; Goldmann, *Voluntary Medical Care Insurance*, p. 114. Serbein states that the Oregon plan was a Blue Shield plan but that the one in Washington was not. *Paying for Medical Care*, p. 135.

[23] Goldmann, *Voluntary Medical Care Insurance*, pp. 123, 125–26. Cash-indemnity plans also contained many of the limitations here discussed that restricted their usefulness.

[24] *JAMA*, 124 (January 15, 1944), 169; *JAMA*, 126 (October 7, 1944), 337.

operated in 1,074 counties at the end of June, 1942. Participants in the program generally made annual prepayments for care that covered an impressive list of medical, hospital, and dental services. The American Medical Association won its contention that all medical services must lie entirely under professional control, and local physician groups drew up fee schedules under the plans.[25]

The AMA also watched the development of a few federal experiments with rural insurance plans. These schemes adjusted the prepayment principle to the family's ability to pay and provided for federal supplements sufficient to bring the annual payment for medical services to about $50 for each participating family. Although the AMA later recognized serious rural medical needs, it looked with disfavor upon the launching of these experiments, believing that "emergency measures in the distribution of medical services do not appear to be longer needed." Even before Congress discontinued federal funds for the experiment in 1946, the AMA had concluded that voluntary insurance offered little hope for solving the medical problems of marginal farm groups, while authorities in the Department of Agriculture found voluntary insurance largely unsuited for all farm classes.[26]

Although the war years moved the AMA toward more enthusiastic support of several programs for meeting the financial problems of medical care, its opposition to compulsory health insurance remained unshakeable. It correctly predicted that compulsory insurance advocates would not relax their agitation during the national emergency. The Association not only expected advocates of compulsory health schemes to propose legislation specifically designed to install a federal compulsory system, but also to seek its establishment by indirection. It remained ever alert to detect threats to private medical practice in any proposed legislation.

Indirect Compulsory Insurance Threat

These threats, as viewed by the Association, were soon forthcoming. Only three months after the Pearl Harbor attack, the Association pointed

[25] Goldmann, *Voluntary Medical Care Insurance,* pp. 130–34; HD, *Proceedings* (Annual Session, June, 1943), p. 35.

[26] Goldmann, *Voluntary Medical Care Insurance,* pp. 145–46; quotation, HD, *Proceedings* (93 Annual Session, June, 1942), pp. 29, 71; HD, *Proceedings* (94 Annual Session, December, 1945), pp. 60, 90.

with much alarm to alleged dangers in the President's recommendation for an extension of social security benefits. While not opposing the administration's proposal for wage-loss insurance to offset the burden of illness, it considered the recommendation for a three-dollar daily hospitalization allowance "as part of a movement toward complete plans for compulsory sickness insurance on either a cash or medical service basis." The Association also raised the objection that the public would likely equate the federal hospitalization payment with the actual value of hospital care and feared the loss of local initiative in handling health problems that fell under federal control.[27]

The AMA found even in the military legislation of the war years cases of encroachment on professional rights. No legislation disturbed the AMA more than that which established the Emergency Maternity and Infant Care Program in the Children's Bureau. This program provided funds for obstetric and pediatric care and hospitalization of expectant wives of men in grades four through seven of the Armed Forces. Initiated in March, 1943, the program allowed maximum benefits of $80 for maternity cases, $40 of which could go in direct payment for physicians' services. By August, 1943, 29,910 wives of servicemen had received benefits under the program, and by the middle of June, 1944, the government had appropriated $24,200,000 for its maintenance.[28]

The Association raised no objection to the purposes of the plan which the House of Delegates endorsed in 1943, but strongly opposed the direct payment of funds to physicians. It urged the payment of allotments directly to the wives of servicemen and resented the intrusion of a third party into the arrangement. Despite the Association's acceptance of the program, outspoken critics within the AMA did not remain silent. L. Fernold Foster of Bay City, Michigan, suspected that the government had launched it as a "trial balloon for complete federalization of medical practice." The editor of the *Journal* later condemned the head of the Children's Bureau for operating "a bureaucracy that functions in a totalitarian manner" divorced from all restraints.[29] Since the AMA worked unsuccessfully to secure a revision in the fee schedule

[27] Editorial, *JAMA,* 118 (March 7, 1942), 821. This editorial was authorized and approved by the Board of Trustees.

[28] J. D. Laux, *JAMA,* 124 (April 8, 1944), 1057; HD, *Proceedings* (94 Annual Session, June, 1944), p. 24.

[29] HD, *Proceedings* (Annual Session, June, 1943), pp. 82–83; see also John H. Fitzgibbon's resolution, p. 70; quotations, *JAMA,* 124 (January 15, 1944), 171; Editorial, *JAMA,* 129 (November 10, 1945), 741.

and to prevent direct payment to physicians, the issue remained a source of trouble for the organization for several months after the war.

Direct Compulsory Insurance Threat

The Association confronted not only what it considered to be indirect movements toward a compulsory health insurance system, but direct assaults upon traditional forms of medical practice as well. Forces arrayed against the AMA before the war seemed to have increased in strength before its close. Within the government the Social Security Board continued to press for a compulsory system supported by Henry Morgenthau, Jr., the Secretary of Treasury. President Roosevelt's friendliness toward the compulsory principle seemed to express itself in outright support when his congressional message of January 11, 1944, called for a "second bill of rights" that included federal aid in providing the public with adequate medical care.[30] Some of the labor unions had begun to show greater interest in compulsory schemes, while among farm organizations the weak but active Farmers' Union continued its support. The Association was particularly shocked when the Governing Council of the American Public Health Association, an organization of nearly 7,500 members which included many physicians, endorsed the compulsory health insurance principle on October 4, 1944.[31] It watched the activities of the Committee on Research in Medical Economics through which Michael Davis and other reputable scholars attempted to lure even portions of the medical fraternity from paths of orthodoxy. Nor did it ignore within the profession the work of the Physicians' Forum that openly endorsed compulsory health insurance. On the world front, the Association also observed the support given by the International Labor Organization to the compulsory insurance principle.[32]

[30] HD, *Proceedings* (94 Annual Session, June, 1944), p. 29.

[31] HD, *Proceedings* (Annual Session, December, 1945), p. 60; *JAMA,* 128 (June 23, 1945), 604. The editor of the *Journal* declared that the action of the Governing Council of the American Public Health Association was undemocratic and did not represent the views of the membership. *JAMA,* 126 (October 14, 1944), 434–35. For a refutation of the editorial see reply of Edward S. Godfrey, Jr., Commissioner of Health, Albany, New York. *JAMA,* 126 (November 18, 1944), 789.

[32] *JAMA,* 120 (November 21, 1942), 922; Mott and Roemer, *Rural Health and Medical Care,* p. 558; Editorial, *JAMA,* 126 (November 4, 1944), 640–41. *JAMA,* 126 (September 2, 1944), 32.

Throughout the war, the AMA found considerable agitation for the adoption of compulsory health insurance on the state level. Compulsory insurance advocates submitted 82 bills in the legislatures of 13 states in the four years from 1941 to 1944, concentrating most of their efforts on California, Massachusetts, New York, and Rhode Island. They achieved a measure of success only in the latter state, however, where legislation enacted in 1942 provided for wage-loss sickness compensation.[33] In April, 1945, the AMA's Bureau of Legal Medicine and Legislation noted that since January 1, bills providing for some form of compulsory insurance had appeared in the legislatures of 12 states and, while classifying these bills as either dead or in committee, added five new states to the list of those in which wartime compulsory insurance bills had been submitted. In addition the bureau observed that the state legislatures of West Virginia and California had recently authorized a study of health insurance systems. The bitter strife over the compulsory health insurance issue in California had not subsided and, although the state medical association had held closely to the AMA's policies, the outcome of the struggle remained in doubt.[34]

Wagner-Murray-Dingell Bill, 1943

While the Association found the agitation for statewide systems of compulsory health insurance too serious to ignore, it was far more disturbed by the reappearance of the issue on the national level. On June 3, 1943, Senator Robert F. Wagner of New York introduced a comprehensive measure (S. 1161) with Senator James E. Murray of Montana as co-author, which according to the AMA, threatened to destroy the foundations of medical practice. Representative John D. Dingell of Michigan introduced a similar bill (H.R. 2861) in the lower house. In brief, the so-called Wagner-Murray-Dingell bill proposed great extensions in the federal social security system. It called for increased unemployment compensation benefits and for the reorganization of the system on a federal basis. It provided for substantial increases in old age and survivors' benefits, for the establishment of temporary and permanent disability insurance, and for a uniform public assistance pro-

[33] Wilson, *Compulsory Health Insurance,* pp. 8–10, see table.

[34] *JAMA,* 128 (May 5, 1945), 41; *JAMA,* 127 (January 20, 1945), 169; *JAMA,* 127 (February 17, 1945), 398; HD, *Proceedings* (Annual Session, December, 1945), p. 19. The five states were Colo., Mich., Mont., Nev., and N.M.

gram. Section 11 of the Senate bill, which touched off an explosion in the ranks of the AMA, provided for a federal system of compulsory medical and hospitalization insurance which excluded only the cost of drugs, dentistry, and home nursing from its coverage. This measure, financed by a six per cent tax from both employers and employees on wages and salaries up to $3,000 a year, anticipated also the inclusion in the system of some 15,000,000 members of other professional, self-employed, and laboring groups.[35]

It would serve no worthwhile purpose to follow closely the Association's bitter and repetitious attacks upon the compulsory insurance forces from the time the Wagner-Murray-Dingell bill was introduced until the end of the war. Never did the *Journal* allow the profession to forget the issue and never did the Association exert greater effort to win public support for its position. It requires no more than a summary of the Association's attack to reveal the substance of its case and the intensity with which it fought.

AMA's Opposition

No argument served better to win support for the Association's cause than the charge that the proposed legislation would establish dictatorial control over medical practice and open the way for a completely socialized state. Less than a month after the introduction of the Wagner-Murray-Dingell bill the editor of the *Journal* charged "it is doubtful if even Nazidom confers on its 'gaulieter' Conti the powers which the measure would confer on the Surgeon General of the U. S. Public Health Service." On November 19, 1943, Louis Bauer warned the Association to offer no amendments to a measure that so fundamentally imperiled sound medical standards.[36] At the same time Olin West charged that federal regimentation generally started with "the mother and baby, or with the poor, downtrodden and underprivileged" and ended with the complete socialization of a nation's economic life. John J. Wittmer, a New York physician, used obstetrical imagery to describe the birth of "the ghost which has haunted American medicine for so many years." Maintaining that most of its body had appeared he asked, "How

[35] *JAMA,* 122 (June 26, 1943), 609; Wilson, *Compulsory Health Insurance,* pp. 13–14.

[36] Editorial, *JAMA,* 122 (June 26, 1943), 601; *JAMA,* 124 (January 15, 1944), 168.

much longer will it take for the legs to appear and for the apparition to materialize into a living Frankenstein, able to walk among us and become the potent dominating factor in our work and in our lives?"[37]

In combating the compulsory health insurance agitation, the Association also pointed to the accomplishments of the nation's unregimented medical system and its voluntary health insurance programs. For the editor of the *Journal,* the system of medical practice in the United States largely explained its high health standards that, when measured in terms of life expectancy, stood among the highest in the world and superior to any nation with a compulsory health insurance system. The editor contended that American medical education had moved from a retarded position to world leadership while medical education in most great nations suffered from the degrading influences of regimented medicine. He maintained that the superiority of American hospitals over those of other nations remained unchallenged, and that they stood as objects of admiration by the rest of the world. He also called attention to the growth of voluntary hospitalization plans that insured some 15,000,000 members, and to the development of medical society plans that offered medical care to approximately 1,000,000 people.[38]

Fortunately for the AMA the introduction of the Wagner-Murray-Dingell bill stirred up opposition in other professional quarters. The American Bar Association at its Chicago session passed a resolution on August 26, 1943, calling for a committee to study the measure. The outcome of the committee's findings hardly lay in doubt, however, as the organization passed a resolution at the same time opposing any legislation "that subjects the practice of medicine to federal control and regimentation beyond that presently imposed under the American system of free enterprise." The committee's report which the *Journal* published on March 11, 1944, bitterly assailed the Wagner-Murray-Dingell bill. It supported the AMA's contention that the measure supplied the Surgeon General of the United States Public Health Service with dictatorial powers over the administration of medical care and denied the authors' assertion that the measure left the patient-physician relationship undisturbed. It charged that the bill provided "the instrumentality by which physicians for their practice, hospitals for their continued existence and citizens for their health and that of their families can be made to

[37] *JAMA,* 124 (January 15, 1944), 171; *JAMA,* 126 (October 7, 1944), 344. For an analysis of the bill by the AMA's Bureau of Legal Medicine and Legislation see *JAMA,* 122 (June 26, 1943), 609–11.

[38] Editorial, *JAMA,* 113 (October 16, 1943), 418; *JAMA,* 123 (October 23, 1943), 484; Editorial, *JAMA,* 124 (February 12, 1944), 441.

serve the purpose of a political agency" and that the program which the measure proposed more closely resembled the Russian system than that of any other nation.[39]

While deriving strength from the American Bar Association's support, the AMA proceeded to turn the fight against the Wagner-Murray-Dingell bill into more than a battle of words. It brought into the struggle a number of its agencies at the central headquarters and established other machinery for developing a more constructive approach to the nation's health problems. To the Council on Medical Service and Public Relations and to the Bureau of Medical Economics fell much of the responsibility for defeating compulsory health insurance agitation by convincing the public of the superiority of voluntary plans in meeting medical needs. The Council on Legal Medicine and Legislation, established in 1943 as a successor to a bureau of the same name, and the Committee on Rural Medical Service, established two years later, also assisted in the crusade. The Council on Medical Service and Public Relations, however, performed the most spectacular wartime work in spurring medical societies into action. It urged the publication of a semimonthly bulletin which first appeared in January, 1944, informing medical leaders throughout the nation of the profession's problems and perils. By April, nearly all state associations had fulfilled its request to establish local committees with which it could communicate. Through regional conferences that brought together outstanding leaders of organized medicine and influential laymen for discussions of the problems of medical care, the council attempted to gain public respect for its position. By the end of February, 1945, it had held meetings in Boston, Cincinnati, Washington, D.C., Kansas City, and Atlanta, with another planned for Portland, Oregon.[40]

Findings of "Pepper Committee"

The unsettled domestic scene in the closing months of the war indicated that the Association had prepared none too soon for another phase of the compulsory health insurance struggle. On December 16,

[39] Quotations, *JAMA,* 124 (March 11, 1944), 121. The entire report appears on pp. 716–21.

[40] HD, *Proceedings* (Annual Session, June, 1943), p. 83; HD, *Proceedings* (Annual Session, December, 1945), p. 59; *JAMA,* 124 (April 29, 1944), 1305; *JAMA,* 127 (March 10, 1945), 600; HD, *Proceedings* (Annual Session, December, 1945), p. 53.

1944, a subcommittee of the Senate Committee on Education and Labor concluded more than a year of hearings on problems related to the nation's health and social welfare. This Subcommittee on Wartime Health and Education (popularly known as the Pepper Committee) whose findings embraced more than 2,300 pages, not only pointed up critical shortages of physicians and medical services during the war, but produced evidence that seemed to show widespread deficiencies in prewar medical care as well.[41] The nation learned that of the 22,000,000 men of military age, 40 per cent could not meet the requirements of general military service, and that from the time the United States entered the war to July, 1944, the lowest monthly rejection rate reached 31.4 per cent of registrants examined, and that the highest rate climbed to nearly 47 per cent in December, 1943. The public found no cause for complacency in knowing that up to May 1, 1944, 35.2 per cent of the total number of registrants rejected in World War II failed because of nervous and mental diseases, compared with 12 per cent in World War I, and that victims of tuberculosis and venereal diseases constituted 12.2 per cent of the rejectees in World War II compared with 12 per cent in World War I. The subcommittee revealed that the Services faced shocking dental problems as well. The Army's statistics showed that in this branch alone dental work by July, 1944, included 31,000,000 fillings, 1,400,000 bridges and dentures, and 6,000,000 teeth replacements.[42]

Nor did the committee's picture appear in any brighter relief as it turned to consider classes of the population dragged down by low incomes and overwhelmed by inflation. While the federal Bureau of Labor Statistics set the weekly family income of $50 as about the minimum requirement for a decent standard of living, the committee found many

[41] Seventy-eighth Congress, first and second sessions, *Hearings Pursuant to S. Res. 74* (Washington: Government Printing Office, 1944), 7 parts. This resolution was entitled "A Resolution Authorizing An Investigation of the Educational and Physical Fitness of the Civilian Population As Related to National Defense." Originally the subcommittee consisted of Senators Claude Pepper (Fla.), chairman; Elbert D. Thomas (Utah), James M. Tunnell (Del.), Kenneth S. Wherry (Neb.), and Robert M. LaFollette, Jr. (Wis.). When Wherry resigned, Howard A. Smith (N.J.), filled the vacancy. Later four new members were added, namely, James E. Murray (Mont.), Lister Hill (Ala.), Robert A. Taft (Ohio), and George D. Aiken (Vt.) In March, 1945, the committee consisted of three Republicans, five Democrats, and one Progressive. See Pepper's comments, *JAMA,* 127 (March 10, 1945), 600.

[42] *JAMA,* 127 (January 6, 1945), 36; Maj. Gen. Lewis B. Hershey, Seventy-eighth Congress, second session, *Hearings on S. Res. 74,* Part 5, p. 1841; statement of Maj. Gen. George F. Lull, p. 1667.

struggling families far below that level. It cited the Social Security Board's survey of some 4,500,000 white collar workers whose weekly salaries in 1943 averaged only $28.69 before tax deductions. Approximately 3,500,000 workers surveyed in the retail trades had monthly incomes of only $24.88 in the second quarter of 1943, while 1,000,000 more employees surveyed in insurance, financial, and real estate companies averaged only $38.84 in the same period. The committee also referred to statistics that the National Education Association compiled, showing that more than 250,000 teachers earned less than $1,000 in the school year 1942–1943.[43]

AMA's Response

Although the subcommittee presented damaging evidence against the adequacy of American medical care, the American Medical Association greeted the publication of its reports with evidences of delight. Morris Fishbein became the first to congratulate Senator Pepper upon the completion of his investigations and published extracts of the reports in the *Journal.* The Council on Medical Service and Public Relations invited him to speak before its Atlanta meeting, February 23, 1945, upon the significance of his disclosures. In no small measure the favorable impression that the senator made upon the Association arose from his disavowal of interest in the establishment of a system of "socialized medicine."[44]

Spokesmen of the AMA, however, lost no opportunity to expound their own interpretation of the subcommittee's findings. Even before the completion of the hearings Fishbein claimed that records of induction boards left no indication that the United States had become "a degenerate and weak and flabby nation" and that its military performance in World War II proved this conclusively. Later, while correctly asserting that standards of military fitness changed considerably during the war and that the draft boards finally accepted many whom they first rejected, he ignored the fact that the highest wartime rejection rates occurred after the middle of the struggle.[45]

[43] Seventy-eighth Congress, second session, *Hearings Pursuant to S. Res. 74,* Part 3, p. ix. The Bureau of Labor Statistics set the $50 figure as a general approximation and stressed the fact that living costs varied in different parts of the nation. See p. viii.

[44] Claude Pepper, *JAMA,* 127 (March 10, 1945), 600.

[45] *JAMA,* 127 (January 27, 1945), 229; Editorial, *JAMA,* 129 (December 1, 1945), 951.

Other leaders of the Association, however, had expressed its viewpoint more fully at the subcommittee's hearings. R. L. Sensenich of the Board of Trustees argued convincingly that draft boards rejected a large portion of the registrants for defects that no amount of medical care could cure. He cited an estimate that not more than one rejected draftee out of six failed because of remediable impairments and contended that the presence of remediable defects offered no proof of the draftees' inability to secure medical care. He charged that draftees of this category often displayed an unwillingness to accept treatment or an ignorance of its availability. He also contended that much of the blame for the presence of unmet medical needs must rest upon government agencies created to assist the needy. Although concluding that the "average earner" could pay the cost of "average illness" without hardship, under questioning he conceded that large segment of the population did not have adequate medical, hospital, and dental care.[46] Harvey B. Stone of the Council on Medical Education and Hospitals supported the trustee's position and attributed the high rate of rejections to one or more of the following factors: the draftees' failure to seek medical aid, the incapacity of medical science to correct many impairments, the unbalanced distribution of medical personnel and facilities, and economic difficulties.[47]

Second Wagner-Murray-Dingell Bill

Although the Subcommittee on Wartime Health and Education offered only moderate recommendations for improving the nation's medical care, its findings, nevertheless, served to strengthen the compulsory health insurance movement.[48] The subcommittee's disclosure of widespread prewar inadequacy in medical service confirmed the views of health insurance advocates whom the Association had generally classified as overzealous, impractical, and misguided social reformers. The undercurrents of unrest over prevailing medical conditions that led to the establishment of the subcommittee found a further outlet in the intro-

[46] Seventy-eighth Congress, second session, *Hearings on S. Res. 74,* Part 6, pp. 1891, 1893, 1914.

[47] *Ibid.,* pp. 1898–99.

[48] Among the subcommittee's recommendations were the extension of federal aid to the states for the construction of hospitals and medical centers in the postwar era, federal aid to the states for granting scholarships to deserving medical and dental students, and federal funds to provide medical care for recipients of public assistance. *JAMA,* 127 (Jan. 6, 1945), 43.

duction of the second Wagner-Murray-Dingell bill (S. 1050 and H. R. 3293) on May 24, 1945. As the compulsory health insurance issue reappeared on the national scene, the American Medical Association saw growing threats to freedom in the United States accompany the liberation of suppressed peoples overseas.[49]

Mounting Tension

It found the second Wagner-Murray-Dingell bill, which proposed an extension of social security coverage to nearly 85 per cent of the nation's workers and offered disability and invalidity insurance and benefits for medical care, just as objectionable as the first. It denied Senator Wagner's contention that the bill provided for the free choice of physicians and did not establish a system of "socialized medicine." The *Journal* charged that the bill allowed free choice only of physicians participating in the program, and that by authorizing compulsory health insurance with federal controls, established a system of "state medicine and socialized medicine." It also maintained that no revolutionary changes in medical care should be considered during a war that had removed so many physicians and laymen from participation in public affairs.[50] In contending that the authors of the measure had ignored the Association in drafting the bill, the *Journal* touched off a sharp dispute with Senator Wagner. Unconvinced by Wagner's replies, Fishbein charged that the senator and the Social Security Board accepted compulsory health insurance as the only method for providing adequate medical care and that this position represented "the apotheosis of stubbornness and obstinacy and with it a complete lack of willingness to confer, to consult or to reason."[51]

Fourteen-Point Platform

The percussions from the introduction of the second Wagner-Murray-Dingell bill not only touched off a series of intemperate verbal exchanges

[49] Editorial, *JAMA*, 128 (June 2, 1945), 364. For a critical analysis of the bill see Wilson, *Compulsory Health Insurance*, pp. 19–25.

[50] *Ibid.*, pp. 19–23; Editorial, *JAMA*, 128 (June 2, 1945), 364; Editorial, *JAMA*, 128 (July 21, 1945), 880.

[51] Editorial, *JAMA*, 128 (June 2, 1945), 365; *JAMA*, 128 (June 9, 1945), 461; *JAMA*, 128 (June 30, 1945), 672–74.

that largely obscured the issues, but revived a compulsory health insurance fight that outlasted the war. No prospect for the reconciliation of opposing sides appeared. The American Medical Association sought to chart the nation's course along lines that would improve medical care without disrupting conventional procedures, while the compulsory health insurance advocates sought far-reaching changes in the provision of medical service. Recognizing the zeal of its opponents and the concreteness of their program, the AMA resolved not to be outdone. On June 22, 1945, the Board of Trustees approved a 14-point plan which it hoped the nation would accept as embodying legitimate health goals for the postwar years. This program that the House of Delegates approved in December proposed a broad attack upon the nation's health problems, but called for no abrupt changes in the Association's policies.[52]

The platform stressed the urgency of a survey by competent personnel of the medical needs of every state, and for the improvement of the living conditions of the population through "progressive action" directed toward achieving "sustained production." It emphasized the importance of extending programs of preventive medicine and for a fuller development of public health services. It called for the growth of voluntary sickness insurance schemes, and for their extension to the "needy" along principles that the Association had already endorsed. Without reference to the problem of payment, it urged the use of voluntary insurance plans for providing the indigent with hospitalization and medical care and recommended the disposal of federal funds for health activities only to states in need of such assistance with provision for administration by local agencies in consultation with the medical profession. The platform also touched on the need for a more balanced distribution of doctors returning from the Services and the idea of increasing the supply of physicians. Although the platform spoke in rather vague terms of worthy objectives, it strangely omitted reference to one goal that the Association had already endorsed. The program did not mention the need for state plans of income-loss insurance as a supplement to the state-administered unemployment compensation systems.[53]

While the revival of the compulsory health insurance issue forecast mounting postwar political troubles, the eastward thrust of American troops in the Pacific left the Association hopeful that its enormous

[52] HD, *Proceedings* (Annual Session, December, 1945), p. 53.

[53] For the complete platform see Appendix, p. 410.

military responsibilities might be nearing an end. On the same day that the trustees approved the new health program, American forces completed the conquest of Okinawa on a course that reached within 370 miles of the crumbling homeland defenses of Japan. The collapse of Germany and the surrender of its forces in Italy in early May left the Pacific empire fighting alone until the threat of total nuclear destruction made further resistance hopeless. Long before the Japanese surrender of September 2, the Association began preparing for the immediate problems facing the profession in the postwar era.

Preparation for Peacetime

One of the Association's most urgent tasks was in aiding discharged physicians in the resumption of private practice or in securing additional training first. The AMA performed a service of inestimable value in removing some of the obstacles that confronted physicians in this transitional period. In February, 1943, it joined with the American College of Physicians and the American College of Surgeons in creating the Committee on Postwar Medical Service which sought to determine the plans and needs of a discharged army of physicians. At the Chicago headquarters, the Association established a Bureau of Information that handled innumerable inquiries from doctors in the Armed Forces and conducted an extensive national survey to determine areas of postwar physician shortage.[54] In a preliminary study that the Committee on Postwar Medical Service conducted, the *Journal* reported in June, 1944, that out of 400 physicians replying to the questionnaire who had graduated between 1937–1943, 207 definitely desired to begin practice in a new locality, and 177 of these wanted to locate in towns of over 2,500. It also found that 73 per cent of the group canvassed who obtained licenses between 1930 and 1936 did not care to relocate. Those who sought a new location, however, generally restricted their choices to areas with adequate hospitals, diagnostic facilities, and sometimes those that would offer beginning subsidies. When the committee completed a more comprehensive study, it found that of the 21,029 doctors canvassed,

[54] *JAMA,* 125 (August 19, 1944), 1099. Other organizations represented on the Committee on Postwar Medical Service were the Catholic Hospital Association, the American Hospital Association, the Association of American Medical Colleges, the Veterans Administration, the Advisory Board for Medical Specialities, and the Procurement and Assignment Service.

4,310 or nearly 21 per cent wished to relocate and 8,379 ignored the question, some of whom apparently had not decided.[55]

The Bureau of Information through its survey of the nation's physician resources became well prepared to advise returning physicians on problems of relocation. By June 27, 1945, it had complete returns on local medical conditions from the professional societies of 18 states and partial returns from 24 others. While the bureau's services probably directed many physicians to new locations, the early trend set by discharged doctors in Indiana indicated that very few moved to areas of acute physician shortage. While many turned away from less attractive areas, state licensing laws also hindered the movement of physicians to localities of greatest need.[56]

The Association found a great demand for refresher courses and additional training among physicians in the Services. On the day before the Japanese surrender, the *Journal* reported that out of 21,029 returns, 4,563 physicians wanted training of six months or less, while 12,534 desired training for a longer period.[57] The AMA reminded discharged physicians of the benefits they could claim under the Servicemen's Readjustment Act ("G. I. Bill of Rights") of 1944, that allowed a year's additional training at federal expense, and loans by which returning doctors could purchase supplies and equipment for practice. The *Journal* also published data on the opportunities for refresher courses and training in hospitals and medical schools that appealed particularly to wartime graduates whose medical education consisted largely of accelerated courses and shortened internships. In addition representatives of the AMA pressed the case for physicians regarding the purchase of surplus military equipment that could be used in private practice and took up the complaints of medical officers who feared assignment to the Veterans Administration before securing release from military service.[58]

[55] *JAMA,* 125 (June 24, 1944), 559; *JAMA,* 128 (May 12, 1945), 138; Harold C. Lueth, "Postgraduate Wishes of Medical Officers," ACMEL, 1945, *Papers and Discussions,* p. 34. Lt. Col. Lueth, who was the Surgeon General's Liaison Officer, Medical Corps, Army of the United States, made this study for the committee.

[56] *JAMA,* 128 (July 7, 1945), 740; *JAMA,* 129 (September 29, 1945), 369. HD, *Proceedings* (Annual Session, December, 1945), p. 60; *JAMA,* 126 (September 23, 1944), 243; *JAMA,* 127 (January 13, 1945), 108.

[57] Victor Johnson, Harold C. Lueth, and F. H. Arestad, "Educational Facilities for Physician Veterans," *JAMA,* 129 (September 1, 1945), 28.

[58] Editorial, *JAMA,* 126 (November 18, 1944), 770; Editorial, *JAMA,* 128 (May 19, 1945), 206; *JAMA,* 128 (June 16, 1945), 565.

The Association had many special reasons for rejoicing when the Japanese surrender ended World War II. The war had claimed the lives of many physicians, and some of the rest were returning physically impaired. The end of the struggle brought some relief for civilian practitioners who labored under staggering burdens in protecting the nation's health. While the AMA looked upon a political scene allegedly overcast with threats to professional freedom, it could now concentrate more fully on domestic issues.

Chapter 15 BACKWASH OF WAR

When the United States moved from the tortuous war years into an era of precarious peace it assumed responsibilities almost as bewildering as those which it had borne in World War II. The postwar era presented a picture of world wreckage, threatening international tensions, and rising internal social and economic pressures, long suppressed by wartime restraints. While the readjustment after World War I had unveiled a similarly disquieting picture, the feeble response of the United States to the earlier crisis bore little relationship to its dimensions and offered no blueprint worthy of adoption after World War II. As the nation struggled hopefully to construct a peaceful world from the ruins of war and to check the advance of Communism, it also faced many domestic problems that the war had either created or magnified.

Problems of Readjustment

Long before the war ended the American Medical Association began to prepare for its professional and public responsibilities in the postwar era. Among its most urgent tasks was that of steering the profession through the rough channels of postwar readjustment. To thousands of returning physicians who wished to relocate and to many others who planned their first civilian practice, the Association offered valuable assistance. For nearly three months after the Japanese surrender, the Bureau of Information received an average of about 675 letters and personal calls weekly from physicians concerned with problems of relocation, licensure, and additional training. With complete files on the medical situation in 2,521 of the nation's 3,072 counties, and with fragmentary information on the rest, the bureau shortened the route to relocation for many physicians. When the AMA placed the bureau on a permanent basis in December, 1945, and recommended that all state societies establish similar agencies, its action held promise of bringing about a more equitable distribution of medical care. Unfortunately, however, precedents set in the last months of the war continued and returning physicians generally shunned the more remote and retarded areas.[1]

State licensing laws often proved just as obstructive as repelling environmental factors in preventing the movement of doctors into areas of physician shortage. Practitioners, who desired to relocate beyond their own state boundries, but whose detailed knowledge of textbook material had long since escaped, vainly registered their complaints against the inflexibility of state examination requirements with the AMA. Believing that the matter largely lay beyond its control, the AMA offered little aid. Nor did it favor the extension of federal control over the licensing of returning physicians as proposed by a bill which Representative Herman P. Eberharter of Pennsylvania introduced in 1945. Physicians who found the AMA generally co-operative in dealing with their relocation problems got little comfort from its position on the licensing issue.[2]

The Association's assistance to discharged officers planning to move directly into private practice accounted for only a part of its aid to returning physicians. It supplied information to many more who sought additional training before commencing civilian practice. For this class of physicians, however, the Association offered more than information. It attempted to co-ordinate and expand the institutional facilities of hospitals and medical schools, and to effect revisions in the Servicemen's Readjustment Act which would allow for a more satisfactory subsidization of their training. From the outset the Association's efforts proved highly successful. Close co-operation between its Council on Medical Education and Hospitals and the nation's hospitals and medical schools raised the number of residencies from 5,256 held shortly before the war to 15,154, available by April 1, 1948.[3]

[1] HD, *Proceedings* (95 Annual Session, July, 1946), p. 27.

[2] HD, *Proceedings* (Annual Session, December, 1945), pp. 22, 86, 87. The licensing boards of fifteen states issued temporary permits to returning doctors starting civilian practice in their jurisdictions but five of these had discontinued the practice by July 1, 1946. *JAMA,* 131 (May 11, 1946), 124.

[3] HD, *Proceedings* (Annual Session, December, 1945), pp. 55, 78–79; HD, *Proceedings* (95 Annual Session, July, 1946), p. 37; HD, *Proceedings* (95 Annual Session, July, 1946), p. 35; HD, *Proceedings* (96 Annual Session, June, 1947), p. 45; HD, *Proceedings* (97 Annual Session, June, 1948), p. 57. The struggle to

In a negative way also the Association tried to bring the supply and demand for residencies into closer balance. The Armed Forces, in discriminating against general practitioners and rewarding specialists, greatly encouraged the trend away from general practice which threatened to inundate hospitals with demands for specialized residency training.[4] As the AMA saw the growing popularity of specialization imperil postwar medical training and general practice, it moved to check the trend. It warned returning doctors of the congestion developing in many areas of specialization and attempted to put general practice in a more favorable light. Taking an action long overdue, the House of Delegates established a section on general practice in 1945 that created immediate interest.[5] The Association also took up the cause of general practitioners who complained of exclusion from hospital practice and urged hospitals adopting discriminatory policies to establish general practice sections on their staffs. The AMA gave further encouragement to general practice by establishing the "General Practitioners Award," given annually to some worthy physician in unspecialized practice and continued the conferences begun during the war that brought the Association in contact with problems of local physicians.[6]

The Association also responded to the appeals of returning physicians who wanted only refresher courses rather than extensive training. Although most of the work involved in promoting the organization of refresher courses in medical schools fell upon the Association of American Medical Colleges, the AMA took much of the responsibility for en-

---

keep the number of residencies ahead of demand led the council to negotiate successfully for the establishment of residency programs in federal hospitals, and in February, 1946, to begin granting temporary approval of hospital residency programs pending inspection. HD, *Proceedings* (97 Annual Session, June, 1948), p. 57.

[4] Wingate M. Johnson, "Will the Family Doctor Survive?" *JAMA,* 132 (September 7, 1946), 1; Charles F. Wilkinson, "The General Practitioner," *JAMA,* 137 (July 10, 1948), 947. The war only encouraged a movement toward specialization that was already well advanced by 1940. The number of doctors engaged exclusively in specialized practice jumped from 24,826 in 1931 to 36,880 in 1940. Joseph W. Mountain, Elliott H. Pennell, and Vance M. Hoge, "Health Service Areas," Federal Security Agency, U. S. Public Health Service, *Public Health Bulletin No. 292* (Washington: Government Printing Office, 1945), p. 2.

[5] HD, *Proceedings* (Annual Session, December, 1945), p. 69; Wilbert C. Davidson, ACMEL, 1944, *Papers and Discussions,* p. 12; HD, *Proceedings* (96 Annual Session, June, 1947), p. 49.

[6] Wingate M. Johnson, *JAMA,* 137 (May 1, 1948), 107–8; *JAMA,* 135 (November 1, 1947), 581.

couraging hospitals and medical societies to institute such training. In addition, the matter of publicizing the character of refresher courses was assumed largely by the AMA. The Council on Medical Education and Hospitals, which normally published in the *Journal* an annual list of brief courses offered by medical schools, began bringing out this information semiannually in the latter part of the war. So rapidly did these courses develop, however, that only through the issuance of supplementary listings could the council keep the profession adequately informed of training opportunities. Its records showed that in the year that followed July 1, 1947, medical organizations and institutions offered 1,679 refresher courses that some 60,000 physicians attended.[7]

As the AMA moved effectively to provide adequate training opportunities for medical officers, it also succeeded in bringing the veterans' program closer in line with the profession's needs. Finding provisions in the Servicemen's Readjustment Act which it viewed as serious shortcomings, it secured modifications in the measure that appeared in Public Law 268 signed by the President on December 28, 1945. The amending law removed the requirement that veterans over 25 years of age must prove that the war had interrupted their education in order to receive federal payments for additional training and made veterans eligible for educational benefits during terminal leave. It also permitted payment of the maximum annual tuition allowance for refresher courses of less than a school year's duration and recognized accredited hospitals as institutions entitled to federal tuition payments.[8]

Less effectively did the AMA represent the profession in matters related to the disposal of surplus government property after the war. The Association hoped that much of the government's medical equipment would be made available at heavy discount to physicians faced with the burdensome expense of beginning practice. Through processes ill-adjusted to individual purchase methods, however, the government turned over most of its surplus medical equipment for institutional medical needs. Late in 1946, leaders of the AMA expressed their dissatisfaction with the government's disposal program and with public

[7] HD, *Proceedings* (Annual Session, December, 1945), p. 44; HD, *Proceedings* (95 Annual Session, July, 1946), p. 36; HD, *Proceedings* (97 Annual Session, June, 1948), p. 58.

[8] 59 Stat. 623–32 (1945); HD, *Proceedings* (95 Annual Session, July, 1946), p. 19. The Committee on Postwar Medical Service also got the Veterans Administration to recognize that residency and fellowship training constituted "institutional training" rather than "training on the job." *Ibid.*, p. 49.

sales that attracted large numbers of physicians who generally found that they could purchase nothing.[9]

While assisting the medical profession with the immediate problems of postwar adjustment, the AMA did not neglect medical schools that were facing the possibility of severe enrollment losses. Shortly after the war the House of Delegates adopted a resolution branding as "indefensible" the government's policy allowing no deferments to premedical students. Through telegrams to the nation's capital the Association set its views before the President, the Secretary of War, the Director of the Selective Service, and other government officials concerned with the problem as well as before members of the House and Senate Committees on Military Affairs.[10] As the Association sought to guard the source of medical school enrollment through an adequate deferment system, it also tried to broaden the source by assisting prospective medical students in military service. Not only did the AMA furnish information on medical education which the United States Armed Forces Institute distributed, but also encouraged prospective students to take some essential course work under military auspices. In addition, the Council on Medical Education and Hospitals worked with medical schools and appropriate governmental agencies to minimize the friction involved in terminating the wartime accelerated medical program.[11]

The hordes of prospective students that pressed for admission to the nation's medical schools in the early postwar era quickly discredited the Association's prediction of a student shortage. Although the government continued its policy of allowing no deferments for premedical students, the total enrollment in approved medical schools in April, 1946, did not fall far behind the 24,028 enrolled during the preceding year, and showed an irregular rise throughout the rest of the decade. The AMA's fears had long before subsided when the Council on Medical Education and Hospitals found the medical schools in 1948 operating at "maximum capacity."[12] However great may have been the Association's

[9] *JAMA,* 133 (January 4, 1947), 41.

[10] HD, *Proceedings* (Annual Session, December, 1945), pp. 79, 81.

[11] *Ibid.,* p. 45; HD, *Proceedings* (96 Annual Session, June, 1947), p. 48 and (95 Annual Session, July, 1946), p. 37.

[12] *JAMA,* 144 (September 9, 1950), 115; quotation, HD, *Proceedings* (97 Annual Session, June, 1948), p. 55. While freshman enrollment fell from 7,307 in 1944–1945 to 5,796 in 1945–1946, it rose to 7,221 in 1946–1947 but dropped to 6,759 in 1949–1950. *JAMA,* 129 (September 1, 1945), 46–47; *JAMA,* 131 (August 17, 1946), 1284–85; *JAMA,* 134 (August 16, 1947), 1310–11; *JAMA,* 144 (September 9, 1950), 112–13.

miscalculation on postwar student supply, it did assist medical institutions in making the transition to peacetime service.

While dealing with the profession's readjustment problems, the AMA also faced issues of broader scope. Into this class fell several important matters, rising in a large measure from problems created or made more urgent by World War II. Chief among these were questions concerned with national security, increased veterans' demands, reforms in medical education, and international medical progress.

Challenge of National Security

When atomic terror hastened the end of World War II and opened up the nuclear age, the AMA became quickly aware of its implications upon problems of national security. As the government yielded to overwhelming pressures and largely dismantled its military establishment, the AMA urged consideration of measures for more adequate defense. Only three months after the Japanese surrender, the House of Delegates created the Committee on Military Medical Service, with authority to investigate the administration of military medical care during the war as a step toward improving the utilization of medical services in any future national emergency. Not only did the committee launch a study that involved the canvassing of some 50,000 medical officers and hundreds of others concerned with the problems of military medical service, but also proceeded to study civilian medical care in wartime as well.[13] This committee, soon known as the Committee on National Emergency Medical Service, drew a frightening picture of the character of modern warfare after canvassing some 5,000 physicians engaged in civilian practice during World War II. Stating that civilian populations would be targets of attack in future conflicts, it asserted that medical problems would assume "an importance co-equal to the military aspects of national security."[14]

[13] HD, *Proceedings* (Annual Session, December, 1945), pp. 37, 79–80; HD, *Proceedings* (Supplementary Session, December, 1945), p. 24.

[14] Quotation, HD, *Proceedings* (Supplemental Session, December, 1946), p. 24. See also HD, *Proceedings* (96 Annual Session, June, 1947), p. 33. The trustees allowed the committee to change its name to Committee on National Emergency Medical Service to indicate the widening scope of its work. On the original committee, two physicians, Perrin H. Long and Harold C. Lueth represented the Army physicians; Edward L. Bortz and James C. Sargent, the Navy physicians; Harold S. Diehl, the Procurement and Assignment Service; and O. O. Miller and V. C. Tisdal, civilian physician groups.

Upon the basis of records that summarized the wartime experience of some 28,300 physicians and 400 laymen participating in the surveys, the Committee on National Emergency Medical Service drew up recommendations for improving medical service in national emergencies. These recommendations as modified by the House of Delegates sought to bring governmental medical policies in line with the needs of the postwar era. The committee proposed that the Surgeons General of the armed services participate during "peace and war" on a level of "commensurate rank" with the "Chiefs of Staff and Chiefs of Naval Operations of the armed forces" in dealing with all military matters that concerned health and medical care. It also proposed the creation of an agency to be known as the National Emergency Medical Service Administration which would include representation from 13 national medical, health, and related organizations, charged with much of the responsibility for the procurement, mobilization, and allotment of "medical and allied personnel" in national emergencies. Still another recommendation called upon cabinet officials responsible for national defense to revise procedures that had been employed for the mobilization of medical resources in World War II to assure their more effective use. Besides these proposals that the committee asked the AMA to press upon the President and Congress, it also suggested that its own services be continued until it had completed its work.[15]

Although the House of Delegates adopted the report and made the Committee on National Emergency Medical Service a standing committee, the AMA could not move fast enough to influence the administration's efforts to reorganize the defense structure. The National Security Act of 1947, passed within a month after the committee had made its recommendations, created the Department of Defense, the Joint Chiefs of Staff, and subordinate agencies, but failed to organize the nation's medical resources as the committee had proposed. Although the committee considered the measure inadequate, it found some reason for hope. It noted the prospect of attaching a national emergency board to the National Security Resources Board created by the act and observed with satisfaction that the Department of Defense planned to appoint a medical adviser who would be supplied with civil and military medical consultants.[16]

[15] HD, *Proceedings* (96 Annual Session, June, 1947), p. 105. For the committee's unamended recommendation, see *ibid.*, pp. 33–34.

[16] HD, *Proceedings* (97 Annual Session, June, 1948), p. 16.

The Committee on National Emergency Medical Service worked enthusiastically with many organizations and government agencies on problems of defense. Its program called for the evaluation and co-ordination of all the nation's medical resources and for the stockpiling of medical supplies for meeting the perils of nuclear, bacteriological, and chemical welfare. It conducted several surveys to determine the adequacy of the nation's emergency medical resources. Defense preparations brought no serious friction between the AMA and the government until 1948, when the administration proposed universal military service and a doctors' draft. While the Association offered no objection to the proposal for compulsory military training, it bitterly attacked the idea of a physicians' draft and spokesmen for the AMA set its views before the House and Senate Committees on Military Affairs. In successfully resisting the physicians' draft, the AMA made no concessions to the proposal other than to suggest that in case of serious physician shortage the committee on emergency medical service be authorized to perfect plans for the selection of former V-12 and ASTP students and others deferred from service to complete medical training.[17]

The AMA's contribution to national security consisted of more than its effort to strengthen the nation's medical resources against the hazards of a nuclear attack. Late in the war it joined with the government's Committee on Physical Fitness in launching a nationwide health emphasis program and continued much of this work through its own agencies after Congress starved the committee out of existence. The Association co-operated in the establishment of the privately sponsored "Keep Fit Foundation" and extended the services of the Council on Industrial Health and the Bureau of Health Education.[18] It kept in contact with health problems developing in educational institutions through a joint committee that brought leaders of the AMA into collaboration with officials of the National Education Association, and in 1946 organized a "Health and Physical Fitness Project" in the Bureau of Health Education which concentrated on improving school health programs. Within a few months directors of the project had compiled material on health programs from schools in nearly all of the states and had revised some of the Association's literature on youth health problems. They also prepared a number of radio transcriptions on physical fitness, ap-

[17] *Ibid.; JAMA,* 140 (July 2, 1949), 800.

[18] HD, *Proceedings* (Annual Session, December, 1945), p. 30; HD, *Proceedings* (96 Annual Session, June, 1947), pp. 20–22.

peared at several health conferences, and identified themselves with several committees and councils concerned with health improvement. Their activities served as a fitting complement to the service performed by *Hygeia,* which carried the Association's health message to many more than its 200,000 subscribers by 1947.[19]

Impact of Veterans' Issues

While the AMA joined in the search for national security with emphasis on adequate medical reserves readily convertible to wartime use, it confronted a second major problem greatly magnified by World War II. The Association fully supported federal programs providing adequate medical care for veterans with service-connected disabilities and for other ex-servicemen unable to pay for needed medical treatment, but resisted the much broader demands of some pressure groups.[20] Much of the ill will that it incurred in the early postwar era arose from its opposition to what it considered to be reckless programs of demonstrable waste launched by the Veterans Administration.

It stubbornly opposed plans of the Veterans Administration in 1948 to add 54,000 beds to its hospital system in which 5,600 remained unoccupied because of insufficient staff. The *Journal* observed that the government, on October 31, had 89 new veterans' hospitals under construction, but that 68,992 of the 105,762 hospitalized ex-servicemen claimed only nonservice-connected disabilities.[21] It was also aware of the pattern of extortion set by many private contractors who usually ran up the construction cost on federal hospitals to a range of from $20,000 to $51,000 per bed, compared with similar construction costs in voluntary hospitals of about $16,000. It saw the possibilities of

[19] HD, *Proceedings* (96 Annual Session, June, 1947), pp. 23–24; HD, *Proceedings* (Supplemental Session, December, 1946), pp. 6–7; HD, *Proceedings* (97 Annual Session, June, 1948), p. 8.

[20] See pp. 158–60, 164–68 above.

[21] The Committee on Federal Medical Care, The Commission on Organization of the Executive Branch of the Government, *Task Force Report on Federal Medical Services: Appendix O* (Washington, D.C.: U.S. Government Printing Office, 1949), p. 17; The Commission on Organization of the Executive Branch of the Government, *Reorganization of Federal Medical Activities,* March, 1949 (Washington, D.C.: U.S. Government Printing Office, 1949), pp. 8, 10; *JAMA,* 139 (January 1, 1949), 42.

unnecessary duplication of services in areas where the federal government supported the construction of veterans' hospitals and civilian medical projects as well.[22]

Since alleged unmet medical needs of veterans with nonservice-connected disabilities gave the program for the expansion of veterans' hospitals its chief support, the AMA offered another plan for providing their medical care. This plan, closely resembling a program that the Association had recommended during the depression, sought to reduce the staggering cost of the veterans' hospital expansion program and prevent further inroads on private medical practice. It proposed that the government provide hospital and medical service contracts to indigent veterans with nonservice-connected disabilities, entitling them to receive medical care and hospitalization at public expense in any institution approved by the Veterans Administration. Moving swiftly to make its voice heard, it submitted the program to the proper officials of the American Legion and brought its plan and grievances to the attention of the Commission on Organization of the Executive Branch of the Government (Hoover Commission), which had the government's handling of veterans' problems under investigation.[23]

In other ways as well the AMA moved against the alleged extravagance of the veterans' program and its threat to private medical practice. It proposed that Congress clarify its restrictions on the use of veterans' hospitals that excluded nonservice-connected disability cases able to pay for medical care, and which authorized service to indigent veterans only when existing facilities could accommodate them. It supported the means test that required applicants with nonservice-connected disabilities to affirm their inability to pay for medical service before receiving hospitalization in the veterans' system. The AMA also proposed in 1948 that the hospitals of the veterans' system be restricted to a 140,000-bed capacity and advanced a plan whereby veterans with service-connected injuries could receive medical care in their home areas, often avoiding the inconvenience and expense of recourse to government facilities. Nevertheless, while crusading for greater economy in the operation of the veterans' hospital program, it upheld the right of state societies to set fees governing civilian doctors' charges in veteran cases and

[22] *Task Force Report on Federal Medical Services, Appendix O,* p. 17; *JAMA,* 138 (December 25, 1948), 1240.

[23] *JAMA,* 138 (December 18, 1948), 1166–67. For an account of the AMA's depression program see pp. 165–66 above.

resisted suspected efforts of the Veterans Administration to set up a nationwide schedule of its own.[24]

Although the AMA never endorsed many aspects of the veterans' program, it seems to have had considerable influence on its development. About the time the Veterans Administration announced plans for the enlargement of its hospital system to include 156,219 beds, the House of Delegates proposed that the maximum number not exceed 140,000. Shortly thereafter the President ordered the Veterans Administration to eliminate 16,000 beds from its construction plans which brought the program almost in line with the Association's proposal. The AMA also saw a task force of the Hoover Commission confirm its fears that the veterans' hospital construction plan would bring about disastrous competition with the government's program of civilian hospital construction. It won a partial victory in the early postwar era over opponents of the means test who made no greater headway against the so-called "pauper's oath" than to prevent government investigation of alleged abuses.[25] Furthermore, the AMA partially succeeded in checking encroachments on private medical care that appeared in the veterans' program, keeping part of the program in the area of private practice under arrangements largely of the profession's making.

Upon problems involving veterans' rehabilitation the AMA and the Veterans Administration stood in closer agreement than upon issues related to nonservice-connected disability benefits. While the Association had little to do with formulating the rehabilitation program, it cooperated with the government in its operation. This program, which included the mental and physical reconditioning of ex-servicemen and a system for their vocational rehabilitation, far outstripped the government's limited efforts to assist disabled veterans after World War I.[26]

[24] Resolution, Medical Society of the State of New York, HD, *Proceedings* (97 Annual Session, June, 1948), pp. 72, 96. See also pp. 92, 93, and HD, *Proceedings* (96 Annual Session, June, 1947), pp. 54, 95, 96. Since physicians served the government in many capacities, in 1947 the House of Delegates requested the editor of the *Journal* and the Bureau of Legal Medicine and Legislation to "collect, annotate, analyze, interpret and publish a digest of all the rules and regulations of the federal government pertaining to medical practice and medical service fees." Resolution, Thomas D. Cunningham, pp. 67, 94, 95–96.

[25] *Task Force Report on Federal Medical Services, Appendix O,* pp. 17, 39, 44. *Reorganization of Federal Medical Activities,* pp. 8, 10.

[26] Charles M. Griffith, "The Veterans Administration," chapter 15 in Morris Fishbein, ed., *Doctors at War,* pp. 322–28. The Government's vocational rehabilitation program for World War II veterans was created by Public Law 16, approved March 24, 1943, and commonly known as the Barden-LaFollette Act.

Agencies of the AMA that had long dealt mainly with problems of civilian injuries turned to give more attention to military disabilities. Late in 1945 the Council on Industrial Health responded to the "enormous" medical interest in rehabilitation, by creating the Committee on Medical Policy in Rehabilitation and Employment. The council laid plans for the establishment of a clearing section responsible for collecting and disseminating information on rehabilitation work, and for bringing health units of state societies in contact with their local rehabilitation agencies. It conducted its activities in conjunction with the Council on Physical Medicine, which took on a name more expressive of its functions when it became the Council on Physical Medicine and Rehabilitation in 1949.[27]

Crisis in Medical Education

While the American Medical Association attempted to fix limits for the operation of the veterans' program, it struggled with another difficult postwar problem. It watched the foundations of medical education, so seriously undermined by the war, threaten to give way before the impact of peacetime pressures. The AMA not only assisted medical schools in meeting the transitional problems of readjustment, but also helped in formulating new long-range policies which the war made all the more urgent. A glance at the status of medical education in 1945 readily reveals areas of both strength and weakness.

During a half century of struggle, the AMA had assisted immeasurably in raising standards of medical education from the generally low levels of the nineteenth century to a position that no nation excelled or perhaps equalled. The Association's attack on the bastions of sectarian medical practice had been mostly successful, and while schools of osteopathy and chiropractic survived along with numerous nondescript medical organizations, other irregular schools of practice had

See 57 Stat. 43–45 (1943), and Howard A. Rusk, *JAMA,* 140 (May 21, 1949), 287. The success of rehabilitation under the act of 1943 is described by Howard A. Rusk and Eugene J. Taylor, "Rehabilitation," The American Academy of Political and Social Science, *Annals,* 273 (January, 1951), 138–43.

[27] HD, *Proceedings* (Annual Session, December, 1945), pp. 15–16; (95 Annual Session, July, 1946), p. 16; *JAMA,* 140 (May 21, 1949), 292.

all but disappeared. Only five states had homeopathic examining boards in 1945, and these examined only three candidates, while the nation's only eclectic board in Arkansas remained totally inactive. Fourteen states tested osteopaths with examinations offered by standard medical boards, while 17 states required candidates to pass basic science examinations.[28]

Not only had the AMA done much to destroy the divisive forces within American medicine, but it had succeeded in elevating the academic standards of the profession as well. When most medical schools required three years of premedical training for admission in 1944 and when over 80 per cent of their graduates that year held baccalaureate degrees, medical education had advanced far beyond the era of negligible entrance requirements. Furthermore, the broadening of curriculum and the toughening of courses brought on by scientific advance made medical training all the more difficult. Completion of internship which 23 states required before licensure and the demands of specialized training that usually required a minimum of five years additional preparation also demonstrated the rise in medical standards.[29]

Despite spectacular advance, however, medical education had a less impressive side and a seemingly dark future. The postwar era found 18 states without medical schools as demands for medical education mounted, and 15 schools rejecting all out of state applicants in 1949. Within the offerings of medical institutions disturbed authorities pointed out serious deficiencies. Two years after the war not more than five schools had adequately endowed departments of psychiatry to prepare for the needs of battle casualties that were from 30 to 40 per cent psychiatric in character. Almost no exemplary departments of dermatology existed, and training in pharmacolological subjects and preventive, tropical, and industrial medicine languished. Nor did most medical

[28] *JAMA,* 131 (May 11, 1946), 114, 127, 132. These homeopathic boards were in Ark., Conn., Del., La., and Md. *Ibid.,* p. 114. Walter L. Bierring stated that the original purpose of the basic science laws appeared to be that of offering a test in basic sciences as a prerequisite for taking examinations for licensure. But he states that they had become about as comprehensive and advanced as licensing examinations. Wisconsin led the way with such legislation in 1925. ACMEL, 1948, *Papers & Discussions,* pp. 36–37.

[29] *JAMA,* 129 (September 1, 1945), 54–55; *JAMA,* 128 (May 11, 1945), 115, 137–38. By 1940, when the American Board of Neurological Surgery was created, there were fifteen approved training boards on medical specialties. The first of these was the American Board of Ophthalmology established in 1917. *Ibid.,* p. 139.

institutions make any room for courses orienting students to the economic aspects of medical care.[30]

Although academic standards had risen considerably during the twentieth century, there was room for much improvement. While acceptance of applicants to 74 of the nation's medical schools stood at 1 to 3.47 in 1949, 54 of these schools admitted 9.1 per cent of their freshman classes with grade averages of less than "B minus."[31] The passing standards of the state examining boards seemed to allow licensure of the strong and weak alike. Most of them required candidates to have a general average of at least 75 per cent, but called for no more than 50 per cent in any one subject. Examining boards in 16 of the 30 states with medical schools failed no candidates in 1945, and 16 of the boards in the 18 states without medical schools reported no failures. A few medical boards, however, reported heavy casualty rates. The New York board failed nearly 25 per cent of its candidates, which included a 6.6 per cent failure rate for graduates of institutions within the state. Massachusetts failed 11 per cent, and Florida, which had no medical school, failed nearly 15 per cent. For the five years from 1942–1946, nine states failed no candidates, while 12 states had a failure rate of less than one per cent. Yet for these years the failure rate reached nearly 58 per cent in Massachusetts, over 42 per cent in New York, over 27 per cent in New Hampshire, and nearly 25 per cent in Connecticut; rates of failure that are only partially explained by the large number of foreign physicians who sought licensure.[32]

The depression and war revealed deficiencies in medical education and created others, leaving many schools unprepared to bear postwar

[30] *JAMA,* 131 (May 11, 1948), 116; *JAMA,* 141 (September 3, 1949), 35; Alan Valentine, "The Privately Endowed Medical Schools," *JAMA,* 137 (May 1, 1948), 1; John Romano, "Basic Orientation and Education of the Medical Student," *JAMA,* 143 (June 3, 1950), 410, 411. Much of Valentine's information was based on a statement signed by 19 presidents of universities with medical schools.

[31] *JAMA,* 144 (September 9, 1950), 125. In 1944, Harold S. Diehl, Dean of Medical Science at the University of Minnesota, said that, although medical schools were drawing students of higher ability than in earlier years, "most medical schools accept the last 20 to 25 per cent of students with distinct reservations as to their qualifications, intellectual or personal, for the study or practice of medicine." ACMEL, 1944, *Papers and Discussions,* p. 5.

[32] *JAMA,* 131 (May 11, 1946), 116; *JAMA,* 134 (May 17, 1947), 275. Between 1942 and 1946, of the 4,975 foreign physicians who took the New York licensing examinations only 2,878 passed. Jacob L. Lochner, Jr., ACMEL, 1948, *Papers and Discussions,* p. 44.

burdens. Inadequate resources almost closed three or four medical schools between 1933 and 1948, and reduced courses, research, and professors' salaries in many others.[33] In the last year of the war, Roger I. Lee, president-elect of the AMA, spoke of students "whisked through the medical schools" in accelerated programs that definitely lowered standards. In 1947, the eminent authority on medical education, Herman G. Weiskotten, observed that inadequate support left over half of the nation's medical schools unable "to conduct a thoroughly satisfactory undergraduate program. . . ."[34] No less pessimistic were the conclusions of the President's Scientific Research Board headed by John R. Steelman, which submitted its report in October of the same year. It noted that most medical schools faced only the undesirable alternatives of restricting training programs or closing doors, unless the nation met the financial crisis in medical education. Two years later, the Council on Medical Education and Hospitals stated that while tuition fees amounted to only 25 per cent of the budgets of medical schools in 1948–1949, they would account for only 22.8 per cent during the following year in which 42 medical schools saw no prospect of securing as much or more financial support from local sources.[35]

Though faced with a crisis of exceptional gravity, the Association's response embodied little more than an attack upon educational problems through conventional methods. In 1947, it joined with the Association of American Medical Colleges in making plans for an extensive three year survey of medical education that got under way in January, 1949. This study was the first comprehensive survey of medical education since the Weiskotten investigation of the middle thirties, and held promise of pointing out areas of deficiency and strength in the structure and direction of medical training.[36]

For institutions whose survival largely depended upon endowment incomes deeply eroded by inflation and upon the precarious bouyancy of a somewhat unpredictable philanthropy, the Association proposed only a more systematic plan for tapping private sources. Three years

[33] Alan Valentine, *JAMA,* 137 (May 1, 1948), 1.

[34] *JAMA,* 127 (January 6, 1945), 32–33; ACMEL, 1947, *Papers and Discussions,* p. 3. A year later Weiskotten stated that standards of medical education in the United States were higher than in any other country and were not deteriorating. ACMEL, 1948, *Papers and Discussions,* p. 4.

[35] Valentine, *JAMA,* 137 (May 1, 1948), 2; *JAMA,* 141 (September 3, 1949), 43.

[36] John E. Deitrick, ACMEL, 1950, *Proceedings,* 8, 10; Editorial, *JAMA,* 138 (December 4, 1948), 1042.

after the war the Council on Medical Education and Hospitals expressed disapproval of the extension of federal aid to medical education until all methods for securing aid from private sources proved inadequate. On July 22, 1948, the Council on Medical Education and Hospitals and the Council of the Association of American Medical Colleges met in New York City with representatives of industry, business, education, and several philanthropic foundations to discuss the problem of raising adequate funds from private sources. This group created a committee headed by Earl Bunting, managing director of the National Association of Manufacturers, that united with a group of university presidents concerned with the same problem to establish the National Fund for Medical Education the next spring.[37]

AMA's Position

Before the national fund could explore methods for private support, however, congressional pressures for the extension of federal aid forced the AMA to take a position on proposed legislation. In March, 1949, Senator Pepper introduced a bill (S. 1453) calling for federal assistance to medical schools, which passed the Senate on September 23.[38] In the meantime the House of Delegates spoke up on the issue and endorsed the principle of federal assistance for schools whose survival depended upon federal aid, if such support brought no federal control. Spokesmen for the AMA set its views before the subcommittee on health of the Senate Committee on Labor and Public Welfare and secured several changes in the original bill. While the companion bill (H. R. 5940) and substitute measures vied for the attention of the House, the trustees laid out in greater detail the conditions to which it felt such a measure should conform.[39]

These conditions included the delegation to the states of complete responsibility for determining the eligibility of schools for federal assistance and the accountability of the schools to the government for only the

[37] *JAMA,* 138 (October 30, 1948), 679; Harvey B. Stone, ACMEL, 1951, *Proceedings* (Part II of *Medical Education in the United States & Canada,* 1950–1951), p. 17.

[38] HD, *Proceedings* (Clinical Session, December, 1949), pp. 34, 41.

[39] HD, *Proceedings* (98 Annual Session, June, 1949), pp. 21–22, 52; HD, *Proceedings* (Clinical Session, December, 1949), p. 34. *JAMA,* 144 (October 21, 1950), 638.

general expenditure of funds. The board also maintained that the maximum federal assistance should constitute only a "limited" part of the institution's total budget and that any subsidy system based on a student ratio should encourage no growths in enrollments that could not be adequately accommodated. Other conditions required that any program of federal scholarships leaves institutions completely free in the selection of students and forces upon individual beneficiaries no future regimentation.[40]

Although the Association's influence appeared particularly effective in reducing maximum federal appropriations from 50 to 40 per cent of a school's budget and in introducing safeguards against the reckless issuance of scholarships and the endless perpetuation of the subsidy system, the Association decided to oppose the measure. It resented the fact that the bill made osteopathic schools eligible for federal assistance. While it approved of provisions in the revised bill that offered federal support of $500 per student for a number equivalent to the average of the school's recent past enrollment, and $1,000 per student for an addition to this average up to 30 per cent, it opposed the allowance to new schools of $1,000 per student for their total enrollments. Likewise it opposed the provision calling for an annual appropriation of $5,000,000 for construction and expansion of schools "in the health professions" before the nation's need had been surveyed and long-range plans developed. Nor did it approve of power which the bill conferred upon the National Council on Education for Health Professions to interfere in the administration of institutions receiving assistance.[41]

While the Association watched the House bill die in committee it had time not only to explore at greater length the problem of private support for medical education, but also the question of federal aid for medical research. Out of the war not only came the prospect of dwindling private funds for medical research, but also competent advice calling for federal subsidization. In July, 1945, Vannevar Bush, director of the Office of Scientific Research and Development, submitted a report to

[40] HD, *Proceedings* (Clinical Session, December, 1949), pp. 34, 68.

[41] HD, *Proceedings* (Clinical Session, December, 1949), pp. 34, 41, 67–68. The Board of Trustees charged that the bill gave the national council "rather sweeping authority to investigate the medical schools and to determine their capacity to maintain and expand student enrolments, to establish a uniform method of calculating costs of instruction and to determine the extent to which equal opportunity to gain an education in the health professions is afforded all properly qualified students."

President Harry S Truman on federal aid for scientific research, eight months after a presidential request launched a study under his direction. The report, entitled "Science the Endless Frontier," called for the creation of a federal agency to promote scientific research.[42] Although the AMA found no measure that it could endorse providing for the subsidization of medical education in the half decade after the war, it did give unenthusiastic support to the movement for the subsidization of medical research. Among the bills that included research in medical areas as an object of subsidization, the AMA's Committee on Postwar Medical Service endorsed the Magnuson bill (S. 1285) as providing the best safeguard for medical freedom. Spokesmen for the AMA appeared at Senate hearings on the Magnuson, Kilgore, and Fulbright bills in October and secured several modifications that appeared in a compromise measure (S. 1720) that Senator Kilgore soon introduced in conjunction with four other senators. On February 21, 1946, however, Kilgore, Magnuson, and six other senators replaced the former bill with S. 1850 calling for the creation of a national science foundation which the Senate passed on July 3. The House took no action and the bill died in the Seventy-ninth Congress.[43]

Prospects for the establishment of a foundation appeared bright the next year when on February 7, 1947, H. Alexander Smith of New Jersey and six other senators introduced a measure (S. 526) that closely resembled the bill that the Senate had passed seven months before. Although the bill moved rather quickly through both Houses, it met the President's pocket veto on August 6. Obstructions to the creation of a science foundation proved insurmountable for nearly three more years. In April, 1950, however, the Senate and House accepted a compromise that adjusted differences in measures that the two bodies had recently passed to encourage scientific research. The President's signature on May 10 to the bill creating a National Science Foundation ended years of agitation for the establishment of such an agency.[44]

[42] Kenneth B. Turner, "Federal Aid to Medical Research," ACMEL, 1946, *Papers and Discussions,* p. 31.

[43] *Ibid.,* p. 32; HD, *Proceedings* (95 Annual Session, July, 1946), p. 24; HD, *Proceedings* (Supplemental Session, December, 1946), p. 13; HD, *Proceedings* (96 Annual Session, June, 1947), p. 26.

[44] AMA, Council on Medical Service, Washington Office, *Bulletin No. 4* (February 17, 1947), 2; *Bulletin No. 12* (August 28, 1947), 6, 2; *Comments No. 23* (March 17, 1950), 1; *Bulletin No. 47* (April 27, 1950), 3; *Bulletin No. 49* (May 11, 1950), 2. The Washington Office is hereafter referred to in footnotes as WO, with publication title.

Provisions of the National Science Foundation Act appeared consistent with principles that the AMA had already endorsed. The measure created a Division of Medical Research within the foundation as one of the four original divisions and prohibited the foundation from operating any laboratories or plants of its own. The act authorized federal appropriations limited to $500,000 for the first year, and to $15,000,000 thereafter for the promotion of research in many scientific areas. Institutions receiving grants faced no limitation upon their right to conduct research unhampered by political pressures.[45]

The International Scene

The backwash of war not only left the AMA with difficult domestic problems, but with responsibilities of an international character as well. As the United States moved to assist a ravaged world scourged by disease and hunger, the AMA turned to deal with world-wide medical problems. It caught the spirit of international co-operation that brought the United Nations into existence and supported the movement for a world medical association. The international picture looked somewhat forbidding, with the medical organizations of the major defeated powers largely disrupted, and in Germany, disgraced by infamous war crimes. Nor did the world scene, that reflected as late as mid-century a disparity in physician-population ratio of 17 to 100,000 among two-thirds of the earth's population, to 106 to 100,000 among the most advanced one-fifth, inspire much hope. Nevertheless, the AMA sent observers to a conference that met in London in September, 1946, called by the British Medical Association to discuss world medical problems. The AMA endorsed the assembly's effort to create a world medical organization and the Board of Trustees quickly voted the Association into the international body.[46]

The AMA appears to have been more responsible for the survival of the World Medical Association, however, than with its establishment. It supported a committee formed in the United States that took on the responsibility of meeting the organization's expenses for five years

[45] Public Law 507, 64 Stat. 152–53 (1950-1951).

[46] C-E. A. Winslow, "International Cooperation in the Service of Health," American Academy of Political and Social Science, *Annals,* 273 (January, 1951), 199; *JAMA,* 132 (October 26, 1946), 430; T. Clarence Routley, "I Believe in This—The Aims and Objects of the World Medical Association," *World Medical Journal* (November, 1959), p. 328.

through funds solicited from medical organizations, pharmaceutical enterprises, and individuals. The editor of the AMA's *Journal* became editor of the international association's new quarterly publication, and other prominent figures in the AMA held responsible positions in the World Medical Association before the decade ended. In 1950, the international body honored the American medical profession by holding its fourth general assembly in the city of New York.[47]

During the half decade that followed the war, the AMA contributed significantly to the accomplishments of the world organization. Among these accomplishments none appeared more important than the issuance of an international code of ethics (applicable both in war and peace), which the associations of ten nations had accepted by October, 1949. The world organization attempted to strengthen many weak associations and to establish national organizations in countries where none existed. It also launched a movement to improve medical advertising and to combat nostrums and quackery.[48] Although moving slowly against staggering odds, the international association had made notable progress by the end of the decade.

While undergirding the World Medical Association, the AMA also co-operated with the World Health Organization. Proposals for the establishment of this agency had been made at the United Nations Conference in San Francisco in 1945, but not until 1948 did it officially come into existence. The American delegation attending its first international assembly the next year included James R. Miller of the AMA's Board of Trustees. The Association not only co-operated with the organization directly, but through the World Medical Association as well.[49]

In addition, it feebly supported the International Refugee Organization, although somewhat indirectly. Among hundreds of thousands of refugees that had gathered under the agency's supervision in September, 1948, 2,500 had registered as physicians. When Congress widened op-

[47] Ernest E. Irons, *JAMA,* 138 (September 18, 1948), 219; Editorial, *JAMA,* 138 (October 2, 1948), 366; *JAMA,* 143 (June 10, 1950), 561; *JAMA,* 144 (September 23, 1950), 316. In 1949 the world organization elected Elmer L. Henderson of Louisville, Kentucky, president-elect, who later served as president of the AMA, while R. L. Sensenich, former president of the AMA, was elected to the council of the organization. In 1950, Louis H. Bauer, chairman of the Board of Trustees, held the office of secretary general. *JAMA,* 141 (November 12, 1949), 784; *JAMA,* 144 (September 23, 1950), 316.

[48] *JAMA,* 141 (November 12, 1949), 782, 783; *JAMA,* 138 (December 17, 1948), 1165.

[49] Winslow, *Annals,* 273 (January, 1951), 195; Editorial, *JAMA,* 139 (January 1, 1949), 37; Edward J. McCormack, "Report on the Third World Health Assembly of the World Health Organization," *JAMA,* 144 (October 7, 1950), 454.

portunities for immigration to the United States in June with the passage of legislation allowing admittance of a maximum of 202,000 displaced persons within two years, the Association anticipated the arrival of a growing number of physicians.[50] The Council on Medical Education and Hospitals, assisted by the Association of American Medical Colleges and an advisory council representing a number of private and governmental agencies, began to acquire information on foreign medical schools for use in assessing their educational standards. Four years later it secured authorization from the House of Delegates to prepare a list of foreign medical schools whose educational programs appeared adequate. By July, 1950, it had compiled a list that included 44 medical schools in eight countries whose programs allowed the council to approve their graduates as trained according to acceptable American standards.[51]

Obstructive state statutes, however, largely nullified the Association's effort to clear the way for the employment of at least some foreign trained alien physicians. Although a few states made room for immigrant doctors in the less desirable positions of public institutions, restrictive legislation in most states at mid-century deprived society of their services. Twenty-two states refused to recognize foreign medical degrees, and none allowed immigrant physicians to become licensed without examination. Eight required procurement of first papers for citizenship, 20 required full citizenship, and 20, internships. Seven states required additional training.[52] Despite the physician shortage appearing in some areas and the urgency of the immigrant location problem, neither the AMA nor state associations made much if any effort to secure modifications in the licensing laws.

Although licensing problems remained as a barrier to the employment of alien physicians, the AMA made a little progress in removing color barriers within the profession, at a time when the world was increas-

[50] Alexander Manlius Burgess, "Resettlement of Displaced Physicians in the United States," *JAMA,* 143 (June 3, 1950), 413; 62 Stat. 1010 (1948). The Displaced Persons Act of 1948 was amended in 1950 to bring in an additional 139,000 persons making a total of 341,000 to be accepted within three years after July 1, 1948. 64 *Stat.* 221 (1950–1951). For problems involved in the employment of refugee physicians who sought to practice in the United States during World War II, see Morris Fishbein, ACMEL, 1942, *Papers and Discussions,* p. 50 and Ernest P. Boas, pp. 25–26.

[51] *JAMA,* 144 (September 9, 1950), 131–32; HD, *Proceedings* (98 Annual Session, June, 1949), pp. 25, 50. In the period between 1934 and 1949 about 10,000 physicians came to the United States. *Ibid.,* p. 25.

[52] Burgess, "Resettlement of Displaced Physicians," *JAMA,* 143 (June 3, 1950), 415.

ingly disturbed by racial tensions. Even though many Northern societies had long included Negro physicians, not until 1949 did a Negro doctor (Peter M. Murray of New York) reach the Association's House of Delegates. Strong prejudice in many areas, however, prevented the Association from making much headway against the segregation problem and from strengthening the nation's position on the diplomatic front.[53]

The AMA seemed more concerned with another matter more directly related to the international scene than with the segregation question. As nations rose from the wreckage of war to find their health insurance systems largely destroyed, they re-established compulsory programs. Even during the war at least eight nations adopted compulsory schemes and three others quickly followed. For the AMA, however, the most alarming development was the expansion of the British system with the establishment of the National Health Service in 1948.[54] Although the Association could do little to turn the international tide, it resisted efforts to impose a highly centralized national system of medical care on Japan during the Allied Occupation. So vigorously did it oppose some of the recommendations made by an American social security commission that the Department of the Army invited the Association to send an advisory group of its own to Japan. The AMA accepted the invitation and in early August, 1948, the commission began its study.[55]

Although the Commission did not advise the rejection of state-administered medical programs after its investigation, it did urge the inclusion of voluntary features. Maintaining that the social security group called for a plan "covering the entire Japanese population with a maximum of uniformity or standardization and administered by a centralized authority," it emphasized the importance of decentralization and local freedom of choice. The commission saw serious threats to the development of democratic processes in Japan in the centralization that the social security group recommended. It also urged that the system be financed when possible by worker and employer contributions rather

[53] *JAMA,* 140 (August 20, 1949), 1278.

[54] "Benefits and Contributions under National Compulsory Health Insurance Programs," *Social Security Bulletin,* 14 (January, 1951), 17. During the war Australia, Belgium, Costa Rica, Mexico, Panama, Paraguay, Spain, and Venezuela adopted compulsory systems, and shortly thereafter, Albania, Colombia, and the Dominican Republic adopted compulsory plans. For an example of the AMA's concern over the inauguration of the British system, see Editorial, *JAMA,* 137 (July 24, 1948), 1132–33.

[55] *JAMA,* 138 (October 30, 1948), 663–64; "A Report to General Douglas MacArthur," *JAMA,* 139 (April 30, 1949), 1279.

than by taxation. The Association's commission did not make its study in vain. The medical programs soon established in Japan were based on the principle of local option and allowed considerable decentralization.[56]

The last half of the turbulent decade not only reached back to World War II, but nearly to the Korean conflict as well. It set before the AMA serious problems that the war created or greatly magnified. It broadened the Association's domestic responsibilities and enlarged its role in international affairs. It required that the Association modify positions that it had formerly taken, and occasionally pioneer along new paths. Yet the demands of this convulsive era did not move the Association very far from the basic principles of its faith.

[56] "A Report to General Douglas MacArthur," *JAMA,* 139 (April 30, 1948), 1281, quotation, 1279; Crawford F. Sams, "Medical Care Aspects of Public Health and Welfare in Japan," *JAMA,* 141 (October 22, 1949), 531. The AMA did not interfere with the re-establishment of a social insurance program in West Germany after the war. West Germany, however, moved with unprecedented speed in getting the system revived and the United States had only partial control over developments there. For the inauguration of the system see Rudolph Wissell, "Social Insurance in Germany," American Academy of Political and Social Science, *Annals,* 260 (November, 1948), 128–29.

Chapter 16

AMA AND THE FAIR DEAL, 1945–1948

WORLD WAR II HAD HARDLY ENDED when President Truman proposed to extend the Progressivism of the Roosevelt Administration through a program that he eventually labeled the Fair Deal. This program, for the most part arising out of the pains of the nation's social and economic growth, quickly revealed to the AMA many of the problems it would face in the postwar era. Only four days after the Japanese surrender the President informed Congress that he would soon present plans for providing the nation with adequate medical care, and these he submitted ten weeks later.

Truman's Health Program

On November 19, in the first presidential message to Congress ever devoted exclusively to health issues, the chief executive laid out the administration's conception of national health goals and methods of achievement. He urged the inauguration of a federally supported program of hospital and health clinic construction and called for the extension of federal programs of medical research and recommended the establishment of a national research foundation. In addition, he called for the provision of medical care through a national system of compulsory sickness insurance, along lines proposed by measures that appeared in Congress during the war.[1]

[1] Seventy-ninth Congress, first session, House Document No. 380, pp. 6–11; Watson B. Miller, ACMEL, 1942, *Papers and Discussions,* p. 53; Editorial, *JAMA,* 129 (November 24, 1945), 874; Harry S Truman, *Years of Trial and Hope* (Vol. 2 of *Memoirs,* Garden City, N.Y.: Doubleday & Company, 1956), pp. 19–20.

Floodlights thrown upon the Association's opposition to portions of the administration's program have left obscure the AMA's part in meeting the health challenges of the early postwar era. Its reaction to the program varied from complete acceptance of some features to total rejection of others and included as well its readiness to accept some proposals with modifications. Yet the Association never accepted the adequacy of political action on the federal level in meeting the nation's health problems. It sought to balance the growing power of the federal government over health affairs with a strengthening of local responsibility for the improvement of health programs and the encouragement of individual initiative. While the early postwar era engendered much friction between the administration and the AMA on health issues, a consideration of the Association's own program for meeting the nation's health problems is first in order.

AMA's Health Program

Only ten weeks after the President announced his health program, the Board of Trustees adopted a ten-point platform that summarized the Association's policies and objectives. While stressing the necessity of providing the indigent with adequate medical care, the board assigned responsibility for this undertaking at the local level. It called for the provision of maternal, infant, and child welfare programs through funds provided by local governments and preferred that localities look for no outside support in providing hospital and clinical facilities. In no area of health and welfare service did the board approve of federal assistance until after the resources of local areas had proved inadequate. The platform also reaffirmed the Association's faith in the voluntary health insurance principle as the only legitimate collective method for distributing the costs of medical care. Point nine recognized the necessity of federal assistance for medical research, but urged the continuance of research activities through private foundations.[2]

Stress on Voluntary Plans

At the time the Board of Trustees adopted the ten-point platform it took other steps to make it effective. The board joined with members of

[2] *JAMA,* 130 (March 9, 1946), 641; Editorial, 130 (February 23, 1946), 494. The Board of Trustees adopted this platform called "The National Program of the American Medical Association," February 14, 1946. See Appendix pp. 411–12.

the Council on Medical Service and Public Relations and representatives of prepayment systems operated by state societies in creating the Associated Medical Care Plans and an agency called the Division of Prepayment Medical Care Plans to administer the system. Before the AMCP lay the responsibility of co-ordinating the various medical society prepayment programs, and providing for the easy transfer of subscribers among the plans. This group also drafted standards to which all plans, meeting the approval of the AMCP, must conform. Compliance with the requirements allowed participating societies to display the Association's "Seal of Acceptance" on their policies and advertising literature.[3]

The Association's growing emphasis upon the extension of medical society plans raised the lagging levels of wartime enrollment appreciably and greatly widened the national area of coverage. The year 1946 added to the 59 plans functioning on January 1, 17 more by December and raised the number of states in which they operated from 25 to 33. The number of society plans affiliated with Blue Shield increased in membership from approximately 4,436,000 in 1946 to 8,399,000 in 1948. During the same interval Blue Cross extended its population coverage from about 18,881,000 to 30,448,000.[4] When to these impressive gains the AMA added the growing enrollments of commercial plans, its faith in the voluntary principle of health insurance increased correspondingly.

[3] HD, *Proceedings* (95 Annual Session, July 1946), p. 43; Editorial, *JAMA,* 130 (February 23, 1946), 494; prepared statement of R. L. Sensenich, Senate Committee on Education and Labor, Seventy-ninth Congress, second session, *Hearings on S. 1606* (Washington, D.C.: Government Printing Office, 1946), Part 2, p. 554. The Council on Medical Service and Public Relations is hereafter referred to as Council on Medical Service, the title that came into general usage late in 1946. Participating societies had to secure a renewal of their seals of acceptance every three years. The AMCP also required that approved plans have the endorsement of medical societies in the areas where they were started and that the profession assume responsibility for providing service under the plans. It ruled out all misleading promotional activities and, while allowing either cash indemnity or service-unit benefits, called for premiums adequate to cover risks. It also required that they provide free choice of physicians and a confidential relationship between patient and physician. CMS, *News Letter,* 5; (November 23, 1948), 5; HD, *Proceedings* (95 Annual Session, July, 1946), pp. 46–47, 70–71; Editorial, *JAMA,* 130 (February 23, 1946), 494.

[4] CMS, *News Letter* (February 1, 1946), 1; HD, *Proceedings* (Supplemental Session, December, 1946), p. 18; U.S. Bureau of the Census, *Historical Statistics of the United States: Colonial Times to 1957,* p. 677. The Council's report to the House of Delegates in December, 1946, appears slightly incorrect in stating that more than 80 plans had been started. In June, 1948, the council set the total number covered by hospitalization insurance at over 40,000,000, and listed 17,000,000 covered by surgical benefits and 6,000,000 by medical benefits. In addition, it noted that 30,000,000 were protected by insurance covering income loss due to disability. HD, *Proceedings* (97 Annual Session, June, 1948), p. 63.

The AMA offered no objection when many state societies tried to protect their plans from competition with lay-administered programs. It watched societies in 22 states secure legislation by 1949 forbidding any group but physicians from establishing insurance plans for the provision of medical care.[5] While it did allow several Blue Cross plans to utilize the administrative services of commercial companies, it always insisted that the profession retain control. The AMA favored close co-operation between the Blue Shield and Blue Cross plans, but opposed the movement to create an insurance company rather than a reciprocal enrolling agency to handle national accounts. Nor would it agree to support an organizational structure co-ordinating the functions of the two plans that deprived the medical profession of control.[6]

Uniting the Profession

While the profession cleared the ground for the advance of medical society plans, the AMA moved to establish better contacts with the profession and public. Through the work of the Council on Medical Service, the Council on Industrial Health, and the Committee on Rural Medical Service, it hoped to promote better co-operation with local physicians. By January, 1948, the Council on Medical Service, often in conjunction with the other two agencies, had sponsored or participated in 16 widely scattered conferences within four years and by December had conducted several more. While the council held most of these meetings to find methods for dealing with regional professional problems, it opened up the Atlanta conference of October, 1947, to laymen as well.[7] Whatever else the AMA may have accomplished by these meetings, it left behind the impression that it shared concern for health improvement with all localities.

As the strains of the postwar era demonstrated the need for greater cohesion within organized medicine, the Association made more effec-

[5] "Restrictions on Free Enterprise in Medicine" (New York: The Committee on Research in Medical Economics, 1949), p. 4.

[6] "Statement of the Council on Medical Service of the American Medical Association Relative to Proposal for the Blue Cross-Blue Shield Association and Blue Cross-Blue Shield Health Service, Inc." [October 2, 1948]; HD, *Proceedings* (Interim Session, November–December, 1948), pp. 52–53, 73, 74.

[7] HD, *Proceedings* (Interim Session, January, 1948), p. 9; HD, *Proceedings* (Interim Session, November–December, 1948), p. 48; *JAMA,* 135 (December 6, 1947), 926.

tive use of its annual and interim sessions for promoting unified action among constituent societies. Although the AMA had sponsored winter conferences of secretaries and editors of state associations at Chicago for many years, it held its first conference of county medical officers just before the Atlantic City session of the House of Delegates opened in June, 1947. This meeting attended by 378 physicians launched the so-called "Grass Roots Conferences" that held promise of increasing the activities of local societies.[8]

Reaching the Public

Complaints about the unmet medical needs of rural areas fixed the Association's attention more fully on the medical problems of farming regions in the postwar era. Through the Committee on Rural Medical Service (established in 1945) and through annual conferences that brought together representatives of farm groups and spokesmen for other interests, it encouraged the formation of local health programs. It promoted a movement that brought about the creation of rural medical service committees within the associations of every state and started another which led to the establishment of a growing number of health councils. It also sought to bring the advantages of professionally sponsored medical plans to rural areas. By the middle of 1948, the committee had made plans for the appointment of a field representative who would travel widely and report on the status of rural health projects.[9]

Tending to balance the work of the Committee on Rural Medical Service was the attack that the Council on Industrial Health maintained against the occupational health problems of urban industrial workers. While the council had long waged a largely unknown battle against employment health hazards, the postwar era only increased its problems. The council added to its normal work the investigation of the new health and welfare programs of labor unions. It co-operated with other organizations in attempting to improve the operation of workmen's compen-

[8] HD, *Proceedings* (95 Annual Session, July, 1946), p. 6; HD, *Proceedings* (96 Annual Session, June, 1947), p. 7; HD, *Proceedings* (96 Annual Session, June, 1947), p. 34; CMS, *News Letter,* 4 (July 9, 1947), 3.

[9] HD, *Proceedings* (97 Annual Session, June, 1948), p. 30; H. B. Mulholland, *JAMA,* 138 (September 18, 1948), 217. After 1948 this committee is referred to as the Committee on Rural Health. HD, *Proceedings* (98 Annual Session, June, 1949), p. 7.

sation systems and remained in close contact with official agencies concerned with vocational rehabilitation. It also attempted with little success to attract more physicians into the less lucrative areas of industrial medical practice.[10]

In the task of unifying professional policy on major health issues and gaining public support for its position, the AMA worked tirelessly to publicize its views to professional and lay groups alike. In 1946, it employed the Raymond Rich Associates to assist in developing a more effective public relations program.[11] The same year it prepared six 15-minute radio transcriptions that sounded out the theme "The Public Comes First," and in the following centennial year chose as the theme of its twelfth annual series of broadcasts "A Century of Progress by American Medicine." It also tried with disappointing results to create speakers' bureaus in state and local societies and in 1948 established the national Medical Public Relations Conference, as the renewed threat of compulsory health insurance made the public relations policies of the AMA all the more important.[12]

As the Association widened its contacts with the profession and public, it also set up machinery adequate for the task. It strengthened the Bureau of Health Education and created an Office of Executive Assistant that functioned under the direction of the Secretary and General Manager. This office soon absorbed the Association's Bureau of Press Relations and launched a new weekly publication, the *Secretary's News Letter* that reported informally to medical leaders all over

[10] HD, *Proceedings* (97 Annual Session, June, 1948), pp. 13–14.

[11] HD, *Proceedings* (96 Annual Session, June, 1947), p. 39; HD, *Proceedings* (Supplemental Session, December, 1946), pp. 34–35. Relations between the AMA and the Raymond Rich Associates appeared to have been strained almost from the beginning. The AMA rejected many of the agency's recommendations and in a short time the two organizations severed relationship. The firm found the AMA's public relations program very unsatisfactory and complained that it had reduced its budget to a point that prevented development of an effective program. See copy of letter of Raymond Rich Associates to R. L. Sensenich, April 8, 1947, submitted with statement of J. Howard McGrath, Subcommittee of Senate Committee on Labor and Public Welfare, Eightieth Congress, first session, *Hearings on S. 545, S. 1320* (Washington: Government Printing Office, 1947), Part 3, p. 1526.

[12] CMS, *News Letter* (March 19, 1946), pp. 2–3; *JAMA,* 132 (December 28, 1946), 1095; *JAMA,* 133 (January 25, 1947), 250; HD, *Proceedings* (Supplemental Session, December, 1946), pp. 18, 46; *JAMA,* 138 (September 18, 1948), 230; American Medical Association, *Secretary's Letter No. 69* (July 26, 1948), p. 1; HD, *Proceedings* (Clinical Session, June, 1947), pp. 8–9. The *Secretary's Letter* is referred to hereafter with title, number, and date.

the nation on the AMA's activities. In addition it started publication of the bimonthly *PR Doctor,* through which it disseminated ideas for the improvement of public relations among local societies. To this list may also be added the *American Medical Association News,* through which the press relations bureau in 1948 reached some 1,300 newspapers, magazines, radio stations, and other media of public information with an account of the Association's work.[13]

The increased emphasis that the AMA placed on public relations and the growing complexity of many postwar issues required that the organization give greater attention to the political and economic aspects of medical care. On September 1, 1944, the AMA opened its Washington Office to keep in closer contact with political developments on the national scene. In September, 1946, it expanded the work of the Bureau of Medical Economics and changed its name to Bureau (later Department) of Medical Economic Research. At the same time the trustees announced the appointment of a professional economist as director, Frank G. Dickinson of the University of Illinois, who filled a vacancy left by R. G. Leland two years before. Under the guidance of the new director, the bureau undertook its most impressive work and greatly strengthened the Association's position against forces calling for far-reaching changes in the provision of medical care.[14]

Threats From the Coal Industry

While the AMA moved vigorously to win public support for its health plan that stressed the extension of hospitalization and medical care insurance and the encouragement of local initiative in providing adequate medical facilities, its program was being threatened from within and without the profession. It found the principles which it had long considered essential to the operation of successful programs often violated or endangered by organizations promoting various kinds of health insurance plans. When the crisis in the coal industry of 1946 brought on federal seizure of the mines and the establishment of the United Mine

[13] HD, *Proceedings* (96 Annual Session, June, 1947), pp. 8–9; HD, *Proceedings* (Interim Session, November–December, 1948), pp. 9–10; *Secretary's Letter, No. 73* (August 30, 1948), 2.

[14] HD, *Proceedings* (Annual Session, December, 1945), p. 51; HD, *Proceedings* (Supplemental Session, December, 1946), p. 9; Fishbein, *History of AMA,* p. 1069.

Workers of America Welfare and Retirement Fund, the Association showed great concern. This fund, raised through royalties on coal production, provided medical care and hospital benefits for miners and dependents as one of its principal services.[15]

The AMA had no objection to the plan offering adequate medical service to mining groups often living in squalor and misery, but attempted to bring the program in line with its policies. The Council on Medical Service sought through conferences with union and employer representatives to place local and professional controls over the plan through the creation of appeal boards representing the union, management, and the profession. It also hoped to separate medical service from the other aspects of the program and approved of a flexible payment schedule, easily adjustable to the requirements of adequate medical care. When the council saw its recommendations partly disregarded with the establishment of a centralized plan financed through the general welfare fund, it viewed the program with much misgiving.[16] It feared the growth of industry-wide plans that weakened local control, and which seemed to open the way for infractions on the Association's principles. Yet had the council considered the degrading welfare programs that management had long operated in many mining areas, it might have been convinced that almost any change would have been an improvement.[17]

Impact of Independent Medical Programs

Not only did the Association disapprove of the way in which the miner's program functioned, but found objectionable features in other

[15] Serbein, *Payment for Medical Care in United States,* pp. 212–15.

[16] HD, *Proceedings* (96 Annual Session, June, 1947), p. 51; HD, *Proceedings* (97 Annual Session, June, 1948), pp. 61–62; HD, *Proceedings* (Interim Session. November–December, 1948), pp. 24–25.

[17] HD, *Proceedings* (Supplemental Session, December, 1946), pp. 45, 46; United States Department of Interior, Coal Mine Administration, *A Medical Survey of the Bituminous-Coal Industry* (Washington: Government Printing Office, 1947), see especially pp. 123–27. Following the crisis of 1946 the government conducted an extensive survey of living and working conditions in the coal regions through a medical survey group headed by Joel T. Bone, Rear Admiral (M.C.), U.S. Navy. The report pointed out the devious methods by which management often awarded contracts to physicians complying with their terms, the occasional practice of medicine by men who were not physicians, the frequent elimination of choice of physicians, and the frequent failure to account for union medical funds.

medical schemes. Its attitude toward programs providing comprehensive medical service, through methods that combined group practice with group prepayment, had not changed since its unsuccessful court struggle with the Group Health Association of Washington, D.C. before World War II.[18] It feared the effects of any program that threatened the future of the individual practitioner, restricted the choice of physicians practicing in the program, promised unlimited medical care for specified periodic payments, stirred up unrest within the profession, or that solicited patients. Nor did it look with favor on the expansion of medical care plans that competed with its own society programs for membership. While the prospect of federal prosecution under the anti-trust laws possibly made the AMA reluctant to launch overt attacks on a number of thriving plans, some local societies and physician groups were less reluctant to engage in both open and guerilla warfare.

Storm centers of professional strife developed in several areas as new medical programs advanced. The Health Insurance Plan of Greater New York that recruited the services of 700 physicians and brought medical care to 200,000 residents by 1949 fought its way against the opposition of many nonparticipating doctors. On the West Coast smoldering professional friction burst into open flame over the growth of plans that competed with those sponsored by medical societies. In 1948, the federal government started unsuccessful prosecution against the Oregon State Medical Society, the Oregon Physicians' Service, and several local societies and individuals whose alleged efforts to monopolize the business of expanding prepaid medical care insurance touched on interstate commerce. The indictment cited the ends to which the profession had gone in expelling physicians from society membership and subjecting them to the pressures of complete professional ostracism for affiliating with unapproved plans. In the same year a nonprofit medical plan and three individuals filed suit under California law against a combine that included the San Diego Medical Society for allegedly engaging in similar monopolistic practices with the AMA's support.[19]

[18] See pp. 247–49 above.

[19] Robert E. Rotherberg, Karl Pickard, and Joel F. Rothenberg, *Group Medicine and Health Insurance in Action* (New York: Crown Publishers, 1949), p. 34; Dean A. Clark and Cozette Hapley, "Group Practice," The Academy of Political and Social Science, *Annals,* 273 (January, 1951), 48; *JAMA,* 138 (November 13, 1948), 825–26. In the Oregon case the Supreme Court stated in dismissing the case that the government had proved "no concerted refusal" among physicians of the state "to deal with private health associations." WO, *Bulletin No. 49—82 Congress* (May 1, 1952), p. 1.

In announcing the litigation, the *Journal* made no effort to conceal its sympathy for the defendants. Expressing no surprise that physicians held divergent views on whether some plans "were good for the patient or for his exploitation," it associated the government's prosecution with the administration's effort to secure the establishment of a national compulsory insurance system. To the *Journal* the issue hinged upon a society's right to determine its own membership, to expel members no longer acceptable, and "to oppose any group of physicians organized to practice as an agency rather than as individuals. . . ."[20] The *Journal* also found the right of hospitals to bar unacceptable persons from their staff involved in the issue.

Health Legislation Favored

The Association, in attempting to strengthen professional control over medical care programs and to revive local initiative in meeting health problems, faced groups that sought to deal with health issues largely through increased federal assistance. Contrary to a popular view, the AMA actively supported a significant portion of Truman's health program. When the war ended before Congress had passed legislation establishing the Hill-Burton hospital construction program, the AMA's support contributed to its enactment in 1946. The Association also watched over the expenditure of funds under the program and urged state societies to see that subsidies provided reached localities of greatest need. Although doctors in some areas resisted the public's effort to secure adequate hospital facilities, they followed a policy out of line with the AMA.[21]

Not only did the AMA support the hospital construction program, but it also got behind the movement to expand the nation's public

[20] *JAMA,* 138 (November 13, 1948), 824.

[21] Prepared statement of R. L. Sensenich, Subcommittee of House Committee on Interstate and Foreign Commerce, Seventy-ninth Congress, first session, *Hearings on S. 191* (Washington: Government Printing Office, 1946), pp. 102–5; Thomas Parran, "Hospitals and the Health of the People," *JAMA,* 133 (April 12, 1947), 1047. *Secretary's Letter No. 30* (September 1, 1947), 2. The Council on Medical Service noted in 1948 that the program was "reaching into areas really in need of additional facilities" and that by July 1, 347 projects had been approved. CMS, *News Letter,* 5 (July 22, 1948), 6. For an example of the opposition that some doctors raised to the program see Chester G. Starr's account of his experience in southeast Missouri while serving as Director of Rural Health of the Missouri Farm Bureau. *JAMA,* 133 (March 15, 1947), 780.

health units through federal assistance to the states. Having long recognized the inadequacy of public health operations in many areas, the Association supported identical bills to extend local health units introduced in the Eightieth Congress by Representatives James Percy Priest and James I. Dolliver. On April 9, 1948, James R. Miller of the Board of Trustees stated the Association's position before the House Committee on Interstate and Foreign Commerce. Heartily endorsing the purposes of the bill, he offered criticisms only of details. To safeguard private medical practice, he called for a clearer definition of the basic health services which the federal government would subsidize and sought to curb the power that the bills conferred upon the Surgeon General of the Public Health Service by allowing appeals to a health advisory council, which he proposed, or to the courts, or to both. Despite considerable support for the program and the committee's favorable report of June 12 on the Dolliver bill (H. R. 5644), the House took no action and the measure died with the expiration of the Eightieth Congress.[22]

More successfully did the Association support the extension of a type of federal medical research that dated from the establishment of the National Cancer Institute in 1937. While the AMA showed little interest in the passage of the National Mental Health Act of 1946, which created the Mental Health Institute, it did support the measure (S. 2215), establishing the National Heart Institute two years later.[23] Although recognizing the insufficiency of funds available for research on heart diseases, it endorsed the measure somewhat cautiously. Its president, Edward L. Bortz, sent a statement to the subcommittee on health of the Committee on Labor and Public Welfare that, while endorsing the bill, urged the establishment of greater limitations on the power that the measure granted to the Surgeon General of the Public Health Service, and stricter requirements for membership on the proposed national health council. He also warned against the further proliferation of health institutes that diffused rather than unified federal health functions. As enacted, this bill represented some concession to the Association's views.[24]

[22] Eightieth Congress, first session, *Hearings on H.R. 5644 and H.R. 5678: Local Health Services* (Washington: Government Printing Office, 1948), pp. 77–79.

[23] For the National Mental Health Act and its operation see 60 *Stat.* 421–26 (1946), and Joseph W. Mountin, Emily K. Hankla, and Georgie B. Druzina, "Ten Years of Federal Grant-in-Aid for Public Health; 1936–1946," *Public Health Bulletin No. 300* (Washington, D.C.: Government Printing Office), pp. 74–75.

[24] Eightieth Congress, second session, *Hearings on S. 720 and S. 2215* (Washington: Government Printing Office, 1948), pp. 115–16; 62 Stat. 464–70 (1948).

Health Legislation Opposed

The American Medical Association not only contributed to the passage of some of the health legislation of Truman's first administration, but just as effectively worked for the defeat of other measures. While it endorsed as a step in the right direction that part of the President's Reorganization Plan Number II of 1946, which transferred to the Federal Security Agency the Children's Bureau and most of its functions as well as the work of the Department of Commerce in the area of vital statistics, it stood against many of the proposed structural changes in the administration of federal health activities.[25] Having long advocated the establishment of a federal department with cabinet status devoted exclusively to health activities, it opposed the Fulbright-Taft bill (S. 140) and the Aiken bill (S. 712) in 1947, which called for the establishment of a federal department of health, education, and security. On May 21, R. L. Sensenich told a subcommittee of the Senate Committee on Labor and Public Welfare that federal health activities stood comparable in importance with the functions of established cabinet departments and deserved separate departmental status. Miller maintained that health functions would probably be neglected under a secretary concerned also with other matters, declaring that "it would be difficult for such a parent to be dispassionate among his children."[26] Although the Association wished to see the establishment of a health department, it preferred to have all federal nonmilitary health functions consolidated in an agency below cabinet level, rather than grouped with other functions in a cabinet department. Sensenich showed preference for that part of another bill (S. 545) which called for the creation of an agency that administered health activities exclusively. Despite widespread support for the bills proposing the creation of a department of health, education, and security, the AMA's opposition appears largely

[25] Editorial, *JAMA,* 131 (May 25, 1946), 288–89; statement of R. L. Sensenich, House Committee on Expenditures in Executive Departments, Seventy-ninth Congress, second session, *Hearings on H. Con. Res. 151, H. Con. Res. 154, H. Con. Res. 155* (Washington: Government Printing Office, 1946), p. 214.

[26] Gerhard Hirschfeld and E. M. Wood, "A Cabinet Department of Health, Education and Security," *JAMA,* 136 (January 10, 1948), 115; Eightieth Congress, first session, *Hearings on S. 545 and S. 1320* (Washington: Government Printing Office, 1947), Part 1, pp. 91–92; quotation, Senate Committee on Expenditures in Executive Departments, Eightieth Congress, first session, *Hearings on S. 140 and S. 712* (Washington: Government Printing Office, 1947), Part 2, p. 105.

responsible for their failure to reach the Senate floor in the Eightieth Congress.[27]

Dealing with measures that proposed broad structural changes in federal health administration, the AMA could not ignore others that appeared to endanger the foundations of private medical practice. It opposed a bill (S. 1318) that Senator Pepper and nine colleagues introduced in 1945, calling for first year appropriations by the federal government of $50,000,000 to finance maternal and child health services and $20,000,000 for child welfare benefits. Finding in this proposal the projection on a permanent basis of the wartime Emergency Maternal and Infant Welfare Program, the AMA raised a bitter protest. It maintained that no need for the plan existed and that it called for federal control of matters properly falling within the province of the state. It also contended that the program challenged the American pattern of life by removing parental responsibility for child welfare. Attacking what it called a "super E. M. I. C. bill" proposing payment of medical care for women and children "irrespective of financial needs," and which included in its classification of children persons under 21, the AMA urged state societies to support its efforts to defeat the measure.[28] Pressure that the Association exerted at the national capital had much to do with blocking the bill, but the AMA moved on to face similar threats in different forms.

In 1948 the Association strongly opposed a measure (S. 1290) which called for federal assistance to states in providing for medical examination of school children and children of school age. To the Association, advocates of the measure, which included the national Parent-Teachers Association, rested their case on untenable assumptions. At a Senate committee hearing on March 9, Miller charged that their bill assumed a considerable need for medical care among school-age groups that could not be met on a family basis because of economic limitations. He contended that it also assumed the incapacity of the states to finance health programs without federal assistance. Charging that the measure made no attempt to relate medical care to other health problems and complaining of its vagueness regarding administrative detail, he main-

[27] Eightieth Congress, first session, *Hearings on S. 545 and S. 1320,* Part 1, p. 92; Hirschfeld and Wood, *JAMA,* 136 (January 10, 1948), 115.

[28] Quotations, HD, *Proceedings* (Annual Session, December, 1945), pp. 57–58, 23; *JAMA,* 130 (March 9, 1946), 640. For Pepper's defense of this bill see the *Congressional Record,* Seventy-ninth Congress, first session, Vol. 91, Part 6, pp. 8052–58.

tained that it would start the nation on a new course "by projecting the schools into the field of curative medicine." Before the nation accepted any part of the program, he felt that at least it should conduct a survey of the health conditions that the measure proposed to improve. The Association found its views on the bill largely in line with prevailing congressional sentiment and watched the measure die in the committee with no regret.[29]

Just as vigorously did the AMA oppose another measure (S. 678) at a Senate hearing five weeks later, which allegedly brought extensive federal encroachments on private medical practice. This bill introduced by Senator Henry Cabot Lodge, Jr., called for federal assistance to the states for the supply of standard medicines and medical services in cases where excessive cost sometimes prevented their use. While the bill represented a revision of a similar measure that Lodge had offered a year earlier, the Association found many of its provisions unacceptable. It did not repudiate the principle of federal aid to states unable to assist residents who could not pay for medical care, but deplored the vague and elastic character of the measure. The Association found no adequate specification of medical services for which the bill proposed subsidies nor any clear identification of income groups that might receive assistance. It believed that upon the Surgeon General of the Public Health Service the bill conferred power unbalanced by specified appeal procedures. J. W. Holloway, Jr. of the AMA's Bureau of Legal Medicine and Legislation emphasized that "The wisdom of a particular provision in a law is not to be determined solely by what will be done under it but more importantly by what can be done." He also urged the committee to decide on some definite philosophy, setting forth the extent of federal responsibility in areas of curative medicine before taking action on the bill. The committee did not comply with this request, but did decline to commit itself in favor of the measure which possibly pleased the Association just as much.[30]

[29] Subcommittee of Senate Committee on Labor and Public Welfare, Eightieth Congress, second session, *Hearings on S. 1290* (Washington: Government Printing Office, 1948), pp. 42–43; WO, *Bulletin No. 19* (March 15, 1948), 1; WO, *Bulletin No. 24* (November 9, 1948), 3. Miller submitted a prepared statement.

[30] Letter from Holloway to H. Alexander Smith, April 12, 1948; Subcommittee of Senate Committee on Labor and Public Welfare, Eightieth Congress, second session, *Hearings on S. 678* (Washington: Government Printing Office, 1948), p. 36; WO, *Bulletin No. 23* (July 12, 1948), 5.

Compulsory Insurance Agitation

While postwar health issues created small political flurries that agitated the Association, they also brought on turbulence of cyclonic intensity. Over a peacetime period a little longer than the span of the nation's participation in World War II, the AMA moved desperately to brace the public against the recurring storms of compulsory health insurance that gathered, spent their force, and passed. Although a new version (S. 1050) of the Wagner-Murray-Dingell bill of June, 1943, appeared in Congress nearly two years later, not until after the war did the issue renew as much strife as it had engendered during the depression decade. Conflict did, however, quickly develop when the President delivered his health message on November 19, 1945, and when a new Wagner-Murray-Dingell bill (S. 1606) was introduced the same day.[31]

The Association's leaders quickly launched an attack on Truman's health insurance program. The *Journal* charged that after rapacious bureaucracy had made "slaves" and "clock watchers" out of the nation's doctors, it would move from the conquered ramparts of medicine upon industry, utilities, finance, and the labor force itself. Louis H. Bauer found the compulsory health insurance specter cast in a feminine mold, but the same disreputable "old sister with the addition of occasional new cosmetics applied not only to allure but to conceal age and status." Nor did the House of Delegates meeting in December neglect to condemn the measure.[32]

Not until the spring of 1946 did the Association have the opportunity to voice opposition in Congress to the newest compulsory health insurance bill. In the meantime, however, it sought to acquaint the public with the evils it found in the measure and to build up a solid resistance to the bill within the profession. Only a few days after the House of Delegates closed its December session, the Association's president, Herman Kretschmer, carried the AMA's position to the public in a radio debate with Senator Wagner, broadcast from WGN in Chicago.[33] The

[31] Wilson, *Compulsory Health Insurance,* p. 19. The House bill accompanying S. 1050 was H. R. 3293 and the bill accompanying S. 1606 was H. R. 4730.

[32] *JAMA,* 129 (December 1, 1945), 950, 953, last quotation, p. 948; HD, *Proceedings* (Annual Session, December, 1945), pp. 74–75, 86, 87.

[33] See Northwestern University, *The Reviewing Stand,* 6 (December 9, 1945), for the complete debate. John Pratt, administrator of the National Physicians Committee for the Extension of Medical Service, also upheld the AMA's position on the program, and Joseph Lohman, chairman of the Department of Sociology, American University, sided with Wagner.

Council on Medical Service sought the assistance of medical leaders throughout the nation in waging the fight, suggesting preparatory materials that they might read. The Washington Office also encouraged action by making somber forecasts about the federal armies of inspectors, auditors, and statisticians that would sweep over the nation after the adoption of a compulsory plan. It also offered aid to any medical leaders wishing to testify at hearings on the Wagner-Murray-Dingell bill, which it announced would begin on April 2.[34]

Hearings before the Senate Committee on Education and Labor highlighted the year's activity in the health insurance struggle. Already important opinion surveys had sensed growing popular support for compulsory health insurance which seemed to undermine the Association's view that its popularity lay largely with self-seeking bureaucrats. Not long before the hearings, a statewide survey which the New York State Medical Commission conducted showed 52 per cent of the people polled in favor of a compulsory system, while a survey which the *Washington Post* conducted in the District of Columbia about the same time showed 70 per cent willing to endorse Truman's compulsory insurance proposal. Even the survey conducted by the National Physicians' Committee for the Extension of Medical Service found 55 per cent in favor of a federal prepaid medical plan. The hearings brought out for public notice significant support for compulsory insurance even within the profession itself.[35]

Spokesmen representing the AMA before the Senate committee included Sensenich, Victor Johnson of the Council on Medical Education and Hospitals, and Walter V. Kennedy, President of Indiana Medical Care, Inc. As their testimony largely repeated points that the Association had long advanced, a summary will suffice. Sensenich emphasized the accomplishments of voluntary plans in meeting the cost of hospitalization and medical care and deplored the regimentation that a compulsory system would establish. He placed primary responsibility for the improvement of health conditions at the local level and maintained that most localities needed no federal assistance in solving their own health problems. Johnson contended that the nation had made rapid strides in building up its health resources for medical service and

[34] CMS, *News Letter* (December 18, 1945), pp. 4–5; WO, *Special Bulletin* (January 14, 1946), p. 1; WO, *Special Bulletin* (March 8, 1946), p. 1.

[35] John D. Dingell, Seventy-ninth Congress, first session, *Hearings on S. 1606* (Washington: Government Printing Office, 1946), Part I, pp. 66–70; *Social Security Bulletin,* 9 (May, 1946), 14.

indicated that no great shortage of hospitals existed. In opposing the Wagner-Murray-Dingell bill, Kennedy drew upon his own experience with European compulsory systems to warn that the adoption of a national plan would greatly lower the high quality of medical care.[36]

Professional strength behind the Association's spokesmen at the committee hearings diminished the political stature of representatives of small medical groups that endorsed the bill. Physicians speaking in support of the measure for the National Medical Association (Negro), the Physicians' Forum, and the Committee of Physicians for the Improvement of Medical Care added length to the hearings, but no great strength to their cause. Furthermore, lay groups, offering testimony against the bill, outweighed in voting power organizations speaking in favor of compulsory health insurance. The hearings indicated that national sentiment had not tilted decidedly in favor of a compulsory program.[37]

While the Association looked upon the revival of interest in compulsory health insurance as probably a temporary manifestation of postwar confusion, it dared not proceed on that assumption. The AMA's president, Roger I. Lee, told the San Francisco session of the House of Delegates in July, 1946, that the Wagner-Murray-Dingell bill appeared to have no chance of passing the Seventy-ninth Congress, but cautioned members against relapsing into a state of overconfidence and indifference. President-elect Harrison Shoulders warned the session that "political crackpots, the yearners for political power, the enemies of freedom and the importers of alien philosophies of government" would work strenuously during the unsettled era to advance their cause. To the Association fell the task of offsetting the exertions of compulsory health insurance advocates with greater activity of its own.[38]

Attack on British System

The Association attempted to meet the threat of compulsory health insurance in the United States by discrediting the international movement as well. Although compulsory systems operated in many countries after the war, the AMA concentrated most of its attack on the British scheme.

[36] Seventy-ninth Congress, second session, *Hearings on S. 1606,* Part 2, prepared statement by Sensenich, pp. 553–59, and 461–63; Johnson's statement, pp. 698–701; Kennedy's statement and exhibits, pp. 703–34.

[37] *Ibid.,* pp. 787–94, 735–68, 981–1016.

[38] HD, *Proceedings* (95 Annual Session, July, 1946), p. 3, quotation, p. 4.

Even before the passage of the national health act of 1946, which established the National Health Service two years later, the AMA denounced the proposed legislation. In January, 1946, the *Journal* published an article in which an American doctor, Paul K. Maloney, bitterly attacked the limited compulsory program that had long been in operation. The British Medical Association found the report so full of error that its Secretary Charles Hill replied:

> The article contains so many inaccuracies and misleading statements and gives such a false impression of National Health Insurance in Great Britain that I cannot let it pass without protest. It is quite obvious that Captain Maloney has entirely misunderstood the British scheme: both his facts and his inferences are wrong. In almost every line there is some statement that could be challenged. . . .[39]

Two weeks after the British Medical Association responded, the *Journal* employed familiar language in charging that the nation, after having gallantly resisted continental tyranny, now planned "to enslave its medical profession and to make every one of its physicians a clock-watching civil servant."[40]

The *Journal* made still other attempts to discredit the British program that both the Conservative and Labor parties supported. It continued to publish the London Letter, in which its English correspondent (an obscure physician without authority to represent the profession) denounced the compulsory health insurance movement.[41] The British Medical Association, however, did not allow all of the AMA's critical reports to go unchallenged. When the *Journal* in August published a condensed record of Senate hearings on the current compulsory insurance bill that included comments of a physician, Edward H. Ochsner, on the alleged mass treatment of patients under the British system, Secretary Hill again replied:

> This is not the first time I have had occasion to protest against the misleading and inaccurate accounts given, evidently at second hand, by certain American doctors who are endeavoring to avert the introduction of any health insurance scheme into their country by denouncing the British

[39] *JAMA,* 130 (March 16, 1946), 724; see *JAMA,* 130 (January 26, 1946), 226–27 for Maloney's article. The *Journal* added with the publication of Hill's letter that "as was subsequently pointed out, this article was actually written by Major Clifford L. Graves to Captain Maloney."

[40] Editorial, *JAMA,* 130 (March 30, 1946), 858.

[41] Although the AMA had long known that its London correspondent did not speak for the British Medical Association, it retained him as correspondent until his death in 1949. *JAMA,* 141 (November 5, 1949), 667. See pp. 198–99 above.

scheme. In the present instance Dr. Ochsner appears to have accepted as fact a story that must surely have passed round as a joke, and it is most deplorable that he should have repeated it in public as responsible evidence to a Senate Committee. It is gross libel.[42]

Protests, however, did not deter the *Journal* which continued to strike at the British system.[43]

Alternative Legislation

The AMA attempted to counter the compulsory insurance movement not only by vigorous verbal attacks, but also by at least partial endorsement of proposed programs that held promise of weakening agitation for a national compulsory insurance system. It looked with considerable favor on the Taft-Smith-Ball bill (S. 2143), introduced by Senator Taft on May 3, 1946. This measure, which the sponsors drafted as an alternative to the Wagner-Murray-Dingell bill, provided among other things for annual appropriations of $200,000,000 for five years to states in need of assistance for providing low-income groups with adequate hospital, surgical, and medical service. Since the bill unified and expanded federal health functions while retaining a large measure of local control over the administration of medical care, stimulated voluntary insurance plans, and repudiated altogether the compulsory principle, the AMA found in the measure much to commend. On May 25, the *Journal* remarked that since the bill attempted to meet the nation's health requirements without "nationalizing the medical profession" or "revolutionizing medical care," the measure was preferable to the Wagner-Murray-Dingell bill.[44]

[42] *JAMA,* 132 (November 9, 1946), 600. The case of mass treatment supposedly involved a panel physician just before World War II, who upon seeing a large number of patients in his office asked all with headaches to stand. When six stood up he gave six identical prescriptions. When Hill challenged this account, Ochsner maintained that the episode had been related by a then prominent Chicago doctor but would not reveal his name. See *JAMA,* 13 (August 3, 1946), 1150.

[43] These attacks intensified in 1948 when the British system began operation. While the British Medical Association did not oppose the national medical program, it did object to some administrative aspects of the program. This controversy is treated in Harry Eckstein, *Pressure Group Politics: The Case of the British Medical Association* (Stanford, Calif.: Stanford University Press, 1960), pp. 92–112.

[44] *JAMA,* 131 (May 25, 1946), 338–41; HD, *Proceedings* (95 Annual Session, July, 1946), p. 22; quotation, Editorial, *JAMA,* 131 (May 25, 1946), 290.

The House of Delegates meeting in San Francisco two months later did not endorse the measure, nor did the Chicago session which met in December. Instead the July session authorized proper officials of the AMA to establish contact with sponsors of the bill for discussion of its provisions. The Council on Medical Service also called upon state societies for suggestions about the measure, and before the year ended the Board of Trustees had conferred with sponsors of the bill.[45] In the meantime, however, political developments appeared to have reduced the compulsory health insurance threat at least temporarily. The Republican party, increasingly antagonistic to the President's program, captured both houses of Congress for the first time in 16 years.[46]

Despite a political shift that appeared to identify public sentiment more definitely with the Association's views on the role of the government in health affairs, the AMA entered its centennial year (1947) under threatening political skies. Even before the new year began, a Nebraska congressman and physician, Arthur L. Miller, told the AMA's conference of secretaries and editors of medical societies that upon the Eightieth Congress fell the task of "deflating the overstuffed Frankenstein, bureaucratic monstrosity of government" that had undermined professional freedom for so many years. Yet, while forces attempting to reverse, halt, or moderate the administration's program planned their strategy, the chief executive moved with equal determination to carry it through. The *Journal* showed no surprise when the President's first message to the new Congress stressed the urgency of establishing a national health insurance system.[47]

Soon after the Eightieth Congress opened, however, opponents of the administration's health program again challenged the President's leadership on health issues. On February 10, Senator Taft introduced S. 545 (Taft-Smith-Ball-Donnell bill), a revision of S. 2143, more than three months before Senator Murray introduced the so-called "1947 Wagner-Murray-Dingell Bill" (S. 1320), which embodied the administration's

[45] HD, *Proceedings* (95 Annual Session, July, 1946), p. 71; HD, *Proceedings* (Supplemental Session, December, 1946), p. 19; HD, *Proceedings* (Supplemental Session, December, 1946), p. 12. The AMA also consulted the American Hospital Association and the American Dental Association on the bill. HD, *Proceedings* (96 Annual Session, June, 1947), p. 27.

[46] The Republicans gained 12 seats in the Senate and 54 in the House raising their strength in the upper house to 51 and in the lower to 246. William Frank Zornow, *America at Mid-Century,* paperback ([Cleveland], Howard Allen, Inc., Publishers, 1959), p. 34.

[47] Quotation, *JAMA,* 133 (February 22, 1947), 555; Editorial, *JAMA,* 133 (January 18, 1947), 180.

program. Alterations made in the Taft-Smith-Ball bill indicate that the Association, whose spokesmen had at least twice consulted with sponsors of the measure, figured prominently in drafting S. 545.[48]

Although the revised measure fell short of the AMA's objectives in failing to give to the national health agency departmental status, it restricted, more than the earlier bill, the authority of the United States Public Health Service, whose growing powers the Association feared. It took from the health service responsibility for the administration of the Hospital Survey and Construction Act and lodged it elsewhere within the agency. The new measure swept away the requirements of administrative, teaching, or research experience for a doctor heading the agency and demanded no more than appointment of an outstanding licensed physician. Of the director of the proposed office of medical and hospital care services, it required a licensed physician with five years or more of practice. On the proposed eight-member national medical care council, the measure stipulated that four must be physicians. Unlike the original bill, S. 545 called for an appropriation of $3,000,000 for a survey of health needs before the authorized expenditure of federal funds began, which appeared in line with the Association's policies.[49]

Despite the influential part the Association apparently had in the revision of the original measure, its favorable attitude toward the Taft-Smith-Ball-Donnell bill fell short of actual support. In recoiling before the compulsory health insurance threat, the AMA was driven toward rather than attracted by a measure that held promise of providing deliverance. At committee hearings in May, Sensenich showed little enthusiasm for the measure, but stated that it was preferable to the latest version of the Wagner-Murray-Dingell bill. The following month the centennial session of the House of Delegates declared that the measure "approximates the legislative background" needed in developing the type of health program the Association recommended.[50]

[48] HD, *Proceedings* (Supplemental Session, December, 1946), p. 12; WO, *Bulletin No. 1* (January 10, 1947), 1. The "1947 Wagner-Murray-Dingell Bill" had, besides the original sponsors, backing from Dennis Chavez (N.M.), Glenn Taylor (Ida.), and J. Howard McGrath (R.I.). Wilson, *Compulsory Health Insurance,* p. 99.

[49] *JAMA,* 133 (March 22, 1947), 868–69; Subcommittee of Senate Committee on Labor and Public Welfare, Eightieth Congress, first session, *Hearings on S. 545 and S. 1320* (Washington, Government Printing Office, 1947), Part 1, pp. 1–14.

[50] *Ibid.,* p. 89; quotation, HD, *Proceedings* (96 Annual Session, June, 1947), p. 101. In January, 1948, the Board of Trustees said that the AMA "has not endorsed this bill in toto but has approved it in principle." HD, *Proceedings* (Interim Session, January, 1948), p. 24.

The indifference of the Eightieth Congress to social legislation made it unnecessary for the AMA to choose between the bills. Only the grave threat of the passage of compulsory health insurance legislation could have brought the AMA behind the Taft-Smith-Ball-Donnell bill and this threat did not exist. In its final form the bill contained provisions that the AMA had long considered dangerous. Section 2, which referred to the government's policy of providing aid to the states for medical and hospital services without regard to "economic status," flatly contradicted the Association's views. The provision that called for dental care for school children and medical examinations set up precedents that the Association feared. Even in legislation offered as an alternative to compulsory health insurance dangers to private medical practice appeared.[51]

The AMA found that the last half of 1947 constituted an interlude of little political turbulence on health issues. It had reason to rejoice that neither the revised Wagner-Murray-Dingell bill or the Taft-Smith-Ball-Donnell bill had reached the floor of the Senate when Congress recessed on July 27. When it convened in special session on November 17, the Association found that matters of principal concern bore only indirectly on health problems. As the President pressed upon a stubborn Congress a ten-point anti-inflationary program, the conflict over the principles embodied in the AMA's ten-point health program temporarily subsided.[52]

The quietness that reigned on the battlegrounds of compulsory health insurance during much of 1947 lasted into the next year but gradually gave way to growing tension. In the *Journal's* first issue of 1948 a Kansas City physician warned against the "serpent of regimentation" and added that because of the profession's long indifference to many economic problems doctors were "perilously close to reaping the just reward of their social sinfulness and neglect."[53] The House of Delegates seemed to prefer precarious tranquility to political disturbance, however, and rejected resolutions at the Cleveland session on January 6 that reaffirmed the Association's position of providing federal subsidies to the states only on the basis of demonstrable need, stating that "these resolutions at this time would be politically inexpedient and might alienate

[51] Eightieth Congress, first session, *Hearings on S. 545 and S. 1320,* pp. 1, 6.

[52] *New York Times,* November 18, 1957, pp. 1, 3.

[53] F. L. Feierabend, "Philosophy of a Medical Service Plan," *JAMA,* 136 (January 3, 1948), 57, 58.

valuable congressional support of our organization."[54] A day later President Truman's message stirred the calm as he again urged the establishment of a national comprehensive insurance system. The *Journal* soon replied, finding in the message "not the slightest evidence that he has departed from his previous insistence on compulsory sickness insurance federally dominated, as an answer to the sickness problem."[55]

National Health Conference

The President's determination to press the compulsory health insurance issue left the Association disturbed over his decision to convene a national health conference in May. Nor were its fears allayed, when the administration appointed to the executive committee of 38 members responsible for planning the conference, three prominent leaders of the AMA, and another as chairman of one of the assembly's 14 sections. Although the assembly had as its purpose the consideration of broad national health goals, officials of the AMA, recalling the health conference of 1938, feared that the administration would find in the assembly a means for attacking the Association and propagandizing for a comprehensive insurance system.[56]

The National Health Assembly did not produce the stormy sessions that the AMA had expected. While it uncovered much evidence of widespread deficiencies in medical facilities and service, it made no recommendations that offended the Association. Agreeably surprised by the character of the conference, the *Journal* reported that "bizarre and weird recommendations" for radical changes in the system of medical care "fell by the wayside" and the Council on Medical Service believed that "American medicine" emerged from the conference "with added friends, prestige, influence and stature."[57] However, George F. Lull,

[54] HD, *Proceedings* (Interim Session, January, 1948), p. 14. The House of Delegates reaffirmed the principle of the resolution of the Chicago session nearly six months later. Resolution by J. Wallace Hurff, HD, *Proceedings* (97 Annual Session, June, 1948), pp. 72, 95, 96.

[55] Editorial, *JAMA,* 136 (January 17, 1948), 178.

[56] National Health Assembly, *America's Health: A Report to the Nation* (New York: Harper & Brothers, Publishers, 1949), pp. x, xi, xii; *Secretary's Letter No. 72* (August 23, 1948), 2; Editorial, *JAMA,* 136 (March 6, 1948), 694; *Secretary's Letter No. 61* (May 11, 1948), 1.

[57] Editorial, *JAMA,* 137 (May 8, 1948), 146; HD, *Proceedings* (97 Annual Session, June, 1948), p. 65.

secretary of the Association, viewed the work of the conference less favorably. Observing that it had "caused about as much noise, nationally, as a ray of moonlight falling on a cup of custard," he implied that the principal contribution of the $45,000 "show" was conversation.[58]

Democratic Victory

While the National Health Assembly brought on no scenes of turbulence between spokesmen for the AMA and the federal government, it stood at the forefront of another stormy era. Less than three months after the session ended, the Association saw the Philadelphia national Democratic convention nominate Truman for a second term and watched as he quickly revived interest in the compulsory health insurance issue. As the President stormed the nation, frequently assailing the AMA, the Association also remained alert to developments at the nation's capital. There, in September, the Federal Security Administrator, Oscar R. Ewing, released his report to the President, which embodied in a large measure the recommendations of the National Health Assembly. He added to the recommendations, however, a proposal for a national system of health insurance which had been so lightly treated at the health conference in May.[59]

As the leader of the shattered Democratic party pressed the national health insurance issue, the Association held somewhat reluctantly to its traditional policy of avoiding political alignment. With the publication of Ewing's report, however, the *Journal* immediately noted that the Republican nominee, Thomas E. Dewey, had expressed unalterable opposition to a federal compulsory system.[60] Nor did it fail to remind the profession of the decisive effect congressional elections might have on the outcome of the health insurance struggle.

Although the *Journal* skirted the tense area of national politics with some restraint, the AMA drew support from an aggressive and effective ally. Established during the turbulent health insurance battle of the depression decade, the National Physicians' Committee for the Extension of Medical Service brought to the crisis of 1948 years of experience in political mechanics and the art of moving the masses. With

[58] *Secretary's Letter No. 61* (May 11, 1948), 1.

[59] *The Nation's Health: A Ten Year Program* (1948), pp. iii, 75–114. *New York Times,* September 3, 1948, pp. 1, 22.

[60] *JAMA,* 138 (September 25, 1948), 298.

methods that often did not reach higher ethical levels, the committee tried to reach the public. In March it launched a national cartoon contest that promised attractive awards for cartoonists whose published pictorial attack on compulsory health insurance seemed most effective. Encouraging a newspaper attack on the compulsory insurance forces, it offered $1,000 for the best cartoon, and $500 for the second, in a scale that descended to $100 each for the nine winners of the sixth award. To guide the contestants, it furnished a number of grotesque examples particularly palatable to coarser tastes.[61] As the election neared, its attack on the administration's program gathered momentum.

Resisting the embattled doctors' assault, however, was the administration's barrage that well obscured vulnerable stretches in its own defenses. As a confused electorate reached the polls after the many months of agitation, it registered a vote that soon touched off a more furious battle. A short suspension in hostilities seemed in order, however, until the AMA could throw off the traumatic effect of Truman's unexpected victory.

[61] One of the cartoons that the committee displayed pictured an operating room and a British physician with a saw reminding the patient that Bevan (Minister of Health) rhymed with heaven. In H. B. Everette collection, Library of the University of Tennessee College of Medicine, Memphis.

Chapter 17 THE AMA AT ARMAGEDDON

THE RENEWAL OF THE COMPULSORY HEALTH INSURANCE threat in November, 1948, brought the AMA to the brink of its greatest crisis. It found little comfort in knowing that all seven physicians in Congress reclaimed their seats in the general election, when the voters also re-elected an administration committed to the establishment of a national health insurance system and strengthened its position in both legislative bodies with substantial Democratic majorities.[1] After the Association recovered from the stunning effect of Truman's victory, it hastily mobilized its strength for a long, exhausting struggle.

Even before the Eighty-first Congress convened in January, 1949, the AMA had already developed much of its battle strategy. Against the advocates of a federal program of medical care, it planned a swift nationwide offensive. The Board of Trustees hurriedly formed a Co-ordinating Committee for the Protection of the People's Health, which had engaged the services of a prominent public relations agency to conduct its advertising campaign before the end of the year. The committee also strengthened the AMA's capacity to work more effectively on the local level by organizing a group of 53 members, representing all state and territorial societies, to assist in carrying out the Association's policies. The House of Delegates convening in December gave the trustees its full support and concurred in their resolve to exhaust, if necessary, the organization's total financial resources to prevent "the enslavement of the medical profession." The delegates further showed their determination in levying a special membership assessment of $25.00 to be used in resisting the movement, while the *Journal,* greatly disturbed by the election results, launched a furious attack on the administration.[2]

[1] *JAMA,* 138 (November 20, 1948), 893. Four of the physicians returned to the Eightieth Congress were Republicans and three were Democrats.

[2] Editorial, *JAMA,* 138 (December 25, 1948), 1230; quotation, HD, *Proceedings* (Interim Session, November–December, 1948), pp. 24, 72–73; *JAMA,* 138 (December 25, 1948), 1255.

Case for the AMA

Although the American Medical Association combated the compulsory health insurance forces on many fronts, its Bureau of Medical Economic Research waged the most impressive but least spectacular fight. Under the direction of Frank G. Dickinson, it conducted a number of penetrating studies that proved of great assistance to the AMA. Hammering hard and mercilessly against arguments advanced in support of a federally administered compulsory system, the bureau also showed considerable skill in defending private practice.

The report that Ewing submitted to the President in September, 1948, on the health goals of the nation brought an immediate attack from the bureau. This report not only contended that the nation faced a current shortage of physicians and an imbalance in their distribution, but that the shortage would become extremely critical unless the public took appropriate action to increase physician supply. Accepting as an adequate physician-population ratio 150 to 100,000, which prevailed as an average in the 12 states with the highest ratios in 1940, Ewing set this goal as the desirable objective for the entire nation to reach by 1960. The employment of procedures for predicting future physician supply that appeared as no more than guesswork shocked the director of the bureau who, as a former university professor of economics, remarked that "In all my 25 years of teaching I have never had a sophomore student make a poorer case than did Mr. Ewing on the question of the shortage of physicians."[3]

In the controversy that developed over physician shortage and distribution, Dickinson engaged in more than a battle of words. Contending that no serious shortage or imbalance of physicians existed, and predicting a more probable surplus than deficit by 1960, he offered evidence that seemed to satisfy the AMA. As early as December, 1946, he had recognized the need for a national survey that delineated "medical service areas" and had often denied the validity of equating the adequacy of medical care with the physician-population ratio of an area whose political

[3] *The Nation's Health: A Ten Year Program,* pp. 37–42; quotation, Frank G. Dickinson to James C. Sargent (October 28, 1948), BMER, No. M–10, p. 2. Dickinson stated that "If any statistician wishes to project an estimated demand, or shortage, he is compelled to test his hypothesis on his base year before he can claim validity for his estimate for the future. The authors of the Report have not even attempted that task." "An Analysis of the Ewing Report," *Bulletin 69* (Chicago: American Medical Association, 1949), 9.

boundaries bore little relationship to established trade patterns. The bureau itself decided to conduct this elaborate and tedious survey and had brought it far toward completion by the end of Truman's second term. The bureau's findings confirmed the director's view that physician distribution suffered no serious imbalance and supported his contention in 1954 that "The distribution of physicians in the United States in April, 1950, in relation to the persons whom they served, was excellent but not perfect."[4]

Dickinson's defense of the idea of a probable approaching physician surplus rested principally upon the annual percentage of physician increase that kept ahead of population growth, and upon the further advancement in scientific technology that held promise of improving medical care. A bureau study pointed out that the physician-population ratio rose from 131 to 100,000 in 1938 to 135 to 100,000 eleven years later, but contended that medical care increased far beyond this rising statistical ratio. According to the bureau, greater technological efficiency raised the total medical care that 1,000 physicians could deliver during these years by at least one-third.[5] Better roads and improved means of transportation had increased the physicians' output of medical service. When the United States Public Health Service published in 1949 an estimate of a probable physician shortage ranging between 17,000 and 47,000 by 1960, the director called the prediction an unsupported assumption.[6]

[4] Frank G. Dickinson, "Supply of Physicians Services," BMER, *Bulletin 81* (1951), 8; *JAMA,* 133 (February 22, 1947), 548; quotation, Frank G. Dickinson, "How Bad Is the Distribution of Physicians?" BMER, *Bulletin 94 B* (Chicago: American Medical Association, 1954), 11. For the bureau's study of physician distribution see Frank G. Dickinson, *Distribution of Physicians by Medical Service Areas* (Chicago: American Medical Association, 1954). While *Bulletin 81,* which gives Dickinson's view on a probable physician surplus by 1960, was published as not "necessarily" representing the views of the AMA, his position was not challenged by the Association and appeared in line with its policies.

[5] Frank G. Dickinson and Charles E. Bradley in co-operation with Frank V. Cargill, "Comparison of State Physician-Population Ratios for 1938 and 1949," BMER, *Bulletin 78* (Chicago: American Medical Association, 1950), pp. 8, 5. These writers pointed out serious deficiencies in the use of a physician-population ratio. "The number of physicians could serve as a measure of supply of medical care only if all physicians were alike in respect to age, skill, case load, use of auxiliary medical personnel, equipment available for diagnosis and treatment, density of population in the area that the physicians serve, etc. On the population side of the ratio, each group of 100,000 persons should be exactly alike in medical care requirements in order to develop comparable physician-population ratios." *Ibid.,* pp. 3–4.

[6] Dickinson, BMER, *Bulletin 81* (1951), pp. 6–8. Thomas Parran, Surgeon General of the United States Public Health Service, told a medical group in 1947

Dickinson also added complexity to the physician shortage controversy by raising questions about the meaning and determination of adequacy when applied to medical care. Considering adequate medical service as an unattainable goal, he remarked that "Medical care can never be adequate to the family of a dying person." From the bureau's research he also concluded that standards often employed for determining adequate care reflected only feebly the health status of an area. He found that "variations in state physician-population ratios" accounted for not more than "26 per cent of the variations in the measure of health" among the states, when tested by standards that took into account infant and maternal mortality and life expectancy at birth.[7] The bureau's findings did not detract from the need for adequate medical resources, but served as a warning against overemphasis on the connection between the adequacy of medical reserves and the health status of an area.

To no part of Ewing's report did Dickinson raise stronger objections than to that which attributed an alleged needless loss of 325,000 lives annually to deficiencies in the nation's health maintenance structure. Ewing's proposal to prevent this wastage of human life through a national health program Dickinson attacked as "fantastic" and "irrelevant." Denying the validity of such a standard as a national health goal, Dickinson maintained that "The true measure of medical progress in America is not how many people die, but how long they live before they die." He also observed that medical progress saved the American people from some diseases only to have them die of others and wondered with what diseases the Social Security Administrator would have them die.[8]

The bureau countered the administration's attack on more vulnerable health front defenses with mounting emphasis on the nation's spectacular health improvement strides. Closely relating evidence of medical progress with longevity, the bureau cited the nation's infant mortality rate, which dropped from 58.1 per 1,000 live births in 1933 to 29.1 seventeen

---

that the nation would have a deficit "of at least 30,000 physicians by 1960" unless present training programs were changed. ACMEL, 1947, *Papers & Discussions,* p. 21.

[7] Frank G. Dickinson, "The Medical Care Team," The American Academy of Political and Social Science, *Annals,* 273 (January, 1951), 26. For further treatment of the significance of variations in physician-population ratios see Dickinson, Bradley, and Cargill, BMER, *Bulletin 78* (1950), p. 4.

[8] BMER, "An Analysis of the Ewing Report," *Bulletin 69* (Chicago: American Medical Association, 1949), pp. 6, 3.

years later, as among the world's lowest. Dickinson showed that whereas only about 750 of every 1,000 babies reached their twenty-first birthday in 1900, about 950 reached that age a half century later. He also noted that the highest maternal mortality rate among the states in 1949 stood only a little over half the lowest state rate 15 years earlier.[9] With an associate in the bureau he offered statistical proof of the nation's virtual triumph over many diseases, observing that pneumonia, which accounted for 12.9 per cent of total deaths in 1900, claimed a toll of only 3.9 per cent in 1948, and that the figures stood at 10.4 and 3.0 per cent respectively for tuberculosis. Dickinson further showed that while the median age at death was 30 in 1900, it had climbed to 66 fifty years later, and that while 25 per cent of the population in 1900 lived to be at least 62 years of age, by 1948 the same percentage reached the age of 76.[10]

The importance that the bureau attached to studies involving the cost of medical care reflected the Association's increasing sensitivity about a problem that had aroused great public concern. One of Dickinson's earliest studies as director of the bureau showed that whereas medical care took 4.4 per cent of total consumer expenditures in 1932, it took only 3.9 per cent fourteen years later.[11] Just before the Democratic party brought the compulsory health insurance issue into the campaign of 1948, he published material that compared the rising costs of medical care with mounting living costs. Using a scale on which average yearly living costs for 1935–1939 stood at 100, he reported that the consumer price index rose to 159.2 in 1947, but that the cost of general practitioners' services reached only 130.3 and that of surgeons and specialists only 129.4. A few months later he reported that recent expenditures for physicians' services showed a smaller percentage rise than other health and medical costs. Although citing a rise in expenditures for physicians' services of 24.2 per cent between 1944 and 1947, he showed that expenditures for drugs and sundries rose 26.4 per cent; dentists' services,

[9] Frank G. Dickinson and Everett L. Welker, "Mortality Trends in the United States, 1900–1949, and an Editorial and Summary from the Journal of the AMA," BMER, *Bulletin 92* (Chicago: American Medical Association, 1952), 26–27; BMER, "An Analysis of the Ewing Report," p. 6; Frank G. Dickinson, "Significance of Half-Century Decline in Population Mortality," BMER, *Miscellaneous Publication M–50,* p. 2.

[10] Dickinson and Welker, BMER, *Bulletin 92* (1952), p. 12; Dickinson, BMER, *Miscellaneous Publication* M–50, p. 3.

[11] Frank G. Dickinson, "Is Medical Care Expensive?" *Bulletin No. 60* (American Medical Association, 1947), p. 8.

28.1 per cent; and expenditures for hospitalization, 66.8 per cent.[12] In 1951 Dickinson showed that although the price of all goods and services had risen 72 per cent by 1950 over the 1935–1939 average, general practitioners' fees rose only 40 per cent and fees of physicians and surgeons only 41 per cent. During the campaign of 1952 he maintained that the same amount of medical care that a whole week's wages purchased in the period from 1935–1939 could be purchased with 54 per cent of a week's wages in 1951.[13]

The bureau also defended the profession more directly against charges of setting exorbitant fees and receiving excessive incomes. It cooperated with the United States Department of Commerce in an extensive mid-century survey of physicians' earnings that brought out information which it might have found more useful in earlier stages of the health insurance fight. From questionnaires returned by 30,000 doctors, it reported that the average (mean) net income of physicians from medical practice, which reached $11,058 in 1949, had shown about the same rate of increase as the national per capita income. In 1952, it published a report from the Department of Commerce showing that while physicians' net average incomes had risen 136 per cent between 1929 and 1951, the average increase in earnings of the general population had risen 141 per cent.[14] Dickinson also related physicians' incomes to their long and costly training. Maintaining that nine years of training for medical practice normally cost physicians $35,000 (including interest on investment), he showed that it required annual earnings of $2,200 just to amortize training costs. On the difficulty of completing the medical program he contended that, while doctorates in some scientific fields

[12] BMER, "Comparative Increases in the Costs of Medical Care and in the Costs of Living," *Bulletin No. 62* (Chicago: American Medical Association, 1948), p. 2; BMER, "The Cost and Quantity of Medical Care in the United States," *Bulletin 66* (Chicago: American Medical Association, 1948), p. 6. In 1949 Dickinson noted that the latest Department of Commerce estimates gave a much higher percentage increase for these items over a period extending to 1942 rather than 1944. In the years 1942 to 1948 it set percentage expenditure increase for physicians' services at 99.7 per cent; hospitalization, 141.0; drugs and sundries, 62.1; and dentists' services, 58.5. "1949 Supplement to *Bulletin 66*—The Cost and Quantity of Medical Care in the United States," BMER, *Bulletin 72* (Chicago: American Medical Association, 1949), pp. 6–8.

[13] BMER, "Medical Care Expenditures, Prices and Quantity, 1930–1950," *Bulletin 87* (Chicago: American Medical Association, 1951), p. 12; WO, *Capitol Clinic,* 3 (October 14, 1952), 1.

[14] Frank G. Dickinson and Charles E. Bradley, "Survey of Physicians' Incomes," BMER, *Bulletin 84* (Chicago: American Medical Association, 1951), pp. 1, 6; BMER, *M–68,* p. 6.

could be earned in institutions rated from A to D, all medical students had to complete work from class A schools.[15]

Nor did the director withhold his views upon the government's rightful role in the nation's life and upon the character of prevailing social welfare programs. Against those who felt that the services of the medical as well as the teaching profession should be placed under governmental administration, Dickinson argued that the services rendered by the two professions vastly differed. He contended that teachers offered largely standardized products to students who stood on approximately the same level, but that doctors' work took greater account of individual differences and offered services not adapted to governmental regulation. Maintaining that the retirement program of the social security system disregarded many sound economic financing principles, he insisted that " 'cradle to the grave' is a scheme whereby those close to the grave fasten themselves on the pay-checks of those closer to the cradle, and ride piggy-back to the grave."[16]

Throughout the compulsory insurance controversy the bureau's publications served to calm unrest created over health conditions by those whom the Association viewed as prophets of despair. To Dickinson, whatever crisis existed resulted from the nation's progress in conquering disease rather than from its failure to respond to challenging health issues. He insisted that the so-called health crisis was no more than "the social crisis that health progress has created—by allowing so many of us to survive the diseases of childhood, youth, and middle age." He viewed the real health crisis as brought on by scientific advance, the "need for pensions and employment for the aged."[17] Dickinson found many of the nation's medical problems arising from a distorted sense of values and contended in 1949 that:

[15] "Income Tax Discrimination against the Professions," BMER, *Bulletin 74* (American Medical Association, 1949), p. 5; ACMEL, 1953, *Proceedings,* p. 42. Dickinson's reference to "Class A" medical schools was made February 13, 1951.

[16] BMER, Frank G. Dickinson to "Dear Professor ________________," mimeographed letter (June 1, 1949), *Miscellaneous Publication Number M–25;* [BMER], "Social Morality and 'Cradle-to-the-Grave Philosophy' " *Miscellaneous Publication M–30;* [BMER], "Economic Aspects of the Aging of Our Population," [*Miscellaneous Publication M–53*] (Chicago: American Medical Association), p. 76, reprinted from Institute of Gerontology Series, University of Florida Press, *Problems of America's Aging Population,* I, 75–86.

[17] Bureau of Medical Economic Research and Council on Medical Service, "What We Get for What We Spend for Medical Care," in "Five Papers for Financing a Health Program for America," *M. 74,* p. 31; Dickinson, American Academy of Political and Social Science, *Annals,* 273 (January, 1951), 26.

> The decision of the consumers has been to spend 96 per cent of their budgets for items other than medical care. They have decided they can afford one and one half times as much for alcoholic beverages and another one and one half times as much for recreation as for medical care. They have decided they can afford twice as much for tobacco as for physicians' services. They have decided they can afford about as much for jewelry and the repair of watches and clocks as for physicians.[18]

Whitaker and Baxter Crusade

While upon the Bureau of Medical Economic Research fell much of the burden of setting forth the Association's case, the task of reaching the nation with the AMA's political message fell largely on an organization of skilled publicity experts. Only a few days after Truman pressed the health insurance issue in his congressional message of January 5, 1949, and after the administration's spokesmen had introduced a new health insurance measure in the Senate, the Whitaker and Baxter public relations counselors of California laid plans for opening an office in Chicago. To the same agency whose publicity campaign figured so prominently in the election of the future champion of compulsory health, Earl Warren, as Governor of California in 1942, and whose work helped defeat his insurance program, now fell the larger task of discrediting the movement on the national level. Responsible to a profession that cried desperately for action, the Whitaker and Baxter staff moved with a speed that soon brought praise from even the most alarmed and impatient physicians.[19] By April 1, it had replaced the National Physicians' Committee for the Extension of Medical Service, which discontinued its operations altogether. It found itself well prepared for action three weeks later when the President sent his special message to Congress, calling again for the enactment of a compulsory system, and when eight mem-

[18] BMER, "Analysis of the Ewing Report," *Bulletin 69* (Chicago: American Medical Association, 1949), p. 11. Fishbein sets forth much the same argument in *JAMA,* 138 (December 25, 1948), 1255.

[19] Editorial, *JAMA,* 139 (January 15, 1949), 156; *JAMA,* 139 (January 22, 1949), 233; HD, *Proceedings* (98 Annual Session, June, 1949), p. 32; Editorial, *The Nation,* 177 (October 10, 1953), 284; *Who's Who in America* (1960–1961), Vol. 31, pp. 3096–97. The bill introduced in January as S. 5 was sponsored by Senators Murray, Wagner, McGrath, Pepper, Chavez, and Taylor, and the same measure (H. R. 783) was introduced by Dingell in the House. Warren first raised the health insurance issue in California in 1945 and twice again before the decade ended. *New York Times,* January 2, 1949, p. 28.

bers of the Senate introduced a measure (S. 1679) on April 25, incorporating his proposal.[20]

In what soon became one of the most sensational and dramatic campaigns that an organization ever conducted over a particular issue, the professional promoters carried forward the Association's program. Backed by mounting assessment reserves that reached $2,250,000 by December, the Whitaker and Baxter group hastily launched a fourfold offensive. Its bold attack included a nationwide plan of pamphlet distribution, a publicity campaign through public communications media, a speaking program, and a vigorous endorsement drive.[21]

The campaign of pamphlet distribution rapidly picked up momentum and secured enthusiastic support from the profession, the AMA's woman's auxiliary, its Council on Medical Service, allied groups including dentists, druggists, and nursing organizations, and sympathetic laymen. Early in June, the co-ordinating committee announced that the national campaign office had issued 25 different classifications of material and that 25,000,000 copies had been circulated which interested groups extended to 55,000,000 by December. To members of Congress the Association gave special consideration, in providing gifts near the end of the year of *The Road Ahead,* subtitled "America's Creeping Revolution,"[22] John T. Flynn's attack on the policies of the Democratic party.

The press and radio greatly assisted the publicity campaign by providing generous coverage of the Association's struggle and required little prodding from the campaign office. The 65,000 posters of "The Doctor" which the campaign headquarters had mailed by December to physicians for office display also dramatically publicized the Association's fight. These posters, depicting the outdated scene of a bearded physician administering aid by dim lamp glow at a patient's bedside, bore the inscription, "Keep Politics Out of This Picture."[23]

[20] *JAMA,* 140 (May 7, 1949), 125; Editorial, p. 11; HD, *Proceedings* (98 Annual Session, June, 1949), p. 32. These senators were Murray, Wagner, Pepper, Chavez, Taylor, McGrath, Elbert Thomas, and Hubert Humphrey. Dingell and Biemiller introduced an identical bill in the House.

[21] HD, *Proceedings* (Clinical Session, December, 1949), pp. 38, 37.

[22] HD, *Proceedings* (98 Annual Session, June, 1949), pp. 54–55; Leone Baxter, p. 33; HD, *Proceedings* (Clinical Session, December, 1949), pp. 53, 37, 39; *New York Times,* December 9, 1949, p. 25.

[23] HD, *Proceedings* (Clinical Session, December, 1949), p. 36; Leone Baxter, p. 34. To Leone Baxter [Mrs. Clem Whitaker], the picture had enduring qualities that she believed represented the ideals of medicine. "In the doctor's face there is compassion, there is personal concern for the welfare of his patient, there is personal loyalty to the patient as a human being and that is not old fashioned;

The campaign in its scope and swiftness took on the character of a blitzkrieg and demanded the almost inexhaustible energy of its directors. In the early months of the crusade they reported that one week's work included establishment of some form of contact with the following:

12,000	Trade associations
2,700	Chambers of commerce
500	Prominent clubs with civic influence
120	Advertising clubs
1,500	Kiwanis clubs
4,500	Lion's clubs
2,300	Rotary clubs
1,300	Carnegie
900	College libraries
8,000	Public libraries
14,000	School principals and superintendents
9,000	Y.M.C.A. city associations
200	Y.W.C.A. city associations
130,000	Dentists and druggists[24]

Speakers' bureaus created by state societies at the insistence of the campaign office also carried the Association's message. From outside the profession as well as among physicians, several societies built up impressive speakers' panels. During 1949 one organization established a panel of 65 physicians, and many reported widespread demand for the services of their bureaus. The Council on Medical Service rendered valuable aid in supplying lay speakers and medical societies with health insurance materials early in the crusade.[25]

No part of the campaign gave the AMA more encouragement than the favorable results of the endorsement drive. While making strong appeals for organizational support, the Whitaker and Baxter staff did not minimize the importance of individual assistance. By early June it had printed for the use of physicians in reaching their patients some 10,000,000 envelopes and accompanying stickers that compressed the Association's case. These stickers, emphasizing that compulsory health insurance would offer "inferior medical service at high cost," encroach on medical privacy, and force patients and doctors alike under political control, urged convinced addressees to inform their congressional dele-

---

that is something very vital and very enduring." These pictures were also displayed by many drugstores. HD, *Proceedings* (98 Annual Session, June, 1949), p. 54. See also *Who's Who in America* (1960–1961), Vol. 31, p. 185.

[24] HD, *Proceedings* (Clinical Session, December, 1949), p. 54.

[25] *Ibid.*, pp. 39, 53.

gation of their opposition. Although individual response could not be measured, by December the staff's appeal for group assistance had brought 1,829 sympathetic local, state, and national organizations into the fight whose members had already flooded the national capital with thousands of letters.[26]

In addition to the dramatic crusade that the Whitaker and Baxter staff conducted, the AMA attempted to strengthen its position by placing greater emphasis on the expansion of voluntary health insurance programs. Point three of the revised health program that the trustees adopted in February, 1949, called for "further development and wider coverage of voluntary hospital and medical care plans" and their rapid expansion into rural areas.[27] A few weeks later the Council on Medical Service laid plans for determining the total membership of voluntary programs and for enlisting the aid of organizations as prominent as the Farm Bureau and the United States Chamber of Commerce in building enrollments. It also called upon the Association to strengthen its own staff at headquarters for the additional work, and to recruit two field assistants for work in the national enrollment drive. Although the council's accomplishments in 1949 were more modest than its plans, it did not appear discouraged. It noted in December that enrollment in hospitalization plans had increased by 8,500,000 during the year and by 7,750,000 in surgical plans, bringing total enrollments to 61,000,000 and 34,000,000 respectively, but also commented on the difficulty of reaching many groups with voluntary health insurance.[28]

Work of House of Delegates

While the campaign of 1949 proceeded mostly according to administrative decision, the House of Delegates, of course, played an important part. In June, it clearly displayed its hostility to the growth of governmental power in adopting a resolution opposing competition of the federal government with its citizens in any enterprise which the constitution did not specify. It also authorized the establishment of better contact at the nation's capital through a committee empowered to confer with Congress. This committee was established before the end of the year.

[26] Quotation, HD, *Proceedings* (98 Annual Session, June, 1949), p. 55; and (Clinical Session, December, 1949), p. 37.

[27] HD, *Proceedings* (98 Annual Session, June, 1949), pp. 20, 52. See Appendix, p. 413, for other parts of this platform.

[28] HD, *Proceedings* (98 Annual Session, June, 1949), p. 25; HD, *Proceedings* (Annual Session, December, 1949), pp. 55–56.

With no great difficulty, the delegates passed a resolution recommending the establishment of annual membership dues that the December session allowed the trustees to set at no more than $25.00 for 1950.[29]

More noteworthy, however, was the action of the House of Delegates in June, 1949, that for the first time gave approval to the development of commercial prepayment health insurance programs by lay groups. In collaboration with organizations greatly interested in extending lay-sponsored plans, the Council on Medical Service drew up 20 principles regulating their development which the delegates accepted. They voted to submit these principles to state and local societies as a guide in approving plans arising in their jurisdictions, and to make lay-sponsored plans eligible to receive the "Seal of Acceptance." While the attitude of constituent societies toward such plans would greatly affect their growth, the action represented an accommodation to a development that was already well advanced.[30]

The House of Delegates not only adapted itself to the growth of lay-sponsored programs, but also reacted to rising complaints from within and without the profession about the unethical conduct of some physicians. These complaints generally involved excessive professional charges, fee splitting, and the rebate practice. While the Association had long denounced the acceptance of rebates and other violations of professional ethics, in December, 1949, the delegates urged all medical societies to establish grievance committees through which offenders might be disciplined. Three years later President Louis H. Bauer told the House that these committees were "rapidly covering the country," but warned that they would be no more than window-dressing unless given effective power. He also noted that many societies had attempted to make professional services more satisfactory by establishing medical emergency call systems.[31]

[29] Resolution, E. Vincent Askey, HD, *Proceedings* (97 Annual Session, Atlantic City, June, 1949), pp. 29, 47; Resolutions, Andrew A. Eggston, pp. 27, 43; HD, *Proceedings* (Clinical Session, December, 1949), p. 33. Those appointed on the committee to confer with Congress were Harvey B. Stone, chairman, R. L. Sensenich, Louis H. Bauer, R. B. Robins, John W. Cline, F. F. Borzell, and Frank H. Lahey. Ex officio members included James R. McVay, George F. Lull, and E. L. Henderson. HD, *Proceedings* (Clinical Session, December, 1949), p. 7.

[30] *JAMA*, 140 (July 2, 1949), 686, 799; *New York Times*, June 10, 1949, pp. 1, 16.

[31] Arthur J. Patek, *JAMA*, 133 (March 8, 1947), 715; Resolution, William Weston, HD, *Proceedings* (96 Annual Session, June, 1947), 58, 94, 96; *JAMA*, 142 (February 25, 1950), 573; Louis H. Bauer, HD, *Proceedings* (Clinical Session, December, 1952), p. 4; HD, *Proceedings* (96 Annual Session, June, 1947), pp. 39–41.

Embattled Leaders

The campaign that the Association waged against the Truman program in 1949 took on the character of a total effort, as the organization's leading spokesmen joined the fight. When the Association ventured to test the strength of its health insurance program in May with hearings in both Houses on health insurance legislation, R. L. Sensenich upheld the Association's position before a subcommittee of the House Committee on Interstate and Foreign Commerce. Bauer spoke on the same subject before the subcommittee on health of the Senate Committee on Labor and Public Welfare. Bauer condemned as intolerable any plan that financed federal participation in meeting the nation's medical problems through a "direct federal tax," and which placed "primary initiative and control in Washington" and "applied uniform and compulsory features on a nationwide basis." Finding a federal compulsory scheme "wrong in principle" and "impossible of practical operation," both he and Sensenich maintained that voluntary insurance had demonstrated its adequacy in meeting the problems of families unable to bear the cost of serious illnesses. For the "price of a package of cigarettes or a bottle of beer," Bauer contended, a family could secure protection against the "bulk of hospital and in-hospital medical bills."[32]

Other leaders of the Association succeeded in arousing the profession to action and sustaining enthusiasm in the struggle. Years of experience in combating compulsory health insurance agitation left Morris Fishbein particularly fitted for the task. Through the *Journal* and in the public forum this hardened veteran fought strenuously. On February 22, he joined Senator H. Alexander Smith in attacking proponents of compulsory health insurance at close range in a radio debate with Oscar Ewing and Walter Reuther. Less than three weeks later, the *Journal* carried his attack on the British system that summarized his impression of its operation on a recent trip to England.[33] Other spokes-

[32] Eighty-first Congress, first session, *Hearings on H.R. 4312 and H.R. 4313 (Identical Bills) and H.R. 4918 and Other Identical Bills on National Health Plans and S. 1411, H.R. 4660, H.R. 3942 and Other Identical Bills on School Health Services* (Washington: Government Printing Office, 1949), pp. 111–14 and *Hearings on S. 1106, S. 1456, S. 1581, and S. 1697* (Washington: Government Printing Office, 1949), Part 1, pp. 203–4, 209–10.

[33] *JAMA*, 139 (February 12, 1949), 461; *JAMA*, 139 (March 5, 1949), 640–41. For other criticisms of the British system that the *Journal* published in 1949, see *JAMA*, 139 (January 22, 1949), 246; *JAMA*, 139 (January 29, 1949), 325; *JAMA*, 139 (April 2, 1949), 952; *JAMA*, 141 (December 31, 1949), 1301; *JAMA*, 140 (July 2, 1949), 797; and *JAMA*, 140 (August 6, 1949), 1145.

men of the Association joined Fishbein in denouncing compulsory schemes. John L. Bach, director of press relations, warned of "pick-pocket medicine" and George H. Lull pictured the cost of "a sprawling, ever-expanding governmental bureaucracy of clerks, bookkeepers, and administrators." In December, Elmer L. Henderson, Chairman of the Board of Trustees, observed that the Association had passed through a "baptism of fire" and warned that although the compulsory insurance forces had fallen back they had not surrendered and that "the Battle of Armageddon" was still ahead.[34]

Year for Decision

As the Association carried the fight into the threatening fifties, it brought with it growing confidence as well. Watching the administration recoil before its attack and believing that it had settled on a strategy of delay and indirection, the Association, aroused and mobilized, determined to bring the issue to a final decision during the year. Although the President briefly referred to the need for a national insurance system in his congressional message of January 4, 1950, the AMA looked for no very aggressive action and soon witnessed many encouraging counter developments.[35] On January 24, the Washington Office reported that Republicans of the House had established a "G.O.P. Price-Tag Committee," which would publicize the cost of programs proposed by the administration. Nearly three months later it announced overwhelming opposition to compulsory health insurance in three districts where congressmen had conducted limited surveys, and early in May reported

[34] For Bach's statement see *Secretary's Letter No. 95* (February 14, 1949), 2; for Lull's, "The Voluntary Way Is the American Way," in "How Shall We Pay for Medical Care?" *Public Affairs Pamphlet No. 152* (New York: Public Affairs Committee, Inc., 1949), 20; for Henderson's, HD, *Proceedings* (Clinical Session, December, 1949), 36. Adding bitterness to the controversy was the seven-month investigation initiated by the Department of Justice in 1949 of the Association's alleged encouragement of monopolistic practices in providing medical care. The AMA viewed the action as purely a political move since J. Howard McGrath, who had fought for compulsory health insurance in the Senate, had recently been appointed Attorney General. *Secretary's Letter No. 123* (October 17, 1949), 1; *Secretary's Letter No. 147* (May 22, 1950), 3; *JAMA*, 141 (October 15, 1949), 465.

[35] Editorial, *JAMA*, 142 (January 14, 1950), 110, *New York Times*, January 5, 1950, p. 10. In June the trustees told the House of Delegates that the Association must avert a "long drawn war of attrition" and must "find a way to make public sentiment on this issue perfectly clear." HD, *Proceedings* (99 Annual Session, June, 1950), p. 13.

a list of 12 state legislatures to which it later added two others, that had taken action opposing the compulsory principle. No development seemed more encouraging, however, than the defeat of the champion of compulsory health insurance, Claude Pepper, in the Florida Democratic primary, after doctors fought vigorously to elect his opponent with an undistinguished political background, George A. Smathers.[36]

At every turn the Association tried to meet the administration's strategy. In answer to Ewing's favorable report early in 1950 on the performance of European health insurance systems, following six weeks of investigation abroad, the AMA soon responded with the uncomplimentary observations of two professional groups which it had sent to study the operation of the British plan.[37] From bastions even high within the Democratic party the Association also kept up the fight. As a Democratic national committeeman and member of the House of Delegates, R. B. Robins of Arkansas fought the alleged effort of the national committee to circulate compulsory health insurance propaganda. Nor did the Association leave top Democratic leaders alone when they held a "Jefferson Jubilee Celebration" in Chicago. At the session devoted to a discussion of government health insurance, Robins brought along Frank Dickinson and the legal counsel of the Illinois State Medical Society, only to find the discussion closed to all but congressmen and committeemen.[38] The *Journal* denounced a pamphlet that the National Democratic Committee issued commending compulsory health insurance and seemed pleased when it could report that two congressmen had protested the use of federal funds for Ewing's trip to Europe. Neither did the June session of the House of Delegates show any regret when

[36] WO, *Capitol Clinic No. 4* (January 24, 1950), 2; WO, *Capitol Clinic No. 14* (April 18, 1950), 1; WO, *Bulletin No. 48* (May 4, 1950), 1; WO, *Bulletin No. 52* (June 8, 1950), 1; *Secretary's Letter No. 145* (May 8, 1950), 1–2. The 14 states were Ark., Del., Fla., Ill., La., Md., Mass., Mich., Miss., Neb., Tenn., Tex., Utah, and Va.

[37] HD, *Proceedings* (99 Annual Session, June, 1950), p. 9. One group consisting of Harold S. Diehl, Loren R. Chandler, and Stanley Dorst made a preliminary report at a meeting of a professional group in February, 1950. ACMEL, *Proceedings Combined with Medical Education in the United States and Canada,* 1949–1950, pp. 32–39. While Ewing closed his European trip more firmly convinced of the merits of the Truman program, he did say that the British plan was unsuited for the United States. *JAMA,* 142 (February 11, 1950), 426.

[38] *Secretary's Letter No. 138* (February 27, 1950), 4; *Secretary's Letter No. 146* (May 15, 1950), 1. Many months earlier Robins had sent a telegram to Senator McGrath, chairman of the Democratic National Committee, protesting the alleged misuse of his position to attack state medical societies and the AMA as medical dictatorships. *Secretary's Letter No. 102* (April 4, 1949), 1.

the Washington Office telegraphed the body that a congressional investigation had found the Federal Security Agency to be inefficient, mismanaged, wasteful, and overstaffed.[39]

While the early months of 1950 brought minor clashes between the AMA and the administration, the Association reserved its major offensive for the fall. Hoping to force the issue into the November congressional elections, the Whitaker and Baxter group started a new publicity campaign in "American medicine's drive to a decision." Into a movement that had already circulated 77,000,000 leaflets, folders, and pamphlets by June, 1950, and which had received the endorsement of 10,234 groups, the campaign directors and co-ordinators prepared to release more furious energies. With "dramatic, powerful advertisement" in over 11,000 newspapers, they hoped to "give voice to the people's mandate on the issue." They planned an enlarged attack through full-page advertisements in 30 national magazines and a barrage of spot announcements on 300 radio stations.[40]

Case for a Compulsory System

In a struggle that had at last reached the zero hour, the Truman administration had fought stubbornly and against growing odds. Since the beginning of the second term, its spokesmen had parried the Association's attacks and struck effective blows at the AMA's position. In January, 1949, Oscar Ewing debated Fishbein in the *American Druggist,* and during the same year set his views against those of Lull in a discussion published by Public Affairs Committee, Inc., categorically denying in both discussions most of the charges that the AMA made against the Truman health insurance program.

Ewing contended that the Truman plan, instead of centralizing most of the authority over medical care at the nation's capital, called for administration by local boards, which in consultation with local physicians would decide on the "basis for determining the amount they are to be paid for their services."[41] He maintained that the program would place no restrictions on the scientific practice of medicine or interfere with the free choice of physicians or with their right to accept

[39] *JAMA,* 143 (May 27, 1950), 377; *JAMA,* 142 (April 8, 1950), 1081; HD, *Proceedings* (99 Annual Session, June, 1950), p. 62, see also p. 63.

[40] HD, *Proceedings* (99 Annual Session, June, 1950), p. 14.

[41] *American Druggist,* 119 (January, 1949), 80.

or reject patients, and in no sense made doctors government employees. He claimed that the plan proposed no changes in patterns of medical care, but only in method of payment. Answering charges of exorbitant cost that a compulsory system would impose, Ewing contended that such a program added little to the cost of medical care, but mainly transferred expense to a new payment method through machinery of the social security system already in operation. Maintaining that a compulsory system would offer complete medical care and encourage preventive medicine, he believed that the system would reduce substantially the $27,000,000,000 annual loss in national wealth inflicted by sickness and disabilities. In contrast to Fishbein, who charged that the proposed system would constitute the first step to complete socialism, Ewing insisted that it was no more socialism than fire insurance.[42]

Spokesmen for a compulsory program showed as much skill in striking at deficiencies in traditional payment methods as in defending the Truman plan. In a debate with Fishbein, Ewing charged that since about half the nation's population came from families with annual incomes of less than $3,000, adequate medical care was beyond reach, and that voluntary plans, with their practice of excluding bad risks and offering only partial coverage, held no hope for low-income groups. Against Lull he argued that expansion of voluntary insurance inevitably followed the distribution of wealth. He showed that residents of six wealthy industrial states, with only 36 per cent of the population, held 60 per cent of the policies issued by the Blue Cross Plans, and that Southern and Western states, with 43 per cent of the population, held only 17 per cent of Blue Cross membership.[43]

At hearings on S. 1679 in May, Assistant Administrator of Social Security, J. Donald Kingsley, maintained that less than 2½ per cent of the population had voluntary health insurance as comprehensive as that which the administration's measure would provide. In an article appearing several weeks after the November elections but supporting the administration's case, Margaret C. Klem, Chief of Medical Programs Branch, Division of Industrial Hygiene of the United States Public Health Service, showed that in 1948 voluntary health insurance paid

[42] *Ibid.*, pp. 80, 102; "The Why, What, and How of National Health Insurance," in "How Shall We Pay for Medical Care?" *Public Affairs Pamphlet No. 152* (New York: Public Affairs Committee, Inc., 1949), 6–7, 11–12; *American Druggist,* 119 (January, 1949), 102, 104.

[43] *American Druggist,* 119 (January, 1949), 81; *Public Affairs Pamphlet No. 152,* p. 10.

only between 8.2 and 8.8 per cent of the nation's "private expenditure for medical care." At the same time, Isadore Falk, Director of Research and Statistics of the Social Security Administration, maintained that millions of modest wage earners lived in constant dread of the burdensome cost of serious illnesses, and that voluntary health insurance had failed as completely in the United States as in Europe, where it had been supplanted by compulsory programs.[44]

Proponents of compulsory health insurance bore heavily on other weaknesses which they found in voluntary plans. Ewing observed that in 1947 companies offering medical indemnity, surgical, and hospital insurance on a group basis paid only 69 per cent of their premiums in benefits, and that companies which sold to individuals paid only 37 per cent. While noting that a few companies offering group policies paid as high as 88 per cent, he also pointed out that a large part of the population could not secure group coverage.[45] Much in line with his evidence were findings soon published by a committee to which the Senate had assigned responsibility for conducting a study of voluntary plans. This investigation showed that retention charges for Blue Cross in 1949 were 15 per cent; Blue Shield, 21 per cent; and that commercial companies retained 20 per cent of the premiums for group insurance and 45 per cent of the individual premiums.[46]

Not only did Ewing attack the high administrative cost of voluntary plans, but also their failure to promote the development of preventive medicine or to meet the needs of many suffering from long serious illnesses. He confidently asserted that a national insurance system would

[44] Eighty-first Congress, first session, *Hearings on S. 1106, S. 1456, S. 1581, and S. 1679* (Washington: Government Printing Office, 1949), Part 1, p. 85; quotation, "Voluntary Health Insurance," American Academy of Political and Social Science, *Annals,* 273 (January, 1951), 99; "Health Services, Medical Care Insurance, and Social Security," American Academy of Political and Social Science, *Annals,* 273 (January, 1951), 116, 119.

[45] *Public Affairs Pamphlet No. 152,* p. 12.

[46] Senate Committee on Labor and Public Welfare, *Report Pursuant to S. Res. 273 and S. Res. 39: Health Insurance Plans in the United States,* Eighty-second Congress, first session, *Report No. 359* (Washington: Government Printing Office, 1951), p. 7. This completely independent study that the Senate sponsored was directed by Dr. Dean A. Clark, Director of the Massachusetts General Hospital, with the aid of Morris Pike, Vice-President of the John Hancock Mutual Life Insurance Company, who served as assistant director. See foreword by Herbert H. Lehman, chairman of subcommittee on health of Senate Committee on Labor and Public Welfare, pp. vii, ix. The committee also listed many other weaknesses in voluntary health insurance that were in line with the contentions of the administration's spokesmen.

make available medical care for the masses that only wealthier groups could then afford. Under a national program, he contended, the reluctance of the public to seek medical care for diseases in their incipient stages would be removed and the sick could get adequate treatment, free from financial worry.[47]

Although the bitterness of the struggle was frequently concealed, temperamental outbursts occasionally reflected the intensity of the fight. The Secretary of the AMA described Ewing's speech in Houston on September 22 as "something Salvador Dali might have mustered up after a midnight snack of raw onion and Welsh rabbit." To his speech in New York before the American Jewish Congress in which he seemed to implicate the AMA with the alleged practices of some medical schools of discriminating against Jewish students, the Secretary quickly replied, attacking Ewing as a "disappointed, embittered bureaucrat, who should be removed from office before he does further harm to the country."[48]

Election Victories

When the largest number of voters in the nation's history (other than in a presidential election year) had cast votes on November 7, the AMA believed that its campaign had succeeded. A disturbed electorate raised Republican strength from 42 to 47 in the Senate and cut by two-thirds the Democratic majority in the House. With growing opposition from Republicans and disgruntled Southern Democrats, defeat for Truman's health insurance program seemed certain. The election cut deep into Democratic leadership, bringing defeat to majority leader Scott W. Lucas (Illinois), Millard E. Tydings (Maryland), and to the strong health insurance advocates, Elbert D. Thomas and Glen H. Taylor in the Senate and Andrew J. Biemiller in the House.[49] From eight of the newly elected senators, including Richard M. Nixon (Cali-

[47] *American Druggist,* 119 (January, 1949), 102, 104. In May, 1950, the *Journal* published an article that stressed the importance of early treatment in cancer. Guy F. Robbins, Alexander J. Conte, John E. Leach, and Mary MacDonald, "Delay in the Diagnosis and Treatment of Cancer," *JAMA,* 143 (May 27, 1950), 346.

[48] *Secretary's Letter No. 159* (October 2, 1950), 2; *Secretary's Letter No. 160* (October 9, 1950), 2.

[49] *New York Times,* November 8, 1950, p. 1 and November 9, 1950, p. 1; WO, *Capitol Clinic No. 44* (November 14, 1950), 1. Senator Lucas had opposed Truman's compulsory insurance plan but nevertheless his defeat was a significant party loss. *New York Times,* November 9, 1950, p. 36.

fornia), Everett M. Dirksen (Illinois), and George A. Smathers (Florida), the AMA expected strong opposition to Truman's plan. While the prospects of a long war in Korea, brought on by the sudden entrance of regiments totally composed of Chinese troops, partially explain Democratic losses, spokesmen for the AMA preferred to view the election results as a widespread revolt against the drift toward a welfare state.[50]

Scars of Conflict

The Association emerged from its fiercest health insurance battle confident of victory, but nevertheless bearing the scars of conflict. Not only had the administration made the public more conscious of deficiencies in voluntary plans, but the struggle itself had brought disturbing division within the ranks of medicine. As the AMA appealed for a united front in attacking the administration's program, a group of 148 physicians protested its assessment which they feared would be used for "standpat propaganda" rather than "to develop a carefully worked out, comprehensive plan to extend and improve medical care and education." In 1950, the Nevada State Medical Association protested the Board of Trustees' decision to pour large additional sums into the advertising crusade. A few other daring medical groups that had long defied the Association continued their opposition, while apparently some other dissenting physicians became convinced of the futility of protest.[51]

During the struggle the Board of Trustees decided to withdraw from the front ranks and finally remove entirely the AMA's most vulnerable target of attack. For years the able and energetic Fishbein had alienated groups within and without the profession, becoming at the same time the symbol of organized medicine. In June, 1949, overwhelming pressure within the Association compelled the trustees to curb his activities and plan for his retirement. When the editor of the *Journal* severed

[50] WO, *Capitol Clinic No. 45* (November 21, 1950), 1; *New York Times,* November 1, 1950, p. 5; *New York Times,* November 9, 1950, p. 36; Elmer L. Henderson, HD, *Proceedings* (Clinical Session, December, 1950), p. 4.

[51] Quotation, *JAMA,* 139 (February 19, 1949), 532; Resolution, Roland W. Stahr, HD, *Proceedings* (99 Annual Session, June, 1950), p. 42; Editorial, *JAMA,* 139 (January 1, 1949), 36–37. In 1947 Paul A. Dodd, in reviewing *Medicine in the Changing Order,* refers to an eminent California physician who, while wishing to testify before a legislative committee hearing in favor of the proposed state compulsory health bill, declined to do so stating that as a specialist he depended on referrals and could not alienate the profession. American Academy of Political and Social Science, *Annals,* 253 (September, 1947), 238.

official connection with the AMA on December 1, to be replaced by Austin Smith, organized medicine had lost its most daring and adroit leader during its most crucial fight.[52]

Watchful Waiting

As the Association, wearied from two years of incessant conflict, planned to carry its battle against compulsory health insurance into the last half of Truman's second term, it suspected that the insurance threat, although still dangerous, had passed the crisis stage. Remaining prepared for any massive offensive that the administration might launch, it gradually reduced the scale of its own operations and watched for limited attacks. In December, 1950, F. F. Borzell, speaker of the House of Delegates, warned that although the AMA had successfully resisted frontal assaults, it still confronted "more or less insidious flank movements which, if successful, can and may prepare the way for ultimate regimentation and enslavement."[53]

Not until after the Republican presidential triumph of 1952 did the AMA release the Whitaker and Baxter staff. Yet expenditures for the national educational campaign that reached approximately $2,593,000 in 1950 fell to about $529,000 in 1951, and to $255,000 a year later. Compensating somewhat for the reduced activity of the campaign directors, however, was the publicity work started by the Department of Public Relations in 1951. Not only did it begin a widespread campaign distributing materials that set forth the Association's views on many medical issues, but the former director, Lawrence Rember, left the home office in charge of the new director, Leo Brown (who had held a similar position with the Pennsylvania state association) and took up

[52] HD, *Proceedings* (98 Annual Session, June, 1949), pp. 22, 51; HD, *Proceedings* (Clinical Session, December, 1949), p. 35; "Dr. Morris Fishbein Meets the Press," *The American Mercury* (February, 1950), p. 182. For an account of how Fishbein's opposition forced the issue of his retirement before the House of Delegates in June, 1949, see *Northwest Medicine,* 48 (July, 1949), 425, and for an account of his successor, who had served as secretary of the Council on Pharmacy and Chemistry and Director of the Division of Therapy and Research, see *JAMA,* 141 (December 10, 1949), 1061. Earlier protests against Fishbein are found in Resolution, Idaho State Medical Association, HD, *Proceedings* (94 Annual Session, June, 1944), p. 83; Resolution, California State Medical Association, ibid., p. 83; Resolution, S. J. McClendon, HD, *Proceedings* (Annual Session, December, 1945), p. 62, and comments on resolution of the California association that the AMA did not see fit to publish. HD, *Proceedings* (95 Annual Session, July, 1946), pp. 54, 69.

[53] HD, *Proceedings* (Clinical Session, December, 1950), p. 2.

the work as field director assisting medical societies in improving their public relations activities.[54]

Resisting Flank Attacks

While doubtful that the administration would launch a frontal assault in the final years of the second term, the Association remained alert to what it considered to be flanking efforts to secure a compulsory health insurance system, some of which appeared soon after the second term began. Fearful of the eventual establishment of political controls over the profession, it registered its opposition in 1949 to the extension of social security coverage to physicians as proposed by H. R. 2893.[55] A year earlier the House of Delegates had hoped to weaken the appeal of the social security system by approving the principle of physicians' purchasing retirement benefits in private plans by tax-exempt income payments, but the idea created little immediate interest. In 1952, however, Frank Dickinson assisted in revising the Reed and Keogh bills for setting up retirement benefit regulations, which first appeared in Congress the year before.[56] The AMA found that it could not avoid contact with the system, however, by the profession's nonaffiliation. In H. R. 6000, which, as enacted became the "Social Security Act Amendment of 1950," it discovered serious indirect threats to medical freedom. While this measure, liberalizing benefits and greatly extending coverage, excluded physicians, the AMA protested its inclusion of permanent and total disability benefits within the social security insurance system.[57]

Although since 1946 the Association had veered away, somewhat indecisively, from its earlier support of temporary disability insurance

[54] Elmer L. Henderson, HD, *Proceedings* (100 Annual Session, June, 1951), p. 5; HD, *Proceedings* (101 Annual Session, June, 1952), p. 25; HD, *Proceedings* (100 Annual Session, June, 1951), p. 11; HD, *Proceedings* (102 Annual Session, June, 1953), p. 10; HD, *Proceedings* (Clinical Session, December, 1951), p. 39; HD, *Proceedings* (100 Annual Session, June, 1951), p. 9.

[55] *JAMA,* 141 (September 24, 1949), 268; Resolution, L. A. Alesen, HD, *Proceedings* (98 Annual Session, June, 1949), p. 47.

[56] HD, *Proceedings* (97 Annual Session, June, 1948), pp. 22, 99, 100; HD, *Proceedings* (100 Annual Session, June, 1951), p. 33; HD, *Proceedings* (Clinical Session, December, 1952), pp. 45–46; *JAMA,* 149 (July 26, 1952), 1244–47; WO, *Comments No. 7—82nd Congress* (May 16, 1952), 2.

[57] For this complicated act that extended coverage to approximately 10,000,000 persons see 64 Stat. 477–561 (1950–1951), and Wilbur J. Cohen and Robert J. Myers, "Social Security Act Amendments of 1950: A Summary and Legislative History," *Social Security Bulletin,* 13 (October, 1950), 3.

and had kept the whole matter under study, its authorized spokesmen strongly denounced the disability provisions of the bill at hearings on February 28, 1950, before the Senate Committee on Finance.[58] While Sensenich charged that the bill did not make "compensable disability demonstrable by objective tests" and joined with Gunnar Gundersen in contending that the measure placed physicians in a difficult position in passing on the eligibility of their patients for disability benefits, their chief objections lay elsewhere. Sensenich expressed the Board of Trustees' view that the program would be "a forerunner of a completely federalized system of compulsory sickness insurance," and Gundersen predicted that adoption of the disability provision would open the way for a "fullfledged" compulsory system.[59] When the Senate rejected the disability provision, the two houses agreed on revisions that followed the recommendations of the AMA in providing federal aid through state public assistance programs for eligible disability cases.[60]

[58] In response to the health program that the President advanced in November, 1945, the *Journal* maintained that the AMA had "consistently favored" a system of insurance against income loss due to sickness, the principle of which it had accepted in 1938. Yet the AMA appeared to have weakened in support of the idea before 1949 after five states adopted sickness indemnity laws and while others considered passing such measures. Many difficulties attended the operation of the program in Rhode Island, where the first law was enacted in 1942. Editorial, *JAMA,* 129 (December 1, 1945), 953; *JAMA,* 138 (October 30, 1948), 664; HD, *Proceedings* (Clinical Session, December, 1949), p. 53; Wilson, *Compulsory Health Insurance,* pp. 10–11. While the House of Delegates authorized a study of the issue in 1946, the Council on Medical Service reported in December, 1949, that it was not yet in a position to report fully on the implications of the matter. It did announce, however, that it was calling a meeting in which its Correlating Committee on Medical Care would meet with representatives of the medical societies in states where these laws were in operation "to consider the advisability of clarifying the American Medical Association's stand concerning the principle of compulsory cash sickness benefits." The next year the council recommended endorsement of the principle of temporary disability compensation, which it noted had been endorsed in 1938. It also recommended that the program be confined to the private insurance business. The House of Delegates adopted recommendations of a reference committee authorizing the AMA to try to limit the benefits of the system to cash indemnity and to prevent the extension of the principle to other fields. HD, *Proceedings* (96 Annual Session, June, 1947), p. 54; quotation, *JAMA,* 141 (November 5, 1949), 700; HD, *Proceedings* (Clinical Session, December, 1950), pp. 55, 72. It is not surprising that spokesmen for the AMA opposed the operation of a permanent disability system on the federal level even in advance of a clearly defined policy.

[59] *Hearings on H.R. 6000* (Washington: Government Printing Office, 1950), Part 3, pp. 1317, 1319, 1321, 1336.

[60] Falk, American Academy of Political and Social Science, *Annals,* 273 (January, 1951), p. 120; 64 Stat. 555 (1950–1951), Title XIV; WO, *Bulletin No. 59* (July 27, 1950), 3.

Near the end of the Truman era, the AMA discovered what it identified as another crafty effort of the administration to advance compulsory health insurance by flank attack through the social security system. On May 12, 1952, Representative Doughton introduced H. R. 7800 which proposed increases in old age and survivors insurance benefits, and a waiver of premium and freezing of benefit rights for persons during periods of total and permanent disability. While the AMA did not oppose the extension of benefits or allowable monthly earnings, it did object to the power that the bill conferred on the Social Security Administration in enforcing the disability provision. It also protested the administration's effort to secure action on the bill (without hearings) only seven days after its introduction as a "flagrant attempt to railroad through a provision to aid in the socialization of medicine which could not possibly be adopted if considered openly and publicly."[61]

The AMA succeeded in breaking the administration's strategy. On May 17, the Washington Office sent telegrams to all members of the House of Representatives summarizing the enormous power the act conferred on the federal Social Security Administrator. These telegrams aroused the resistance of a number of congressmen to the administration's plan, preventing a vote on the measure two days later.[62] Not until June 17 did the bill pass the House, and then only after powers delegated to the Social Security Administrator had been reduced. The bill which the Senate approved a few days later further weakened the administrator's powers and, as enacted into law, transferred to state officials much of the authority originally delegated to the federal administrator.[63]

[61] WO, *Bulletin No. 50—82nd Congress* (May 23, 1952), 1; quotation, HD, *Proceedings* (101 Annual Session, June, 1952), p. 56.

[62] WO, *Bulletin No. 50—82nd Congress* (May 23, 1952), 1–2. The telegraphed message told congressmen that the bill conferred upon the Federal Security Administration the following "unusual" powers in the medical field: "(1) to promulgate rules and regulations on a national basis for governing medical examinations. (2) To select and approve examiners of applicants. (3) To remunerate for examinations. (4) To refund expense of applicant going to and from examination and most of all (5) To deny application if applicant refuses to take indicated rehabilitation under Vocational Rehabilitation Act." It added "This is socialized medicine and pages 12 to 16 should be stricken from the bill in the interest of the public good."

[63] WO, *Bulletin No. 52—82nd Congress* (June 19, 1952), 1; WO, *Bulletin No. 53—82nd Congress* (June 27, 1952), 1; 66 Stat. 772 (1952). By a strange arrangement the bill provided for the termination of disability benefits on June 30, 1953, one day before anyone was eligible to apply for such. This strategy allowed the bill to go through without additional delays but left the matter open for additional consideration in 1953. WO, *Capitol Clinic* 3 (July 8, 1952), 1.

The AMA watched the general areas of proposed federal health activity for what might be other flank attacks on private medical practice. In 1951, it opposed a measure (S. 1328) that called for a federal investigation of sickness in the United States, maintaining that other studies in progress made a governmental investigation unnecessary.[64] Later in the year it attributed to Truman political motivation in appointing an investigating group, known as the President's Commission on the Health Needs of the Nation, directed by Paul Magnuson, formerly head of the Department of Medicine and Surgery of the Veterans Administration. In 1952, the AMA's president, John W. Cline, offered evidence to show that the establishment of the commission resulted from the President's effort to turn public attention from the "troublesome" compulsory health insurance issue during an election year. As prominent officials in the AMA participated in health discussions which the commission sponsored, a trustee of the Association, after accepting the President's appointment to the group, quickly resigned from the position.[65] Nor did the Association seem to regret having severed official connection with the commission which soon submitted recommendations for the improvement of medical care, which, while fairly moderate, attested to great deficiencies in medical service.[66]

The Association's attitude toward the government-sponsored survey bore some resemblance to its position on several health measures that reached the stage of congressional hearings during Truman's second term. While favorable to the idea of federal assistance to needy states for the provision of adequate public health units, James R. Miller of the Board of Trustees showed in 1949 that the authority S. 522 conferred upon the Surgeon General of the Public Health Service left this official largely in control of the program and provided the states with no procedures for appeal.[67]

[64] WO, *Bulletin No. 29—82nd Congress* (August 24, 1951), 1, and attached statement of AMA.

[65] HD, *Proceedings* (101 Annual Session, June, 1952), p. 6; WO, *Capitol Clinic,* 3 (January 8, 1952), 1; WO, *Bulletin No. 38—82nd Congress* (January 11, 1952), 2. The trustee, Gunnar Gundersen, was replaced by Donald M. Clark of Peterborough, New Hampshire. WO, *Capitol Clinic,* 3 (April 15, 1952), 3.

[66] WO, *Capitol Clinic,* 3 (November 18, 1952), 1–3. For explanations and comments on see Eli Ginzberg, "What Every Economist Should Know about Health and Medicine," *The American Economic Review,* 44 (March, 1954), 107, 116, 118.

[67] Subcommittee of Senate Committee on Labor and Public Welfare, Eighty-first Congress, first session, *Hearings on S. 132, S. 522, Title V of S. 1381, and Title V of S. 1679 Local Health Units* (Washington: Government Printing Office, 1949), pp. 78–81.

The following year the Association resisted pressures placed upon Congress to pass legislation granting loans to co-operatives and nonprofit organizations for hospital construction. On May 9, 1950, Walter B. Martin of the Board of Trustees testified at a Senate subcommittee hearing against S. 1805 which, he contended, broke with the philosophy that guided the federal hospital construction program. He maintained that the bill conflicted with the spirit of the Hill-Burton program which called for public rather than private hospital facilities, and that the measure allowed construction in disregard of surveys that pointed to areas of need. He charged that the bill did not balance the power that it conferred upon Federal Security Administrators with adequate safeguards, stating that it allowed federal officials to regulate the medical care programs that operated in such institutions.[68]

The AMA raised even stronger protests to bills that appeared in Congress in 1949, authorizing diagnostic and therapeutic medical care for students in the nation's public elementary and secondary schools. It did not oppose federal aid to states in need of assistance in providing medical service for school children of medically indigent families, but objected to measures that called for indiscriminate medical care. With arguments closely resembling the Association's attack on a similar bill in the Eightieth Congress, Martin opposed the measures in spirit and detail. Not only did he condemn the uniformity of administration authorized by the legislation but added

> If 29,000,000 children are to be taught that their health service must stem from the Federal Government, then in one generation the road to complete Federal control of medicine will be open.[69]

Just as stubbornly did the Association hold the line in the early fifties against federal control of medical education, while at the same time formulating a policy inviting federal assistance. In June, 1951, the House of Delegates gave its first real support to the principle of federal

[68] Subcommittee on Health of Senate Committee on Labor and Public Welfare, Eighty-first Congress, second session, *Hearings on S. 1805, Cooperative Health Act* (Washington: Government Printing Office, 1950), pp. 52–64.

[69] Eighty-first Congress, first session, *Hearings on H. R. 4312 and H. R. 4313 (Identical Bills) and H. R. 4918 with Other Identical Bills on National Health Plans and S. 1411, H. R. 4660, H. R. 3942 and Other Identical Bills on School Health Services* (Washington: Government Printing Office, 1949), pp. 27–28, quotation, p. 27. For resolutions that the House of Delegates adopted in June, 1949, against S. 1411, H. R. 3942, and H. R. 4660, authorizing medical care for school children see those submitted by R. B. Robins, HD, *Proceedings* (98 Annual Session, June, 1949), pp. 26, 46–47, 58, and HD, *Proceedings* (Clinical Session, December, 1949), pp. 59, 68.

aid to medical schools, accepting the formula laid down for the Hill-Burton program. It approved "one-time federal grant-in-aid" used for "construction, equipment and renovation of the physical plants of medical schools," but condemned the extension of federal grants for salaries and other operational expenses. Only a few months earlier, however, the Board of Trustees created the American Medical Educational Foundation through which it hoped to reduce the need for federal assistance by raising funds from private sources for medical education. The Association itself contributed $500,000 to the total of $1,600,000 raised in 1951, which provided all approved medical schools with an average grant of $20,000. The foundation fell far short of its goal of $2,000,000 for the first year, however, and much further from that of $5,000,000 set for 1952.[70]

In attempting to improve the position of medical schools without incurring federal control, the AMA also tried to raise the efficiency of federal health functions without unduly enlarging areas of operation. Throughout Truman's second term the AMA's attempt to achieve these objectives brought it into further conflict with the administration. Holding out for a federal health department with cabinet status, it joined Senate opposition in 1949 that defeated the President's Reorganization Plan No. 1, which called for the elevation of the Federal Security Agency to cabinet level as a department of welfare responsible for federal health activities.[71] The following year it opposed Truman's Reorganization Plan No. 27, which provided for the establishment of a department of health, education, and security at cabinet level. Condemning the proposal as an effort to elevate the structurally defective Federal Security Agency to cabinet rank with power to extend domination over the Veterans Administration and the private hospital system, the House of Delegates registered an emphatic protest.[72] In 1950 the Association

[70] Quotation, HD, *Proceedings* (100 Annual Session, June, 1951), pp. 41, 43. HD, *Proceedings* (Clinical Session, December, 1951), p. 64; HD, *Proceedings* (101 Annual Session, June, 1952), p. 24.

[71] Editorial, *JAMA,* 140 (August 27, 1949), 1344.

[72] HD, *Proceedings* (99 Annual Session, June, 1950), pp. 13, 54. Louis H. Bauer presented the AMA's case at committee hearings in both Houses and although the House Committee on Expenditure in the Executive Departments approved the plan on June 20, the lower body defeated the proposal nearly three weeks later. See House Committee on Expenditures in Executive Departments, *Hearings on H. Res. 647: Reorganization Plan No. 27 of 1950* (Washington: Govenment Printing Office, 1950), pp. 27–38; *JAMA,* 143 (July 1, 1950), 819; WO, *Bulletin No. 55* (June 30, 1950), 2; WO, *Capitol Clinic No. 26* (July 11, 1950), 1. The President's proposal would have become law had it not been

also raised strong objections to proposed legislation (H. R. 5182 and S. 2008) that embodied the recommendations of the Hoover Commission in providing for the establishment of a united medical administration. While endorsing the idea of co-ordinating federal health activities, on July 11, Walter B. Martin charged that the measures conferred upon the administration enormous power without adequate controls and called for the creation of a weak and ineffective advisory council. He contended that the integration of medical services authorized by the bill failed to meet the goals of the AMA, calling for the co-ordination of the nation's hospital system to promote efficiency and economy. Nor did he feel that the measure properly recognized the special services of the Armed Forces and the Veterans Administration or guaranteed high quality medical care.[73] Believing that the bills possessed more defects than virtues, the AMA showed no regret when they failed to get beyond the committee hearing stage.

Despite the Association's strong insistence on the co-ordination of federal health functions in a national health department with cabinet rank, it entered the last two years of Truman's second term prepared to settle for less. In December, 1950, the House of Delegates, in response to a committee report which concluded that a health department with cabinet rank was not then attainable, urged the co-ordination of federal health functions in an "independent agency with executive status."[74] Yet not even the prospect of the establishment of a health department could bring the AMA to support another bill (S. 1140) in 1952 in which it found hazards to private medical practice. At a Senate subcommittee hearing on March 3, Martin opposed inclusion of the medical services of the Armed Forces and the Veterans Administration in the proposed department. In addition, he called upon Congress to determine first the scope of federal responsibility in medical matters, to carry out the recommendations of the Hoover Commission by clearly defining classes entitled to benefits from federal medical services, and to remove incon-

---

defeated by one of the Houses before July 31. After the lower house rejected the plan, the Washington Office asked the profession not to forget the congressmen who had helped defeat the measure, many of whom disrupted their local campaigns to return to the capitol for the vote. WO, *Capitol Clinic No. 21* (June 6, 1950), 1; WO, *Bulletin No. 57* (July 13, 1950), 3.

[73] Subcommittee on Health of Senate Committee on Labor and Public Welfare, Eighty-first Congress, second session, *Hearings on S. 2008* (Washington: Government Printing Office, 1950), pp. 69–70, see also pp. 75, 77.

[74] HD, *Proceedings* (Clinical Session, December, 1950), pp. 66, 67.

sistencies in the government's hospital construction program. When the Senate Committee on Government Operations rejected S. 1140 on June 10 and supported a substitute measure (S. 3314), calling for the prevention of unnecessary duplication in the functions of federal hospitals and for the elimination of excessive construction costs, the AMA heartily approved and proposed only a few changes in the bill. Its support, however, proved insufficient to get the measure before the Senate. The closing months of Truman's administration found the AMA still urging the establishment of a federal department of health with cabinet status.[75]

While the Association watched federal efforts in dealing with civilian health and medical problems during Truman's second term for evidence of flanking attacks on private medical practice, it found that the greatest threats to the profession came from legislative proposals for expanding the veterans' program. To the veterans' problems that World War II multiplied, the Korean War added others and increased agitation for the extension of medical benefits that encroached on private practice. Although patriotically supporting passage of the doctors' draft bill of 1950 that the President signed on September 9, the AMA just as decidedly opposed measures that appeared to extend dangerously the government's role in medical care.[76] When the Children's Bureau attempted in 1952 to revive and expand the Emergency Maternity and Infant Care program that had expired nearly five years earlier, it met the Association's stubborn opposition. For the bill (S. 2337) that the bureau supported giving wives of enlisted men in the lowest seven grades and their children under five benefit of government medical care, the AMA had only criticism. It challenged the bureau's evidence that indicated considerable need for the program with findings of independent surveys

[75] Subcommittee on Reorganization of Senate Committee on Government Operations, Eighty-second Congress, second session, *Hearings on S. 1140* (Washington: Government Printing Office, 1952), p. 54; WO, *Bulletin No. 52—82nd Congress* (June 19, 1952), 2; Resolutions, Russell V. Lee, *JAMA,* 150 (December 27, 1952), 1703. Within less than three months after the House of Delegates approved the health department resolution it agreed to support Eisenhower's plan for the elevation of the Federal Security Agency to cabinet level as a Department of Health, Education and Welfare, which was accomplished April 11, 1953. HD, *Proceedings* (Special Session, March, 1953), pp. 8, 9; 67 Stat. 18–19 (1953).

[76] HD, *Proceedings* (Clinical Session, December, 1950), p. 13, WO, *Bulletin* No. 65 (September 14, 1950), 2. The AMA's support of the physicians' draft during the Korean War marked a departure from its opposition to such a draft in World War II, possibly because of earlier experiences with the difficulties of voluntary recruitment.

and investigations of its own and contributed greatly to the defeat of bills providing for this program in the Eighty-first Congress.[77]

The AMA raised one of its strongest protests to a provision within another measure (S. 1) introduced in January, 1951, providing for the mental and physical rehabilitation of rejected draftees by the federal government, whose rejection resulted from failure to meet physical and mental induction standards of the Armed Forces. While the Association had long supported the government's rehabilitation work and efforts to unify its rehabilitation services, it looked upon this proposed expansion of activities as another threat to private practice.[78] Believing that rehabilitation for rejected draftees should be offered to them at reasonable expense through existing facilities co-ordinated for this service, Lull strongly attacked the bill charging that:

> Here, in the guise of a national defense measure, is a new health proposal that surpasses, in the extent to which it nationalizes medicine, even the compulsory health insurance bills that have been introduced for so many years. [and added] The effort to utilize an important defense measure to promote a wide expansion of Government medicine is a flagrant attempt to circumvent the will of Congress and of the people. It represents a disregard of public opinion that bodes ill for the future of our country and it must be prevented.[79]

While watching the Korean crisis for growing threats to medical practice, the AMA kept alert to older military encroachments on private medical care. As veterans with nonservice-connected disabilities crowded the facilities of hospitals directed by the Veterans Administration or co-operating with its program, the AMA again raised a cry of alarm. In 1951 it proposed that Congress authorize the Veterans Administration

[77] Statement of Edwin S. Hamilton, Subcommittee on Health of Senate Committee on Labor and Public Welfare, Eighty-second Congress, second session, *Hearings on S. 1245 and S. 2337, Health Care for Dependents of Servicemen* (Washington: Government Printing Office, 1952), pp. 93–94; testimony of Woodruff L. Crawford, *ibid.*, pp. 99–162. See also remarks of Chief of Children's Bureau, Martha M. Eliot. *Ibid.*, pp. 14–38.

[78] In 1950 a spokesman for the AMA had urged the consolidation of the government's rehabilitation work in the Federal Security Agency. See statement of Harry H. Kessler, Subcommittee of Senate Committee on Labor and Public Welfare, Eighty-first Congress, second session, *Hearings on S. 1066, S. 2273, and S. 3465* (Washington: Government Printing Office, 1950), pp. 381–84.

[79] Prepared statement, Preparedness Subcommittee of Senate Committee on Armed Forces, Eighty-second Congress, first session, *Hearings on S. 1: Universal Military Training and Service Act of 1951* (Washington: Government Printing Office, 1951), pp. 1122–23.

to investigate the financial status of exservicemen with nonservice-connected injuries who sought medical care in the veterans' program. A year later it not only urged that veterans with nonservice-connected disabilities be required to sign a statement affirming medical indigency, but that this statement be read to them in advance. Suspecting widespread abuse in the operation of the veterans' hospitalization program in which the daily patient load of nonservice-connected cases in the fiscal year 1950 doubled the number of cases with service-connected injuries, the AMA offered proposals that held little promise of reversing the trend.[80]

Times of Intolerance

As the Association stood on guard against alleged efforts of the federal government to establish a national system of medical care by indirection, it became convinced that the profession's interests were threatened from other sources. Apparently influenced by the national hysteria partially aroused by Senator Joseph R. McCarthy's reckless anti-Communist crusade, the AMA joined some other groups in finding threats to freedom in the nation's schools. In December, 1951, the House of Delegates urged a congressional investigation of the nation's "entire school system" that would expose "teachers and authors of textbooks" undermining "free enterprise" by upholding the "fallacies of collectivism." It urged the removal of teachers and textbooks supporting collectivistic thought.[81]

On the world front also the AMA attempted to check the development of sentiment favorable to the establishment of national medical systems. At the meeting of the International Labor Organization in 1952, it attempted to publicize the position of the World Medical Association that was more sympathetic toward voluntary programs of medical care when it found the World Health Organization circulating material

[80] Resolution, Raymond F. Peterson, HD, *Proceedings* (100 Annual Session, June, 1951), pp. 39, 53; and (101 Annual Session, June, 1952), pp. 38, 53; Paul B. Magnuson, "Medical Care for Veterans," American Academy of Political and Social Science, *Annals,* 273 (January, 1951), 81.

[81] Resolution, Eugene F. Hoffman, HD, *Proceedings* (Clinical Session, December, 1951), p. 70, see also pp. 80, 81. The Board of Trustees at a meeting on August 12, 1950, approved a resolution calling for more emphasis on American history in the nation's schools to awaken interest in the importance of the American heritage. *JAMA,* 144 (September 9, 1950), 188.

supporting national programs. It seemed greatly disturbed when the assembly recommended that most nations adopt a broad social security program that included compulsory health insurance or voluntary programs under governmental administration and supervision. In anticipation of this action, however, the House of Delegates adopted a resolution urging an amendment to the constitution that would invalidate all treaties or executive agreements conflicting with the constitution. Six months later it endorsed the "Bricker Amendment" that sought to place congressional control over executive agreements.[82]

Republican Victory

Important developments, international and domestic, still troubled the AMA near the end of Truman's second term. Despite the defeat of the administration's health insurance program, legislation encroaching on private medical care still threatened. The international scene held before the profession not only the specter of objectionable social legislation, but also the demands and uncertainties of the Korean War. Leaders of the AMA attributed many of their problems to Democratic policy and believed that the national election of 1952 held promise of calming the recurrent political storms that swept wildly over areas of health and medicine. Although Earl Warren's appearance high in Republican ranks repelled the AMA, the party's platform and its presidential nominee, Dwight D. Eisenhower, were irresistible. Doctors in large numbers worked tirelessly for a Republican victory, which Elmer Henderson described as a "reissue of the Declaration of Independence."[83]

[82] Statement, Louis H. Bauer in "Supplementary Report of Board of Trustees," HD, *Proceedings* (101 Annual Session, June, 1952), 22; WO, *Capitol Clinic,* 3 (July 1, 1952), 3; Resolution by Bauer for Board of Trustees, HD, *Proceedings* (101 Annual Session, June, 1952), pp. 23, 51; Resolution, Willard A. Wright, *JAMA,* 150 (December 27, 1952), 1704, 1705.

[83] HD, *Proceedings* (Clinical Session, December, 1951), p. 64; Henderson's statement given by John W. Cline, *JAMA,* 150 (December 27, 1952), 1695.

Chapter 18 SURVEY OF A DECADE

WHEN THE REPUBLICAN PARTY set its eight-year record before the voters in 1960, the American Medical Association had reason to believe that the confidence so many physicians had placed in the Republican nominee in the early fifties was justified. Indeed, by the fall of 1962, as the Association fought the proposal of the Kennedy administration for providing hospitalization for the aged through the social security system, it could look with nostalgia on most of the Eisenhower era as one of relative calm. Although the AMA was not in full agreement with some of the programs that the Republican administration supported and others that it tolerated, it found the President's basic policies largely in line with its own. Somewhere to the right of Eisenhower's "middle-of-the-road" program and generally left of the party's most conservative wing, the AMA followed a course fairly consistent with its earlier policies.

Legislation in Review

Throughout most of a decade the Eisenhower administration stood as a bulwark against the Association's greatest fear—the adoption of a compulsory health insurance system. It also espoused reforms in areas of health legislation that were acceptable to the AMA. Although the Association had long advocated the creation of a national health department with cabinet status, it supported the administration's successful efforts to establish a department of health, education, and welfare in 1953, when convinced that its original goal could not be achieved. In the same year it endorsed a measure which Congress enacted strengthening the power of the Food and Drugs Administration over the inspection of firms preparing food products for shipment in interstate commerce. Nearly a decade later and after years of agitation, it saw the passage of the Self-Employed Individuals Tax Retirement Act that made favorable tax concessions to several self-employed groups in establishing private retirement plans.[1]

On other fronts the AMA's struggles of recent years have brought notable victories. Its opposition to the President's reinsurance plan, calling for federal appropriations to extend voluntary insurance plans and expand their coverage, partially accounted for its defeat. Although the AMA strongly supported the spread of voluntary health insurance, it saw no justification for launching the program and feared the power it would confer on the federal government in the health insurance field. In 1959, it waged a vigorous and successful fight against a bill (H. R. 4700) introduced by Representative Aime J. Forand of Rhode Island that called for the payment of limited hospitalization and medical care costs through the social security system for those entitled to Old-Age and Survivors' benefits. Not only did the AMA find no crisis among the aged that required an extension of the social security system, but it maintained that adoption of the measure would lead inevitably to the establishment of a national medical program for the entire population.[2] Instead, it supported the Kerr-Mills bill, which Congress enacted the following year, providing federal assistance to the states in meeting the medical care costs of the aged, and in 1961 fought successfully to protect the subsidy program by resisting efforts to enact the King-Anderson bill that proposed hospitalization benefits for the aged through the social security system.[3]

[1] HD, *Proceedings* (Special Session, March, 1953), p. 5; prepared statement of George F. Lull, House Committee on Interstate and Foreign Commerce, Eighty-third Congress, first session, *Hearings on H. R. 2769, H. R. 3551,* and *H. R. 3604* (Washington: Government Printing Office, 1953), p. 208; *AMA News* (November 12, 1962), p. 14.

[2] HD, *Proceedings* (103 Annual Session, June, 1954), p. 16; statements of Leonard L. Larson, Frederick C. Swartz, and Joseph Stettler, House Committee on Ways and Means, Eighty-sixth Congress, first session, *Hearings on H. R. 4700* (Washington: Government Printing Office, 1959), pp. 273–310.

[3] Prepared statement of Leonard Larson, Senate Committee on Finance, Eighty-sixth Congress, second session, *Hearings on H. R. 12580* (Washington: Government Printing Office, 1960), pp. 202–20; HD, *Proceedings* (108 Annual Session, June, 1960), pp. 88–89; statements of Leonard W. Larson, Edward R. Annis, Ernest B. Howard, and C. Joseph Stettler, House Committee on Ways and Means, Eighty-seventh Congress, first session, *Hearings on H. R. 4222* (Washington: Government Printing Office, 1961), Vol. 3, pp. 1300–1466.

While the AMA passed through a decade with numerous victories, it wielded no very effective influence in the handling of several issues. The triumph of Modern Republicanism in the early fifties encouraged no attack on the nation's school system to uproot suspected proponents of "totalitarian" views as the House of Delegates had urged in 1951. The administration's spokesmen seemed eager to forget the suspicion partially generated by the McCarthy crusade that brought considerable embarrassment to the party, and agitation for the extension of inquisitorial policies gradually subsided within the profession itself. The Association also lost in its opposition to a measure (H. R. 7225) in 1956, which, while lowering the age of retirement for women and the age of eligibility for total disability benefits under the social security system, also allegedly threatened federal control over medical practice. Against many abuses which it found in the administration of veterans' benefits, it raised a loud but often futile protest.[4]

Minor setbacks, however, must not obscure the enormous influence the American Medical Association has exercised over the development of national programs involving matters of health and medicine. As these programs have evolved for the most part since World War II in line with the Association's views, and since it has prevented the initiation of others of more comprehensive scope, an appraisal of its policies in recent years is first in order, before evaluating its accomplishments through the century. So thoroughly have truth and fiction been mixed in late controversies over the Association's policies that detachment in an appraisal of its position is all the more urgent. Even those, however, who view a national comprehensive program of medical care as the only answer to the nation's health problems will probably find appealing arguments in the Association's stand on many health issues.

Appraisal of Recent Policies

In the political controversies since World War II, the AMA has often placed commendable stress upon the principles of individual responsibility and initiative that appear so essential to the survival of a

[4] See pp. 314–17 above. Prepared statements of F. J. L. Blasingame and David B. Allman, Senate Committee on Finance, Eighty-fourth Congress, second session, *Hearings on H. R. 7225* (Washington: Government Printing Office, 1956), Part 2, pp. 827–31, 833–36. HD, *Proceedings* (Clinical Session, December, 1955), pp. 63–64.

politically free society. It has sometimes stressed that majority policies in the broad areas of social reform must preserve free choice of action for minority groups, insofar as the preservation of minority rights does not injure majority welfare. It has also called for a revival of state and community responsibility for state and local problems, challenging widespread apathy and inertia. At congressional hearings its spokesmen have called for the adoption of a clearer philosophy of the government's role in social and economic affairs, assailing aimlessness in federal policies. It has assisted immeasurably in preventing the nation from drifting almost imperceptably into a system of medical care that the public, if faced forthrightly with the issue, might reject. Espousing the cause of efficiency in governmental operations, it has frequently cited deficiencies in the organization of federal agencies. Moreover, it has often reminded the public that much of the cost of the federal government's economic benefits has been passed on for a future generation to pay.

The AMA has also rendered invaluable service in attacking the loose and vague phraseology of many bills that reached the committee hearing stage, protecting public interest against possible abuses in administrative implementation. Frequently it has pressed proponents of legislation to make a case for their proposals which often did not buttress their demands. In addition, it has conducted many extensive and difficult investigations of its own on the nation's medical problems.

While supporting much of the important health legislation of the postwar era, the Association moved in more indirect ways to guard the nation's health. Its policies retarded influences that weakened standards of medical education after the war and that undermined the educational process in many nonprofessional schools. It has contributed to the impressive growth of voluntary health insurance against opponents who forecast failure for the movement. Through its Department of Investigation, it enlarged the battlefront in an effective warfare on nostrums and quackery. Its publications have also occasionally offered gentle warnings about dangers in rising costs of drugs and physicians' services.

Unfortunately, however, the Association's record in recent years has a less impressive side which is partially attributable to the loose structure of the organization itself. While local societies can wield enormous pressure to force conformity upon deviating physicians (from which the latter usually have no very effective appeal), this pressure generally has only negative results. The Association's legislative body adopts platforms embodying high ideals, but the federated nature of the organization has given it no great control over the implementation of its policies at the local level. Medical society plans initiated as an alternative to compulsory health insurance have experienced only modest success, and the AMA is still trying to bring abuses like the rebate evil under control. At the nation's capital its spokesmen can wield effective influence over the course of legislation, but the Association is less effective in getting professional support for its programs after securing congressional acceptance.[5]

Organizational peculiarities, however, do not explain the Association's somewhat exaggerated suspicion of innovations and its willingness to support some measures only as a deterrent to the adoption of a national health insurance system. Its reserve in accepting innovations in medical practice delayed development of a more friendly attitude toward closed panel systems until 1959.[6] More serious, however, has been its failure to recognize the magnitude of the nation's expanding medical needs. Soon after World War II, the director of its Bureau of Medical Economic Research contended that there was little likelihood of a growing physician shortage and predicted even the possibility of a surplus. Not until 1951 did the AMA formulate a definite policy regarding direct federal assistance to medical schools (outside areas of research), and then only for construction purposes. While it did assist in retarding some erosive postwar influences in medical education, its inclination to minimize the nation's needs partially accounted for a generally recognized physician shortage by 1960 that since then has become increasingly acute.[7]

[5] For methods by which the organized medical profession can enforce conformity and for appeal procedures see "The American Medical Association: Power, Purpose, and Politics in Organized Medicine," *The Yale Law Review* 53 (May, 1954), 949–53; 1018–19. In 1958 Allan M. Butler of the Harvard Medical School said "there are no standards enforced by medical societies as regards medical care except the standard of malpractice." House Committee on Ways and Means, *Hearings on All Titles of the Social Security Act* (Washington: Government Printing Office, 1958), p. 939. See Robert L. Brenner, "Is Medicine's Self-Discipline Program Doomed?" *Medical Economics* (January 1, 1962), pp. 175, 177, 179, 180, 181, for the AMA's recent disciplining efforts.

[6] HD, *Proceedings* (101 Annual Session, June, 1959), pp. 27–30, 60–68.

[7] See pp. 355–56 above. HD, *Proceedings* (100 Annual Session, June, 1951), pp. 9, 43. For evidence supporting a physician shortage see Abraham Ribicoff, then Secretary of Health, Education, and Welfare, Committee on Interstate and Foreign Commerce, Eighty-seventh Congress, second session, *Hearing on H. R. 4999, H. R. 8774, and H. R. 8833* (Washington: Government Printing Office, 1962), pp. 12–16; Joan Braddon, "Tomorrow's Doctors—A Critical Question," *Newsweek* (October 16, 1961), pp. 108, 110–11; Hal Higdon, "The Doctor Drouth,"

As the nation struggled with the problem of physician supply late in the fifties, it could question the great confidence the AMA had placed in voluntary health insurance as a generally satisfactory method for meeting the costs of medical care. Although 72 per cent (nearly 128,000,000) of the population had some type of health insurance at the end of the decade, and 135,000,000 or 75 per cent two years later, and despite a trend toward more liberal benefits, the voluntary system had demonstrated serious deficiencies. Of a national private expenditure for medical care that reached approximately $18,965,000,000 in the fiscal year 1958–1959, voluntary insurance paid only $4,138,-000,000, or a little less than 22 per cent. In 1958 it paid only 54 per cent of the nation's total private expenses for hospitalization and 32 per cent of the "currently insurable" medical care bills.[8]

Moreover, the soaring costs of health protection in the 1950's that far outstripped percentage increases in general prices and wages threatened to retard the development of voluntary plans along lines of wider enrollments and more comprehensive coverage. Although physicians' fees have generally stayed well in line with the standard price index since World War II, a survey in 1962 in 20 cities showed a 16 per cent rise over a decade in charges for appendectomies, 30 per cent for tonsillectomies, 39 per cent for obstetrical care, 35 per cent for office calls, and 42 per cent for house calls. From 1948 to 1958 the expenditure per capita for the total cost of personal medical care rose 82 per cent. Hospital rates that since World War II have shown an annual increase of about 9 per cent stood at 208.9 in 1960 on a scale

---

Commercial Appeal (Memphis), July 10, 1961, p. 15; July 12, 1961, p. 25. Higdon challenges the contention of George Cooley, director of the AMA's Department of Medical Service, that the problem is one of imbalance, not shortage. For an estimate of future physician needs in order to maintain the present physician to population ratio see *Report of the Surgeon General's Consultant Group on Medical Education: Physicians for a Growing America* (U.S. Department of Health, Education, and Welfare, Public Health Service, October, 1959), pp. 1–2.

[8] Statistics derived from *AMA News* (August 22, 1960), p. 15, and (October 15, 1962), p. 9; Somers and Somers, *Doctors, Patients, and Health Insurance,* p. 437; Rita R. Campbell and W. Glenn Campbell, "Voluntary Health Insurance in the United States" (Washington, D.C.: American Enterprise Association, 1960), pp. 16–18; for an explanation of the term "currently insurable" see *ibid.,* pp. 16–17. Reasonable coverage of health insurance for family medical bills has been set at about 80 per cent. Odin W. Anderson and the Staff of the National Opinion Research Center of the University of Chicago, *Health Insurance in Two Cities* (Cambridge, Massachusetts: Harvard University Press, 1957), p. 49.

that set average rates from 1947–1949 at 100. Consequently, family group rates under Blue Cross plans that rose 112 per cent during the decade still generally purchased only rather limited coverage.[9]

Rising costs of hospitalization, physicians' services, and drugs threatened growing numbers in the 1960's with medical indigency. Upon the elderly especially (approximately 17,000,000 over 65 by early 1961) has fallen a heavy burden. An investigation by the National Opinion Research Center showed that 44 per cent of married couples surveyed, headed by men 65 years of age and over, had total annual monetary incomes of less than $2,000 in 1956, supporting findings of the Bureau of Census three years later which showed that "one-third of the families headed by an aged person had a total monetary income of less than $2,000 . . ." and that 30 per cent of the aged families had no liquid assets. By 1960, despite a significant rise over the decade in the income of elderly citizens, less than one in four over 65 had annual monetary incomes of as much as $2,000.[10] As the AMA has correctly demonstrated this low ratio is partially explained by the fact that many aged couples rely largely on the income of one partner, yet less than one-fifth of the elderly are married women and the income of many couples falls even below the $2,000 mark. While some studies of the financial status of the aged tend to discount charges of overwhelming medical indigency in showing the "median net worth of OASI recipients with a wife entitled to benefits" as $9,616 in 1957, and 40 per cent of these couples a year later with liquid assets of over $2,000, much evidence supports the view that a serious economic situation has developed. As insurance companies move desperately to provide the elderly with coverage at unusually low rates and as strong agitation develops for the

[9] Somers and Somers, *Doctors, Patients, and Health Insurance,* pp. 201–2, 403, 195, 545, 312–13; *U.S. News and World Report* (May 28, 1962), p. 71; *Statistical Abstract of the United States* (1960), p. 22; Roland H. Berg, "The Battle for Your Health Dollar," *Look* (April 11, 1961), p. 24.

[10] Special Committee on the Aging, Senate, Eighty-seventh Congress, first session, Staff Report, "Basic Facts on the Health and Economic Status of Older Americans" (Washington: Government Printing Office, 1961), p. 18, and Staff Report, "State Action to Implement Medical Programs for the Aged" (Washington: Government Printing Office, 1961), pp. 6–7; Ethel Shanas, "Meeting Medical Care Costs among the Aging," Health Information Foundation, *Research Series 17* (New York: Health Information Foundation, 1960), pp. 1, 10, 13, Christopher Jencks, "The Unhealthy Aged," *New Republic* (February 5, 1962), p. 17; prepared statement by Wilbur J. Cohen, Subcommittee on Retirement Income of Senate Special Committee on Aging, Eighty-seventh Congress, first session, *Hearings on Retirement Income of the Aging* (Washington: U.S. Government Printing Office, 1961), p. 7.

payment of their hospitalization coverage through social security, some observers believe that the greatest tests for voluntary health insurance are yet ahead.[11]

Groups finding as many defects as virtues in voluntary health insurance also criticized the AMA's response to the compulsory health insurance challenge. While the Association had strengthened the democratic process by retarding the nation's drift toward a comprehensive program of medical care that had no convincing popular mandate, it had failed to provide the electorate with adequate information so essential to the formulation of national policy. By publishing distorted accounts of deficiencies in the operation of compulsory systems abroad, it stood in danger of ultimately damaging its own cause. In finding behind much of the legislation it opposed the spectre of "socialized medicine," it resorted to a use of loose terminology that stood in a sharp contrast to its insistence on clarity of language in the drafting of federal legislation.[12]

Attention must also be given to the Association's frequent charge since World War II that the financial problems of medical care have

[11] The AMA's position is set forth in Arthur Kemp, Leonard W. Martin, and Cynthia Harkness, "Some Observations on Financial Assets of the Aged and Forand-Type Legislation," *JAMA,* 171 (October 31, 1959), 1228–29; quotation, HD, *Proceedings* (108 Annual Session, June, 1960), pp. 41–43; see also prepared statement of Wilbur J. Cohen, Eighty-seventh Congress, first session, *Hearings on Retirement Income of the Aging,* p. 7; Pearl Barland, "Health Insurance for Oldsters? There's Plenty!" *Medical Economics* (January 1, 1962), pp. 164–70. For a favorable report on the condition of the aging see James W. Wiggins and Helmut Schoeck, "A profile of the aging: U. S. A.," (reprint) *Geriatrics,* 16 (July, 1961), 336–42, and for a less favorable view see "Hospital and Medical Economics: A special report on the Michigan study," (reprint), *Hospitals* (August 1, 1961).

[12] See pp. 198–99, 345–47 above. A completely socialized medical system would place the government in charge of four areas of medical care in addition to public health operations: namely, production of medical personnel, provision of medical facilities, administration of medical services, and payment of the nation's medical expenses. Medical care offered in the Armed Forces is a close approach to this system. A simple compulsory health insurance system concentrates on the payment problem and a soundly financed one places the government in the position of an insurer. It falls far short of a thoroughly socialized governmental system. Throughout most of the nation's history a sizable part of the medical profession has been trained largely at public expense in state medical schools. Increasingly the AMA has supported greater governmental assistance in the provision of medical services and has long favored federal aid where need existed in financing the medical expenses of medically indigent groups. Many aspects of American medical care have long been socialized either by the government or through other forms of collective action but the public's attention has generally been turned to the payment aspect. The ambiguity of the term "socialized medi-

risen more from an improper allocation of expenditures for medical purposes than from a shortage of income. It has referred to the enormous aggregate expenditure for tobacco, alcoholic beverages, jewelry, and recreation as evidence of the low priority medical care has held in the family budget.[13] It has failed to note, however, that other legitimate needs given low priority also compete with medical care for the family's income devoted to the purchase of luxury items. Insurance companies claim that a large part of the public is underinsured; dentists call for more adequate dental care; educational authorities lament the impoverished character of many school systems; retail trades cite the consumer's need for greater quantities of goods ranging from clothes to household items; while religious and philanthropic institutions call for more support and greater self-denial. Even memorial gardens stand as constant reminders to many Americans that they have made no provision for a final resting place. The timely and realistic question for a *free* society is not whether the family can have recreation or education or medical care, but whether it can pay for life's basic needs and some of its luxuries as well.

General Evaluation

Generalizations will suffice in summarizing the Association's record over most of the century which has already been described in considerable detail. The AMA moved from political obscurity in the nineteenth century to carry through a major internal reorganization early in the twentieth, and to identify itself with the dynamic reform forces of the Progressive Era. Upon both state and federal levels, it waged relentless campaigns for much reform legislation affecting health and medicine, and was attacked by opposition from within and without the organization for supporting measures that would allegedly fasten upon the nation and profession a system of Russian tyranny and Czarist bureaucracy.[14]

---

cine" and the emotional response it so often creates make its use perhaps unwise. Even the term "voluntary insurance" has become increasing complex. When employees are covered by group payment plans partially subsidized by employers the incidence of cost is shifted rather directly to the public in the form of higher prices for the employers' goods or services and the public bears the cost in compulsory payment, at least for essential purchases.

[13] See pp. 360–61, 366, and see also pp. 146–47.

[14] See pp. 100–1 above and G. Frank Lydston, "The Russianizing of the Medical Profession by the Political Machine of the AMA," *Texas Medical Journal,* 25 (November, 1909), 169–78.

While it allowed the movement for workmen's compensation legislation to advance without its assistance and showed no strong interest in some other forms of labor legislation, it stood in the front ranks battling for state and federal food and drugs legislation, vital statistics legislation, and a national department of health. In addition, it carried the reform crusade into areas of medical education where its effective work was largely responsible for raising the nation's standards to among the world's highest within less than two decades. Nor did the reform spirit that largely spent its force on the national level before the end of Wilson's first term remain as dormant in the AMA, whose leadership developed an interest in reforms as far-reaching as compulsory health insurance.

While the Association shared in the reform spirit of Progressivism, it soon adjusted to the extreme caution and complacency of the 1920's. Not only did it attack forces on the left with a total repudiation of compulsory health insurance at the beginning of the decade, but found no justification for the government's policy allowing federal assistance to the states for infant and maternal welfare benefits. It attacked portions of the veterans' program that infringed on private medical care and looked apprehensively upon the growth of group practice plans. Moreover, it was distressed by the spread of contract practice and later by the development of voluntary health insurance schemes.

The impact of the Great Depression and the drive of Democratic national leadership brought to the AMA new traces of the Progressive spirit. Generally to the right of a "middle" line that gradually shifted leftward, it accepted many reforms of the Roosevelt era. Contrary to a popular view, it did not oppose the first Social Security Act and three years later endorsed the principle of wage-loss insurance.[15] It called for even stronger food and drugs legislation than Congress enacted in 1938 and finally accepted the voluntary health insurance movement, while remaining unalterably opposed to a compulsory system. During the postwar era it gradually accepted the need for greater federal participation in health and medical affairs, also calling for a revival of local responsibility.

The pressing political challenges before the American Medical Association in the 1960's bear only a remote relationship to those it faced when the new century began. To the struggles of an earlier era spokes-

[15] See pp. 194–97, 218–21 above. For recent charges by President John F. Kennedy that the AMA opposed the Social Security Act see Douglas B. Cornell, *Nashville Tennessean,* May 24, 1962, p. 2, and for the AMA's denial and the President's reaction see *ibid.,* June 6, 1962, p. 8. For similar charges by Senator Albert Gore (Tenn.), see Nellie Kenyon, *ibid.,* June 2, 1962, p. 3.

men of the AMA brought the pioneer spirit of daring and adventure, while its critics called for caution and restraint. To the baffling problems of this era medical leadership must bring no less.

For an indeterminate future the Association has set before itself enormous tasks. It seeks not only to provide the nation with adequate medical care, but through methods that have been forcefully challenged in the United States and largely discarded abroad. Its position is further weakened by the nature of the organization itself which sometimes prevents hasty implementation of its positive programs. Furthermore, its resistance to any governmental extension of the compulsory principle in meeting the costs of medical care has alienated many groups that share its own opposition to a comprehensive system. Yet among the Association's assets are the commitment of a large part of the population to most of its basic policies, the vitality and flexibility of the voluntary insurance system, the success of newer forms of private practice, and a growing inclination within the profession to act against abuses.

While the survival of the voluntary insurance system is by no means assured, its strength will depend in a large measure upon the response of the profession and allied groups to present challenges. It will depend on greater adaptability of the system to the nation's needs, including greater encouragement of preventive medicine and broader adjustment to the requirements of low-income classes most in need of its benefits. It will depend on support of efficient forms of medical practice that hold promise of maximizing service and minimizing expense and upon provision of an adequate supply of general practitioners as well as specialists with greater emphasis in their training on the social and economic aspects of medical care and the profession's cultural heritage. The vitality of the movement will require a continuing struggle against such abuses as rebating, fee-splitting, and unnecessary hospitalization through which a small number of physicians weaken the influence of the rest. It will require the profession's vigorous support of measures promoting economy in the drug industry and may demand partial accommodation to the social security system. The profession's strongest critics contend that it cannot meet the complex challenges of this era as they explore the structure and temperament of organized medicine and the dimensions of the task. More friendly observers find no impenetrable barriers in the road ahead. Neither the AMA nor its critics will likely emerge from the struggles of the sixties with total victory, but the balancing influences of both are required if the nation moves on to "New Frontiers."

APPENDIX

ANNUAL MEETINGS OF THE AMERICAN MEDICAL ASSOCIATION IN THE NINETEENTH CENTURY

Year	*Attendance*	*Location*
1847	239[a]	Philadelphia, Pa.
1848	277[a]	Baltimore, Md.
1849	446[a]	Boston, Mass.
1850	255[a]	Cincinnati, Ohio
1851	222[a]	Charleston, S.C.
1852	264[a]	Richmond, Va.
1853	573	New York, N.Y.
1854	260	St. Louis, Mo.
1855	535	Philadelphia, Pa.
1856	200 (over)	Detroit, Mich.
1857	175	Nashville, Tenn.
1858	500 (nearly)	Washington, D.C.
1859	300	Louisville, Ky.
1860	535	New Haven, Conn.
1861	no session	
1862	no session	
1863	200 (over)	Chicago, Ill.
1864	535	New York, N.Y.
1865	616	Boston, Mass.
1866	367	Baltimore, Md.
1867	367	Cincinnati, Ohio
1868	324	Washington, D.C.
1869	193	New Orleans, La.
1870	463	Washington, D.C.
1871	200	San Francisco, Calif.
1872	723	Philadelphia, Pa.
1873	450	St. Louis, Mo.
1874	420	Detroit, Mich.
1875	475	Louisville, Ky.
1876	760	Philadelphia, Pa.
1877	663	Chicago, Ill.
1878	537	Buffalo, N.Y.
1879	320	Atlanta, Ga.
1880	1200 (nearly)	New York, N.Y.
1881	475	Richmond, Va.
1882	1000 (about)	St. Paul, Minn.
1883	900	Cleveland, Ohio
1884	600 (nearly)	Washington, D.C.
1885	650	New Orleans, La.
1886		St. Louis, Mo.
1887		Chicago, Ill.
1888		Cincinnati, Ohio
1889		Newport, R.I.
1890		Nashville, Tenn.
1891		Washington, D.C.
1892		Detroit, Mich.
1893		Milwaukee, Wis.
1894		San Francisco, Calif.
1895		Baltimore, Md.
1896		Atlanta, Ga.
1897	1970	Philadelphia, Pa.
1898	1335	Denver, Colo.
1899		Columbus, Ohio

[a] Apparently includes only delegates classified as such by the constitution.

SOURCE: Davis, *History of AMA*, p. 117; Nathan Smith Davis and others, "Looking Backward," *JAMA*, 32 (June 3, 1899), 1242; Fishbein, *History of AMA*, pp. 1189–90, 1201.

STRENGTH OF THE AMERICAN MEDICAL ASSOCIATION — 1920

	No. of Physicians in State	*No. of Fellows in AMA*	*Percentage of Fellows in AMA*[a]
NEW ENGLAND			
Maine	1,179	326	27.7
New Hampshire	657	279	42.5
Vermont	639	163	25.5
Massachusetts	5,870	2,243	38.2
Rhode Island	759	296	39.0
Connecticut	1,701	653	38.4
Total	10,805	3,960	36.6
MIDDLE ATLANTIC			
New York	15,877	5,302	33.4
New Jersey	3,046	1,187	39.0
Pennsylvania	11,539	4,407	38.2
Total	30,462	10,896	35.8
SOUTH ATLANTIC			
Delaware	264	73	27.7
Dist. of Columbia	1,237	366	29.6
Florida	1,296	285	22.0
Georgia	3,436	539	15.7
Maryland	2,268	708	31.2
North Carolina	2,237	433	19.4
South Carolina	1,237	305	24.6
Virginia	2,509	591	23.6
West Virginia	1,759	481	27.3
Total	16,243	3,781	23.3
EAST SOUTH CENTRAL			
Alabama	2,530	411	16.2
Kentucky	3,503	731	20.9
Mississippi	1,975	281	14.2
Tennessee	3,481	643	18.5
Total	11,489	2,066	18.0
WEST SOUTH CENTRAL			
Arkansas	2,587	380	14.7
Louisiana	2,023	470	23.2
Oklahoma	2,672	610	22.8
Texas	6,236	1,395	22.4
Total	13,518	2,855	21.1
EAST NORTH CENTRAL			
Illinois	10,909	4,584	42.0
Indiana	4,765	1,333	28.0
Ohio	7,802	2,432	31.2
Michigan	4,598	1,685	36.6
Wisconsin	2,783	1,110	39.9
Total	30,857	11,144	36.1

	No. of Physicians in State	*No. of Fellows in AMA*	*Percentage of Fellows in AMA*[a]
WEST NORTH CENTRAL			
Iowa	4,004	1,332	33.3
Kansas	2,683	837	31.2
Minnesota	2,548	1,115	43.8
Nebraska	2,237	652	29.1
North Dakota	605	269	44.5
South Dakota	646	236	36.5
Total	18,785	5,970	31.8
MOUNTAIN			
Arizona	333	160	48.0
Colorado	1,713	582	34.0
Idaho	449	94	21.0
Montana	661	190	28.7
Nevada	152	43	28.3
New Mexico	456	108	23.7
Utah	477	173	36.3
Wyoming	254	73	28.7
Total	4,495	1,423	31.7
PACIFIC			
California	5,929	2,099	35.4
Oregon	1,128	263	23.3
Washington	1,673	535	32.0
Total	8,730	2,897	33.2

[a] The percentages are figured to the nearest one-tenth of one per cent for both the separate states and the averages for each section.

SOURCE: This table is derived from statistics appearing in "Report of Secretary," *JAMA*, 74 (May 1, 1920), 1233. See footnotes in source for minor modifications in meaning of statistics cited.

GROWTH OF STATE ASSOCIATIONS 1911 AND 1920

Constituent Assns. of	*No. of Counties in State*		*No. of Component Societies in State Assn.*		*No. of Counties not Organized*		*No. of Members of State Assn.*	
	1911	*1920*	*1911*	*1920*	*1911*	*1920*	*1911*	*1920*
Ala.	67	67	67	67			1,676	1,728
Ariz.	13	14	7	11	6	3	157	213
Ark.	75	75	63	63	9	12	963	1,042
Calif.	58	57	36	43	21	14	1,972	3,311
Colo.	60	63	25	29	29	34	822	950
Conn.	8	8	8	8			841	1,054
Del.	3	3	3	3			103	123
D.C.							550	567
Fla.	46	54	24	32	22	22	341	572
Ga.	146	154	86	92	52	62	1,169	1,188
Idaho	23	44	4	19	6	25	124	184
Ill.	102	102	95	101	3	1	5,616	7,049
Ind.	92	92	87	91	4	1	3,107	2,331
Iowa	99	99	97	99	1		1,961	2,342
Kan.	105	105	74	67	17	38	1,452	1,760
Ky.	119	119	112	117	6	2	1,863	2,353
La.	59	64	39	40	18	24	893	1,203
Me.	16	16	13	15	3	1	577	712
Md.	24	23	22	21	2	2	1,122	1,143
Mass.	14	14	18	14			3,392	3,840
Mich.	83	83	58	81	6	2	2,092	2,620
Minn.	85	86	38	83		3	1,207	1,335
Miss.	78	81	50	78	8	3	965	499
Mo.	114	114	94	103	15	11	3,073	3,402
Mont.	28	50	10	17	16	33	234	375
Nebr.	91	92	62	64	26	28	1,026	1,116
Nev.	14	16	6	3	8	13	89	73
N.H.	10	10	10	10			540	526
N.J.	21	21	21	21			1,404	1,748
N.M.	26	28	14	12	12	16	246	199
N.Y.	61	61	57	61	3		6,885	9,110
N.C.	98	100	87	86	4	14	1,137	1,377
N.D.	46	52	14	51	5	1	400	431
Ohio	88	88	87	87	1	1	3,866	4,670
Okla.	75	77	68	67	6	10	1,132	1,638
Ore.	34	36	12	33	2	3	445	707
Pa.	67	67	63	63	4	4	5,487	6,687
R.I.	5	5	5	5			357	400
S.C.	41	46	40	41		5	760	640
S.D.	64	67	9	10	7	8	265	385
Tenn.	96	96	63	67	33	29	1,400	1,612

Constituent Assns. of	*No. of Counties in State*		*No. of Component Societies in State Assn.*		*No. of Counties not Organized*		*No. of Members of State Assn.*	
	1911	*1920*	*1911*	*1920*	*1911*	*1920*	*1911*	*1920*
Tex.	243	248	143	178	77	70	3,145	3,102
Utah	27	29	6	4	21	25	195	266
Vt.	14	14	11	12	3	2	410	406
Va.	100	100		59		41	1,604	1,735
Wash.	38	39	23	19	10	20	934	1,096
W.Va.	55	55	31	43	11	12	861	1,078
Wis.	71	71	55	71	2		1,820	1,904
Wyo.	15	22	5	5	10	17	122	92
	2,917	3,039	2,016	2,366	489	612	70,865	82,894

SOURCE: This table is compiled from statistics appearing in "Report of Secretary," *JAMA*, 57 (July 1, 1911), 58, and "Report of Secretary," 74 (May 1, 1920), 1233. Check footnotes in sources for an explanation of figures in a few instances. The figures for 1911 are used rather than for 1910 as the number of counties unorganized in 1910 does not appear in the *Journal*.

CIRCULATION OF THE JOURNAL BY STATES, 1910 AND 1920

	1910			*1920*		
	No. of Physicians in State	*No. Receiving Journal*	*Percentage[a] Receiving Journal*	*No. of Physicians in State*	*No. Receiving Journal*	*Percentage[a] Receiving Journal*
NEW ENGLAND						
Maine	1,198	407	34.0	1,179	481	40.8
New Hampshire	679	288	42.4	666	365	54.8
Vermont	663	211	31.8	653	258	39.5
Massachusetts	5,577	2,365	42.4	5,926	3,459	58.5
Rhode Island	720	317	44.0	752	435	57.8
Connecticut	1,424	675	47.4	1,701	1,071	63.0
Total & Average	10,261	4,263	41.5	10,877	6,079	55.9
MIDDLE ATLANTIC						
New York	14,117	4,858	34.4	15,877	8,452	53.2
New Jersey	2,455	977	39.8	3,153	1,777	56.4
Pennsylvania	11,056	4,686	42.4	11,495	6,608	57.5
Total & Average	27,628	10,521	38.1	30,525	16,837	55.2
SOUTH ATLANTIC						
Delaware	220	78	35.5	264	129	48.9
Dist. of Columbia	1,231	564	45.8	1,237	639	51.7
Florida	786	318	40.5	1,296	510	39.4
Georgia	2,887	762	26.4	3,442	1,084	31.5
Maryland	2,012	1,006	50.0	2,268	1,217	53.7
North Carolina	1,761	586	33.3	2,257	878	38.9
South Carolina	1,141	415	36.4	1,433	565	39.4
Virginia	2,215	843	38.1	2,552	1,068	41.8
West Virginia	1,608	568	35.3	1,759	764	43.4
Total & Average	13,861	5,140	37.1	16,507	6,854	41.5
EAST SOUTH CENTRAL						
Alabama	2,287	648	28.3	2,530	758	30.0
Kentucky	3,708	1,184	31.9	3,483	1,102	31.6
Mississippi	2,054	515	25.1	1,975	507	25.7
Tennessee	3,303	779	23.6	3,481	1,065	30.6
Total & Average	11,352	3,126	27.5	11,469	3,432	30.0
WEST SOUTH CENTRAL						
Arkansas	2,553	595	23.3	2,587	638	24.7
Louisiana	1,798	735	40.9	2,060	786	38.2
Oklahoma	2,703	672	24.9	2,672	872	32.7
Texas	5,789	1,527	26.4	6,246	1,965	31.5
Total & Average	12,843	3,529	27.5	13,565	4,261	31.4

	1910			1920		
	No. of Physicians in State	*No. Receiving Journal*	*Percentage[a] Receiving Journal*	*No. of Physicians in State*	*No. Receiving Journal*	*Percentage[a] Receiving Journal*
EAST NORTH CENTRAL						
Illinois	9,744	5,023	51.6	11,095	6,961	62.7
Indiana	5,306	1,779	33.5	4,765	1,894	39.7
Ohio	7,838	2,807	35.8	8,089	3,751	46.4
Michigan	4,109	1,806	44.0	4,598	2,402	52.3
Wisconsin	2,518	1,360	54.0	2,817	1,703	60.5
Total & Average	29,515	12,775	43.3	31,364	16,711	53.3
WEST NORTH CENTRAL						
Iowa	3,624	1,854	51.2	4,004	2,037	50.9
Kansas	2,650	1,119	42.2	2,668	1,230	46.1
Minnesota	2,204	1,288	58.4	2,566	1,706	66.5
Missouri	6,332	2,047	32.3	6,063	2,355	38.9
Nebraska	1,776	738	41.6	1,960	1,103	56.3
North Dakota	552	341	61.8	604	400	66.2
South Dakota	607	328	54.0	695	406	58.4
Total & Average	17,745	7,715	43.5	18,560	9,237	49.8
MOUNTAIN						
Arizona	246	142	57.7	333	262	78.7
Colorado	1,690	798	47.2	1,713	979	57.2
Idaho	343	161	47.0	458	239	52.2
Montana	417	219	52.5	661	336	50.8
Nevada	177	75	42.4	159	81	50.9
New Mexico	367	172	46.9	456	202	44.3
Utah	359	213	59.3	488	303	62.1
Wyoming	202	86	42.6	254	151	59.4
Total & Average	3,801	1,866	49.1	4,522	2,553	56.5
PACIFIC						
California	4,313	1,871	43.4	5,929	3,491	58.9
Oregon	782	349	44.6	1,157	545	47.1
Washington	1,404	700	49.9	1,698	881	51.9
Total & Average	6,499	2,920	44.9	8,784	4,917	56.0

[a] The percentages are figured to the nearest one-tenth of one per cent for both the separate states and the averages for each section.

SOURCE: This table is based upon those appearing in "Addenda to Trustees' Report," *JAMA*, 54 (June 11, 1910), 1966, and "Addenda to Trustees' Report," 74 (May 1, 1920), 1236–37. Percentages are computed to the nearest one-tenth of one per cent and do not in all cases correspond with the tables in the *Journal*, where the percentages are sometimes only approximately correct.

PHYSICIANS SERVING IN CONGRESS 1774–1789

	Name	*State*	*Term*
1.	Arnold, Jonathan	R.I.	1782–1784
2.	Bartlett, Josiah	N.H.	1775–1776, 1778
3.	Beatty, John	N.J.	1784–1785
4.	Brownson, Nathan	Ga.	1777, 1783
5.	Burke, Thomas	N.C.	1776–1781
6.	Burnet, William	N.J.	1780–1781
7.	Cobb, David	Mass.	1775
8.	Dick, Samuel	N.J.	1783–1784
9.	Elmer, Jonathan	N.J.	1776–1778 1781–1784 1787–1788
10.	Gardner, Joseph	Pa.	1784–1785
11.	Hall, Lyman	Ga.	1775–1778, 1780
12.	Hand, Edward	Pa.	1784–1785
13.	Holten, Samuel	Mass.	1774–1775 1778–1780 1782–1787
14.	Irvine, William	Pa.	1786–1788
15.	Jackson, David	Pa.	1785–1786
16.	Jones, Noble W.	Ga.	1775, 1781–1782
17.	Lee, Arthur	Va.	1781–1784
18.	McHenry, James	Md.	1783–1786
19.	Paine, Ephraim	N.Y.	1774, 1785
20.	Peabody, Nathaniel	N.H.	1779–1780
21.	Ramsay, David	S.C.	1782–1786
22.	Rush, Benjamin	Pa.	1776–1777
23.	St. Clair, Arthur*	Pa.	1785–1787
24.	Scudder, Nathaniel	N.J.	1777–1779
25.	Shippen, William	Pa.	1778–1780
26.	Thornton, Matthew	N.H.	1775–1776, 1778
27.	Tilton, James	Del.	1783–1785
28.	Tucker, Thomas T.	S.C.	1787–1788
29.	White, James*	N.C.	1786–1788
30.	Williamson, Hugh	N.C.	1782–1785 1787–1788

* A student of medicine but apparently did not practice.

SOURCE: Clifford P. Reynolds, Chief Compiler, *Biographical Directory of the American Congress, 1774–1961* (U.S. Government Printing Office, 1961).

Physicians Serving in Congress
1900–1963

Name	*State*	*Party*	*Branch*	*Term*
1. Alford, Thomas D.*	Ark.	D	House	1959–1963
2. Allen, Henry D.	Ky.	D	House	1899–1903
3. Austin, Albert E.	Conn.	R	House	1939–1941
4. Ball, Lewis H.	Del.	R	House	1901–1903
			Senate	1903–1905
			”	1919–1925
5. Barchfeld, Andrew J.	Pa.	R	House	1905–1917
6. Bohn, Frank P.	Mich.	R	House	1927–1933
7. Browne, Charles	N.J.	D	House	1923–1925
8. Burton, Hiram R.	Del.	R	House	1905–1909
9. Copeland, Royal S.	N.Y.	D	Senate	1923–1938
10. Deboe, William J.	Ky.	R	Senate	1897–1903
11. Douglas, Fred J.	N.Y.	R	House	1937–1945
12. Drew, Ira W.†	Pa.	D	House	1937–1939
13. Durno, Edwin R.	Ore.	R	House	1961–
14. Faison, John M.	N.C.	D	House	1911–1915
15. Fenton, Ivor D.*	Pa.	R	House	1939–1943
16. Fernos-Isern, A.	P.R.	D		1946–
17. Ferris, Woodbridge N.‡	Mich.	D	Senate	1923–1928
18. Fitzgerald, William T.	Ohio	R	House	1925–1929
19. Foster, Martin D.	Ill.	D	House	1907–1919
20. France, Joseph I.	Md.	R	Senate	1917–1923
21. Furlong, Robert G.	Pa.	D	House	1943–1945
22. Gaines, John W.‡	Tenn.	D	House	1897–1909
23. Gallinger, Jacob H.	N.H.	R	Senate	1891–1918
24. Griffith, John K.	La.	D	House	1937–1941
25. Hall, Durward G.	Mo.	R	House	1961–
26. Hatfield, Henry D.	W.Va.	R	Senate	1929–1935
27. Hedrick, Erland H.	W.Va.	D	House	1945–1953
28. Henney, Charles W. F.	Wis.	D	House	1933–1935
29. Higgins, William L.	Conn.	R	House	1933–1937
30. Hunter, Whiteside G.	Ky.	R	House	1903–1905
31. Irwin, Edward M.	Ill.	R	House	1925–1931
32. James, Addison D.	Ky.	R	House	1907–1909
33. Judd, Walter H.*	Minn.	R	House	1943–1963
34. Kindred, John J.	N.Y.	D	House	1911–1913
			”	1921–1929

	Name	*State*	*Party*	*Branch*	*Term*
35.	Lane, Harry	Ore.	D	Senate	1913–1917
36.	Larrabee, William H.	Ind.	D	House	1931–1943
37.	Layton, Caleb R.	Del.	R	House	1919–1923
38.	Lazaro, Ladislas	La.	D	House	1913–1927
39.	Massey, Zachary D.	Tenn.	R	House	1910–1911
40.	Miller, Arthur L.	Neb.	R	House	1943–1959
41.	Morgan, Thomas E.	Pa.	D	House	1945–
42.	Mouser, Grant E., Jr.	Ohio	R	House	1929–1933
43.	Neal, William E.	W.Va.	R	House	1953–1955
				"	1957–1959
44.	Norton, James A.	Ohio	D	House	1897–1903
45.	Olpp, Archibald E.‡	N.J.	R	House	1921–1923
46.	Palmer, John W.	Mo.	R	House	1929–1931
47.	Park, Frank‡	Ga.	D	House	1913–1925
48.	Pfeifer, Joseph L.	N.Y.	D	House	1935–1951
49.	Samuel, Edmund W.	Pa.	R	House	1905–1907
50.	Showalter, Joseph B.	Pa.	R	House	1897–1903
51.	Shull, Joseph H.	Pa.	D	House	1903–1905
52.	Sibley, Joseph C.‡	Pa.	D	House	1899–1901
			R	"	1901–1907
53.	Sirovich, William I.	N.Y.	D	House	1927–1939
54.	Smith, Frederick C.†	Ohio	R	House	1939–1951
55.	Stokes, James W.‡	S.C.	D	House	1895–1901
56.	Summers, John W.	Wash.	R	House	1919–1933
57.	Swick, Jesse H.	Pa.	R	House	1927–1935
58.	Tenerowicz, Rudolph G.	Mich.	D	House	1939–1943
59.	Thorkelson, Jacob	Mont.	R	House	1939–1941
60.	Volk, Lester D.	N.Y.	R	House	1920–1923
61.	Weatherford, Zadoc L.	Ala.	D	House	1940–1941
62.	Wilson, Frank E.	N.Y.	D	House	1899–1905
				"	1911–1915
63.	Wise, Richard A.	Va.	R	House	1900
64.	Wood, John T.	Idaho	R	House	1951–1953
65.	Woodrum, Clifton A.‡	Va.	D	House	1923–1945

* Alford did not run for re-election in 1962; Judd and Fenton were defeated.

† Osteopath.

‡ Either did not practice or no record of practice.

SOURCE: Clifford P. Reynolds, Chief Compiler, *Biographical Directory of the American Congress, 1774–1961* (U.S. Government Printing Office, 1961); Eighty-seventh Congress, first session, *Official Congressional Directory* (Washington: Government Printing Office, 1961). For 1962 election results see *New York Times*, November 7, 1962, p. 44; *ibid.*, November 8, 1962, pp. 19, 31; and *Newsweek* (August 13, 1962), p. 19.

Position of the American Medical Association in 1937 on Voluntary Health Insurance Plans

1. The plan of organization should conform to state statutes and case law. The majority of the governing body of the hospital insurance plan should be chosen from among members of official hospital groups and members of medical societies. Great care should be taken to assure the nonprofit character of these new ventures.

2. The plan should include all reputable hospitals. The qualifications of the participating hospitals should be closely supervised. Member hospitals should be limited to those on the Hospital Register of the American Medical Association or to those approved by the state departments of public health or other state agencies in those states in which there is approval, registration or licensing of hospitals.

3. The medical profession should have a voice in the organization and administration of the plan. Since hospitals were founded to serve as facilitating means to the practice of medicine, the medical profession must concern itself intimately with plans likely to affect the relations of hospitals to physicians.

4. The subscriber's contract should exclude all medical services—contract provisions should be limited exclusively to hospital facilities. If hospital service is limited to include only hospital room accommodations such as bed, board, operating room, medicines, surgical dressings and general nursing care, the distinction between hospital service and medical service will be clear.

5. The plan should be operated on an insurance accounting basis with due consideration for earned and unearned premium, administrative costs and reserves for contingencies and unanticipated losses. Supervision by state insurance departments has been advantageous for both the buyer and the seller of insurance contracts. Laws permitting the formation of hospital service corporations should not remove the benefits of such supervision nor violate the principles enumerated.

6. There should be an upper income limit for subscribers. If group hospitalization plans are designed to aid persons with limited means to secure hospital services, they should render such service at less than regular rates. If no consideration in rates is made for persons with limited means, group hospitalization plans lose their altruistic purpose and there may be little justification for an income limit.

7. There should be no commercial or high pressure salesmanship or exorbitant or misleading advertising to secure subscribers. Such tactics are contrary to medical and hospital ethics and are against sound public policy.

8. There should be no diversion of funds to individuals or corporations seeking to secure subscribers for a profit. The moment hospitals lose their traditional character as institutions of charity and humanitarianism the entire voluntary hospital system will break down.

9. Group hospitalization plans should not be utilized primarily or chiefly as means to increase bed occupancy or to liquidate hospital indebtedness. Such plans, if they are necessary, should place emphasis on public welfare and not on hospital finances.

10. Group hospitalization plans should not be considered a panacea for the economic ills of hospitals. They can serve only a small portion of those persons needing hospital services. Hospitals must continue to develop efficient methods of administration and service independent of any insurance method of selling their accommodations.

SOURCE: "Report of Board of Trustees," HD, *Proceedings* (88 Annual Session, June, 1937), pp. 22, 68.

Constructive Program for Medical Care of the American Medical Association, 1945

1. Sustained production leading to better living conditions with improved housing, nutrition and sanitation which are fundamental to good health; we support progressive action toward achieving these objectives.
2. An extended program of disease prevention with the development or extension of organizations for public health service so that every part of our country will have such service as rapidly as adequate personnel can be trained.
3. Increased hospitalization insurance on a voluntary basis.
4. The development in or extension to all localities of voluntary sickness insurance plans and provision for the extension of these plans to the needy under the principles already established by the American Medical Association.
5. The provision of hospitalization and medical care to the indigent by local authorities under voluntary hospital and sickness insurance plans.
6. A survey of each state by qualified individuals and agencies to establish the need for additional medical care.
7. Federal aid to states where definite need is demonstrated, to be administered by the proper local agencies of the states involved with the help and advice of the medical profession.
8. Extension of information on these plans to all the people with recognition that such voluntary programs need not involve increased taxation.
9. A continuous survey of all voluntary plans for hospitalization and illness to determine their adequacy in meeting needs and maintaining continuous improvement in quality of medical service.
10. Discharge of physicians from the armed services as rapidly as is consistent with the war effort in order to facilitate redistribution and relocation of physicians in areas needing physicians.
11. Increased availability of medical education to young men and women to provide a greater number of physicians for rural areas.
12. Postponement of consideration of revolutionary changes while 60,000 medical men are in the service voluntarily and while 12,000,000 men and women are in uniform to preserve the American democratic system of government.
13. Adoption of federal legislation to provide for adjustments in draft regulation which will permit students to prepare for and continue the study of medicine.
14. Study of postwar medical personnel requirements with special reference to the needs of the veterans' hospitals, the regular army, navy and United States Public Health Service.

Source: "Report of Council on Medical Service and Public Relations," HD, *Proceedings* (Annual Session, December, 1945), pp. 53, 85, 87.

National Health Program of the American Medical Association, 1946

1. The American Medical Association urges a Minimum Standard of Nutrition, Housing, Clothing and Recreation as fundamental to good health and as an objective to be achieved in any suitable health program. The responsibility for the attainment of this standard should be placed as far as possible on the individual, but the application of community effort, compatible with the maintenance of free enterprise, should be encouraged with governmental aid where needed.

2. The provision of Preventive Medical Services through professionally competent health departments with sufficient staff and equipment to meet community needs is recognized as essential in a health program. The principle of federal aid through provision of funds or personnel is recognized with the understanding that local areas shall control their own agencies as has been established in the field of education. Health departments should not assume the care of the sick as a function, since administration of medical care under such auspices tends to a deterioration in the quality of the service rendered. Medical care for those unable to provide for themselves is best administered by local and private agencies with the aid of public funds when needed. This program for national health should include the administration of Medical Care, Including Hospitalization to All Those Needing It But Unable to Pay, such medical care to be provided preferably by a physician of the patient's choice with funds provided by local agencies with the assistance of federal funds when necessary.

3. The procedures established by modern medicine for advice to the prospective mother and for Adequate Care in Childbirth should be made available to all at a price that they can afford to pay. When local funds are lacking for the care of those unable to pay, federal aid should be supplied with the funds administered through local or state agencies.

4. The child should have throughout infancy Proper Attention, Including Scientific Nutrition, Immunization Against Preventable Disease and Other Services Included in Infant Welfare. Such services are best supplied by personal contact between the mother and the individual physician but may be provided through child care and infant welfare stations administered under local auspices with support by tax funds whenever the need can be shown.

5. The provision of Health and Diagnostic Centers and Hospitals necessary to community needs is an essential of good medical care. Such facilities are preferably supplied by local agencies, including the community, church and trade agencies which have been responsible for the fine development of facilities for medical care in most American communities up to this time. Where such facilities are unavailable and cannot be supplied through local or state agencies, the federal government may aid, preferably under a plan which requires that the need be shown and that the community prove its ability to maintain such institutions once they are established (Hill-Burton bill).

6. A program of medical care within the American system of individual initiative and freedom of enterprise includes the establishment of Voluntary Nonprofit Prepayment Plans For the Cost of Hospitalization (such as the Blue Cross plans) and Voluntary Nonprofit Prepayment Plans

FOR MEDICAL CARE (such as those developed by many state and county medical societies). The principles of such insurance contracts should be acceptable to the Council on Medical Service of the American Medical Association and to the authoritative bodies of state medical associations. The evolution of voluntary prepayment insurance against the costs of sickness admits also the utilization of private sickness insurance plans which comply with state regulatory statutes and meet the standards of the Council on Medical Service of the American Medical Association.

7. A program for national health should include the administration of MEDICAL CARE, INCLUDING HOSPITALIZATION, TO ALL VETERANS, such medical care to be provided preferably by a physician of the veteran's choice, with payment by the Veterans Administration through a plan mutually agreed on between the state medical association and the Veterans Administration.

8. RESEARCH FOR THE ADVANCEMENT OF MEDICAL SCIENCE is fundamental in any national health program. The inclusion of medical research in a National Science Foundation, such as proposed in pending federal legislation, is endorsed.

9. The services rendered by VOLUNTEER PHILANTHROPIC HEALTH AGENCIES such as the American Cancer Society, the National Tuberculosis Association, the National Association for Infantile Paralysis, Inc., and by philanthropic agencies such as the Commonwealth Fund and the Rockefeller Foundation and similar bodies have been of vast benefit to the American people and are a natural outgrowth of the system of free enterprise and democracy that prevail in the United States. Their participation in a national health program should be encouraged, and the growth of such agencies when properly administered should be commended.

10. Fundamental to the promotion of the public health and alleviation of illness are WIDESPREAD EDUCATION IN THE FIELD OF HEALTH and the widest possible dissemination of information regarding the prevention of disease and its treatment by authoritative agencies. Health education should be considered a necessary function of all departments of public health, medical associations and school authorities.

SOURCE: *JAMA,* 130 (March 9, 1946), 641. This platform appeared as a news release in *American Medical Association News* (February 22, 1946), pp. 1–2.

Program of the American Medical Association for the Advancement of Medicine and Public Health, 1949

1. Creation of a Federal Department of Health of Cabinet status with a Secretary who is a Doctor of Medicine, and the coordination and integration of all Federal health activities under this Department, except for the military activities of the medical services of the armed forces.
2. Promotion of medical research through a National Science Foundation with grants to private institutions which have facilities and personnel sufficient to carry on qualified research.
3. Further development and wider coverage by voluntary hospital and medical care plans to meet the costs of illness, with extension as rapidly as possible into rural areas. Aid through the states to the indigent and medically indigent by the utilization of voluntary hospital and medical care plans with local administration and local determination of needs.
4. Establishment in each state of a medical care authority to receive and administer funds with proper representation of medical and consumer interest.
5. Encouragement of prompt development of diagnostic facilities, health centers and hospital services, locally originated, for rural and other areas in which the need can be shown and with local administration and control as provided by the National Hospital Survey and Construction Act or by suitable private agencies.
6. Establishment of local public health units and services and incorporation in health centers and local public health units of such services as communicable disease control, vital statistics, environmental sanitation, control of venereal diseases, maternal and child hygiene and public health laboratory services. Remuneration of health officials commensurate with their responsibility.
7. The development of a program of mental hygiene with aid to mental hygiene clinics in suitable areas.
8. Health education programs administered through suitable state and local health and medical agencies to inform the people of the available facilities and of their own responsibilities in health care.
9. Provision of facilities for care and rehabilitation of the aged and those with chronic disease and various other groups not covered by existing proposals.
10. Integration of veterans' medical care and hospital facilities with other medical care and hospital programs and with the maintenance of high standards of medical care, including care of the veteran in his own community by a physician of his own choice.
11. Greater emphasis on the program of industrial medicine, with increased safeguards against industrial hazards and prevention of accidents occurring on the highway, home and on the farm.
12. Adequate support with funds free from political control, domination and regulation of the medical, dental and nursing schools and other institutions necessary for the training of specialized personnel required in the provision and distribution of medical care.

Source: *JAMA,* 139 (February 19, 1949), 529. Headings above each of the 12 points have been eliminated. This platform appeared as a news release in *American Medical Association News* (February 18, 1949), pp. 5–6.

BIBLIOGRAPHICAL ESSAY

A brief discussion of the literature related to the development of the AMA must be confined largely to its own publications and to recent books that have given some attention to the organization's policies. While few books have appeared placing the Association's work in historical perspective, the periodical literature related to the profession's struggles with the health problems of the last hundred years is overwhelming. In fact, so large is the volume of the Association's own publications that only those relevant to this study can be surveyed.

Throughout the early years of the Association's history the annual *Transactions* (1848–1882) provide most of the information about the organization's work. Nathan S. Davis's *History of the American Medical Association* (1855) covers only the early years; his history of medical education closes with 1850, and both volumes appeared as independent publications. Supplanting the *Transactions* in 1883 was the *Journal of the American Medical Association,* which has carried a weekly record of many of the Association's activities for nearly eighty years. While the *Journal* alone presented a formidable problem of research, the information it yielded more than compensated for the effort.

Following the Association's reorganization in 1901, the *Proceedings of the House of Delegates of the American Medical Association* record the organization's official actions and give the reports of countless committees. While the *Proceedings* were first published in full only in the *Journal* (where they later appear in sometimes abbreviated form), the Association began to issue separate editions of its official actions about the beginning of the second decade. Future research will be greatly aided by Mrs. Susan Crawford's meticulous compilation, *Digest of Official Actions, 1846–1958,* Vol. I (1959), which appeared after most of the research for this volume was completed. A second volume is now in preparation. Although the records of the Board of Trustees have never been made available for research, some of its work has been carried in the Association's publications.

While the *Journal* and the *Proceedings of the House of Delegates* are indispensable sources of information, their usefulness is supplemented by other important publications. Many of the AMA's organizational activities are recorded in the *Councilor's Bulletin,* first published in 1905, which became the *Bulletin of the American Medical Association,* November 15, 1907. Both of these publications were published nine times each year and the life of the latter extended to December, 1936. *Hygeia* (now *Today's Health*) was first published in April, 1923, and also supplies important information on the Association's work.

Records of the Association's struggles against nostrums and medical charlatanry are voluminous. The Department of Investigation has preserved massive files of material, some of which were consulted in this study. Most of the Association's exposures of quackery have appeared in the *Journal,* and many of these were condensed and published in three volumes—the last, entitled *Nostrums and Quackery and Pseudo-Medicine,* appeared in 1936. The AMA also issued two volumes entitled *Propaganda for Reform in Proprietary Medicines,* publishing the last volume in 1922. These records, when combined with those of the national Bureau of Agricultural and Industrial Chemistry, provide abundant material for the organization's early crusade against exploitative forces in the healing world.

Since the establishment of the Bureau of Medical Economics (later Bureau of Medical Economic Research and now Department) in the early thirties, the Association has published many impressive studies devoted to the economic and social aspects of medical care. A large part of these publications appeared after World War II and some reflect years of careful research. Many of these studies have greatly strengthened the Association's position in the political battles of the postwar era.

The Association's Washington Office has also issued extensive materials since its establishment in 1944. Its releases, including *Capitol Clinic, Bulletin,* and *Comments,* reflect the influence the AMA has exerted in national politics. Its publications have informed the profession's leadership of developments affecting the profession at the nation's capital and of the political activities of the AMA. Supplementing these publications are the government's records of Congressional hearings that present the position taken by the Association's spokesmen on many issues.

A few other publications of the AMA were also useful in the preparation of this volume. The *News Letter,* issued by the Council on Medical Service and Public Relations (later Council on Medical Service), threw helpful light on much of the Association's work with local societies in the middle forties; the reports of the Annual Congress on Medical Education and Licensure were particularly valuable in presenting problems in various areas of medical education during and shortly after World War II. For providing the general picture of medical education throughout most of the century, the annual reports of the Council on Medical Education (later Council on Medical Education and Hospitals), which appear in the *Journal,* were indispensable. Various editions of the *American Medical Directory* were also helpful in supplying information on the Association's growth.

While the reader is referred to the footnotes for secondary materials used in this study, a brief reference to more recent books touching on the Association's work is in order. James Cook in *Remedies and Rackets* (1958) discusses some of its most recent efforts in combating nostrums. Louis Lasagna's *The Doctors' Dilemnas* (1962) deals with many medical problems of recent decades and with some of the Association's policies. Richard Carter in *The Doctor Business* (1958) attributes many of the profession's ills to the structure of organized medicine and bitterly denounces the AMA for the alleged inadequacy of its response to the nation's medical problems. William Michelfelder in *It's Cheaper to Die: Doctors, Drugs, and the A.M.A.* (1960) also offers many criticisms of trends in areas of medical care.

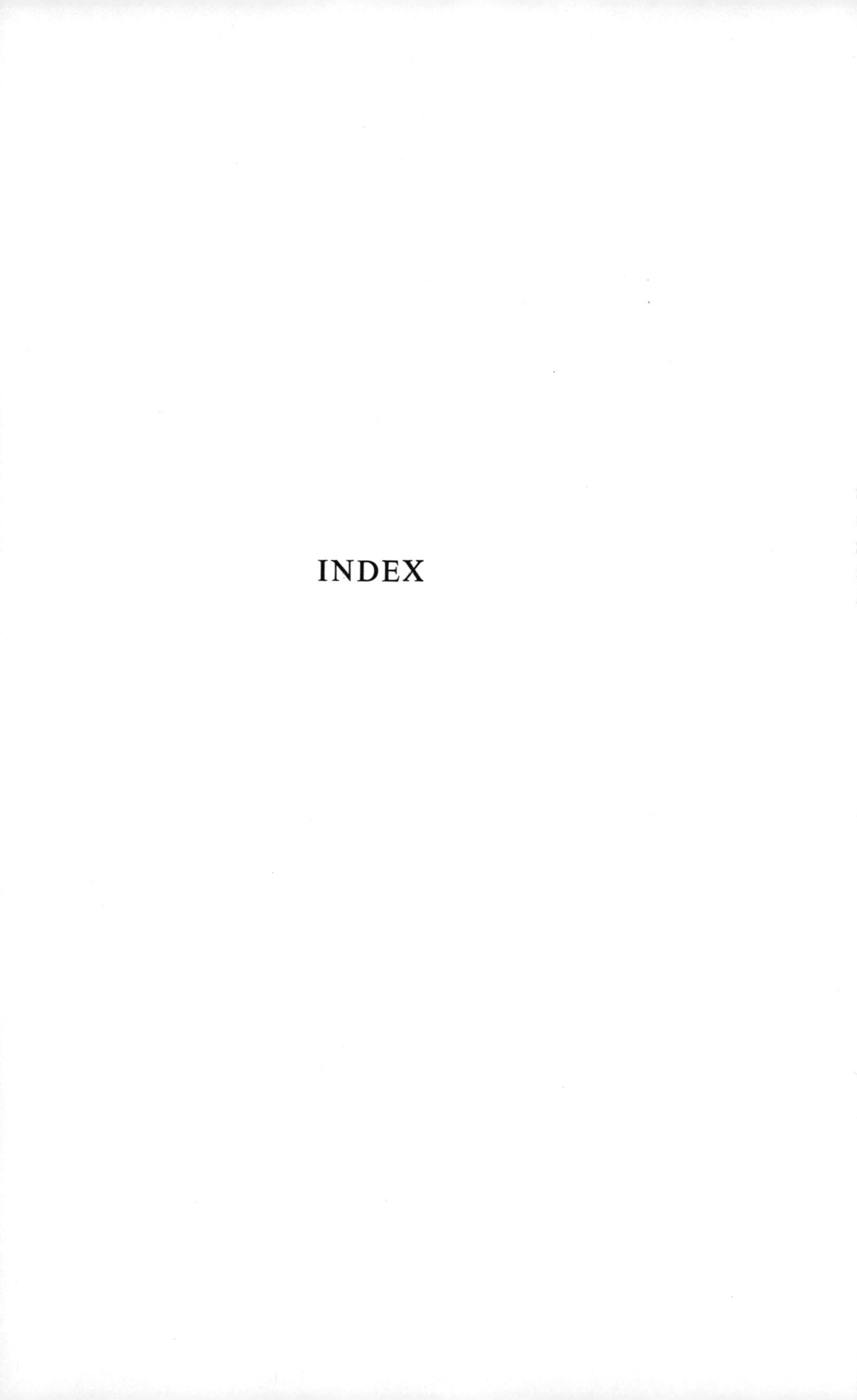

INDEX

A

B

D

E

F

I

J

K

L

M

N

Q

R

S

W